Assessment of Communication Disorders in Children

Resources and Protocols

Assessment of Communication Disorders in Children

Resources and Protocols

Second Edition

M. N. Hegde, Ph.D.
Frances Pomaville, Ph.D.

California State University-Fresno

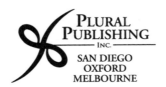

PLURAL
PUBLISHING
INC.
SAN DIEGO
OXFORD
MELBOURNE

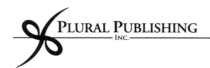

5521 Ruffin Road
San Diego, CA 92123

e-mail: info@pluralpublishing.com
Web site: http://www.pluralpublishing.com

Typeset in 11/14 Stone Informal by Flanagan's Publishing Services
Printed in the United States of America by McNaughton & Gunn
17 16 15   4 5

Library of Congress Cataloging-in-Publication Data

Hegde, M. N. (Mahabalagiri N.), 1941-
  Assessment of communication disorders in children : resources and protocols / M.N. Hegde and Frances Pomaville. — 2nd ed.
      p. ; cm.
  Includes bibliographical references and index.
  ISBN-13: 978-1-59756-487-8 (alk. paper)
  ISBN-10: 1-59756-487-7 (alk. paper)
  I. Pomaville, Frances. II. Title.
  [DNLM: 1. Communication Disorders—diagnosis. 2. Child. 3. Clinical Protocols.
4. Needs Assessment. WL 340.2]
  LC Classification not assigned
  616.85'5075—dc23
                          2012022802

Contents

Preface

Assessment of communication disorders in children needs a precise plan of action based on scholarly information. Clinicians typically find that they have to seek scholarly and background information on assessment in one source and practical assessment tools in another. Most background information on assessment techniques are to be found in more traditionally written textbooks on assessment. More practical assessment tools are typically presented in resource books. Clinicians often find this an inefficient arrangement to gain access to both scholarly background and practical procedures of assessment. Sometimes, the different sources the clinicians have to access may be somewhat inconsistent with each other, creating further problems of integration and validation. Therefore, to solve these practical and technical problems, we have designed an assessment book that includes two chapters each on the most commonly assessed communication disorders in children: one to provide the scholarly background and the other to give practical assessment protocols. Thus, in a single source, the clinicians can find both scholarly information and practical protocols to assess speech, language, fluency, voice disorders, as well as nonverbal communication in children with limited verbal skills. We also have written a single chapter on literacy skills that offers both the background information and assessment parameters and procedures, and a single chapter introducing assessment for augmentative and alternative communication (AAC) systems.

The book has an initial section on the *foundations of clinical assessment*. This section includes chapters on common assessment procedures and major assessment matters and issues. The first chapter gives the outline of a basic assessment procedure. The second chapter then offers all the protocols commonly used in assessing most, if not all, disorders of communication in children. This section includes additional chapters on assessment based on standardized tests, assessment of ethnoculturally diverse children, and alternative assessment procedures along with a model that integrates alternative and traditional approaches. All chapters offer extensive background information and critical review of major issues.

A unique philosophy that has guided the writing of this book is that the *alternative and traditional assessment procedures need to be integrated in assessing all children — including mainstream children*. We do not believe that traditional assessment is good for some children and alternative procedures are needed for others. Certain fundamental limitations of standardized tests do not disappear when they are administered to mainstream children. Many alternative procedures are designed to overcome the limitations of standardized tests and those limitations are evident even when the tests are administered to children included in the standardization sample (mainstream *or* culturally diverse). Most alternative procedures have additional strengths that will enhance the reliability and validity of assessment data obtained on any child, not just an ethnoculturally diverse child. For this second edition, we have added behavioral assessment as an additional alternative approach, a well-established method in applied behavior analysis, but somewhat new to most speech-language pathologists. Behavioral assessment offers several distinct advantages over the traditional linguistically oriented approach popular in speech-language pathology. Our chapter on alternative assessment procedures not only reviews extensive information on alternative procedures, but also describes a model of assessment that integrates the strengths of the traditional approach with those of the various alternative approaches.

The first chapter on each disorder, called the *resource* chapter, is a review of scholarly information on assessment, the kind typically found in traditional textbooks. The chapter gives the research base on the normal skill development when relevant, describes the disorder and its classification, summarizes etiologic information, specifies any associated clinical conditions, and gives a descriptive overview of assessment. Each resource chapter offers critical review of issues related to assessing the particular disorder. In addition, the chapter includes a description of diagnostic criteria, differential diagnosis, and probabilistic prognostic statements. All resource chapters include a section on postassessment counseling in which the clinician gives the parents or other caregivers the assessment results and answers their questions. The most frequently asked questions and the clinician's answers are written in a dialogue format that the student and the beginning clinician can model after.

The second chapter on each disorder and on augmentative and alternative communication is a collection of detailed as well as *practical and precisely written protocols* to make a complete and valid assessment. The protocols go beyond the typical resources offered to speech-language pathologists. Most protocols are detailed enough to be used immediately in assessing any child with a communication disorder. All protocols may be individualized on the CD and printed out for clinical use. In addition, the common and the standard assessment protocols given in Chapter 2 may be combined with specialized protocols given in the respective chapters on disorders of speech, language, fluency, voice, and on alternative and augmentative communication. Therefore, with the help of resources and protocols given in the book and the CD, the clinicians can develop child-specific and individualized assessment packages to be readily and easily used during assessment sessions.

For this second edition, we have updated assessment research and tools throughout the book. As mentioned before, we have added behavioral assessment as an additional, alternative approach to assessment. Furthermore, we have created a new chapter for assessing augmentative and alternative communication systems. This new chapter significantly expands the information included in other chapters in the earlier edition.

We would like to thank Scott Barbour for his excellent editorial support and Joy Heitzmann for her expert copyediting of this book. We also are thankful to Angie Singh and Caitlin Mahon for the fine production of this second edition.

Creating Child-Specific Assessment Packages with Protocols on the CD

Assessment protocols are detailed forms the clinicians can use to complete specific diagnostic tasks. These protocols are time-saving devices for the clinician. The accompanying CD contains all the standard protocols: the child case history form, the orofacial examination and hearing screening form, and the assessment report outline. These protocols are essential in assessing all children with any disorder of communication.

The CD also contains protocols offered in various *protocol chapters* in the book. These specific protocols help assess speech sound production and phonological patterns, various language skills, fluency disorders, voice disorders, and nonverbal and minimally verbal children. Although the protocols are offered as detailed procedures in specific formats, we emphasize that assessment is a dynamic process. No procedure can be applied to a child without modifications. Tailoring assessment procedures to suit the individual child and the family requires both creativity and scholarship; in fact, this is one of the themes of the book. Therefore, we do not expect the clinician to photocopy the protocols from the printed book and use them during assessment. Instead, we expect the clinician to modify the protocols on the CD to suit an individual child and family, print them out, and use them during assessment. Even as they use printed forms during assessment, clinicians will modify certain procedures, change the wordings of questions to be asked, and alter the manner in which information is given to the families.

Individualizing a protocol is accomplished with relative ease because the bulk of the information on the CD will be relevant to most children and families. A few additions and deletions may help individualize each protocol for a specific child. The clinician also can type in the name of the school or clinic, along with all the identifying information needed (e.g., the name and address of the child and the parents, name of the clinician, the date of assessment, etc.). Therefore, the protocols can easily be converted into the clinician's stationery formats. When filled out and printed, they will be appropriate to be placed in a child's clinical folder.

In addition to an opportunity to individualize the protocols, clinicians also are offered the possibility of *putting together a comprehensive assessment package for a child* efficiently and relatively quickly. The clinician can select the protocols needed for a given child's assessment, individualize them, and print them for clinical use. This feature is especially useful when a child needs to be assessed for multiple communication disorders. For example, for a child who exhibits both a speech sound and a language disorder, the clinician may print out all the basic protocols plus the several speech and language protocols. For a child with a diverse ethnocultural background, the clinician may print out the specific speech and language protocols given in Chapters 7 and 9 and attach them to all the other protocols used.

An additional advantage of the protocols is that several of them *help assess speech and language skills without the use of standardized tests* that may not be appropriate for certain children. For example, the clinician can assess apraxic or dysarthric speech features and the production of grammatic morphemes, basic vocabulary, conversational skills, and so forth with protocols designed in the manner of criterion-referencing without normative comparisons.

We encourage clinicians to freely individualize and use the practical and time-saving protocols to design a child-specific and comprehensive assessment package. The assessment report outline given on the CD will further expedite the task of writing an assessment report.

PART I

Foundations of Assessment

CHAPTER 1

Assessment in Speech-Language Pathology

- Assessment, Evaluation, and Diagnosis
- Written Case History
- The Initial Clinical Interview
- Hearing Screening
- Orofacial Examination
- Diadochokinetic Tasks
- Speech-Language Sample
- Standardized Assessment Instruments
- Alternative and Integrative Assessment Procedures
- Assessment of Nonverbal and Minimally Verbal Children
- Assessment of Literacy Skills
- Stimulability
- Postassessment Counseling
- Assessment Report

No communication disorder may be effectively treated without a thoughtful assessment. Treatment is a systematic effort to change an existing condition, and assessment is a first step to determine what needs to be changed, and if possible, why. In medicine, diagnosis of the disease precedes treatment; in communication and other behavioral disorders, efforts designed to understand the nature of the problem precedes treatment.

Treatment may not be offered unless the clinician knows what exactly to treat. On the other hand, treatment may be more effective if the cause of a disorder can be determined. Generally, causes may be better inferred or demonstrated for physical diseases than for communication disorders, especially for the commonly treated speech sound and language disorders in children. A highly correlated clinical condition such as a cleft of the palate, traumatic or congenital brain injury, autism, or similar disorders may suggest causation of communication disorders, but in fact, both the clinical condition and the communication disorder are coexisting conditions. Potential causes of communication disorders, especially of those characterized as *functional*, are inferred, rather than experimentally demonstrated.

Assessment, Evaluation, and Diagnosis

Because of the difficulty in establishing the causes of communication disorders in many cases, speech-language pathologists typically use the term *diagnosis* in a restricted sense. Strictly speaking, diagnosis specifies a cause of a set of symptoms, but because such specification is impractical in many cases of communication disorders, diagnosis often means naming the disorder (e.g., language disorders, stuttering) and describing its characteristics with or without speculation about its causes. Speech-language pathologists have preferred to describe a set of pretreatment activities as assessment or evaluation. The term *assessment* means *to determine the value of something*; but as used in speech-language pathology, assessment is inclusive of several kinds of clinical activities that result in naming the communication disorder of a client (diagnosis), making statements about prognosis for improvement with or without treatment, and offering recommendations for communication treatment, additional assessment, or other kinds of specialized services. The term *evaluation* is often used interchangeably; we make no distinction between *assessment* and *evaluation* in this book. We use the term diagnosis in the restricted sense of naming the disorder and determining its parameters (characteristics).

Communication disorders may be diagnosed in a different sense, too. Although it may be difficult to specify why a child has not acquired speech sounds or language behaviors, it may be possible to find out what maintains the child's current appropriate or inappropriate verbal repertoire. The maintaining causes of the disorders may be studied by what is known as a *functional analysis* in applied behavioral science (Duker, 1999; Esch, LaLounde, & Esch, 2010; Kelley, Shillingsburg, Castro, Addison, & LaRue, 2007; Kelley et al., 2007; Lerman et al., 2005). This kind of functional analysis (assessment) has been demonstrated to be useful in diagnosing the maintaining or currently controlling variables of verbal behaviors of the kind specified by Skinner (1957). Furthermore, an identification of maintaining causes helps design an effective treatment procedure. Regrettably, most speech-language pathologists, being linguistically oriented by their training, have not included a functional analysis in their assessment of communication disorders. The traditional assessment helps identify what needs to be taught, but it does not suggest what might be an effective treatment procedure. We describe the highly useful functional assessment in Chapter 5 on alternative assessment approaches and in Chapter 8 on assessing language skills in children.

Historically, the term *diagnosis* was more commonly used than *assessment*. The classic books of this kind were likely to be called *diagnosis in speech-language pathology* (Darley, 1964; Darley & Spriestersbach, 1978). Even if tentative, subject to later revision, *diagnosis* is the end result of a series of scientific and clinical activities, examinations, and data gathering through various means; adding a functional analysis to these traditional activities will greatly enhance the usefulness of the data collected in planning treatment. In this sense, diagnosis is a part of an overall assessment (or evaluation) strategy. In this book, we use the term *assessment* in this inclusive sense.

As different forms of disorders of communication have come to light through research and clinical observation, assessment also has become an increasingly complex activity. As we learn more about the behavioral, neurophysiologic, genetic, and cultural aspects of communication disorders, we find ourselves expanding the parameters of assessment. In the past, communication disorders in children were viewed with relatively little concern for the cultural and social contexts of speech and language. In most cases, *linguistic deviation* from established norms was sufficient to diagnose a disorder of communication. Clinicians now realize that linguistic deviation cannot be evaluated in isolation and needs to be evaluated in the context of the individual child, his or her family, the culture, the language background, the educational demands and objectives, the future occupational goals, and so forth. A linguistic deviation from some accepted norm by itself is not a basis to diagnose a disorder of communication. This realization is not surprising because communication is always social and cultural; a linguistic deviation may only be a cultural difference. Therefore, more than a linguistic deviation, a concept of verbal behavior deficits may better serve the ultimate purpose of assessment: treatment planning.

Parameters of assessment of communication disorders in adults and children share common elements, but there are significant differences. Not all, but most disorders of communication in adults are due to aging and related disease processes that affect previously mastered speech-language skills. To the contrary, most disorders in children are due to factors that tend to disrupt the speech-language learning process. Furthermore, many clinicians tend to specialize in assessing and treating communication disorders in either children or adults. Therefore, to offer comprehensive assessment information as well as a collection of practical tools, we have devoted this book to communication disorders in children.

We begin this initial chapter with an outline of the basic assessment process. Assessment, as noted, is a series of well-planned activities. These activities strive to be systematic and scientific, but all clinicians know that clinical experience and judgment also play their role. When science can do no more and more still needs to be done, experience and judgment can help.

From a procedural standpoint, assessment includes attempts at understanding the child's past and the present, the current problems, and the family constellation (case history), a face-to-face interview of people concerned (often the parents or other caregivers), and various examinations done in the clinic. When all the activities, including planned clinical examinations are completed, the clinician shares the findings with the family and the child, makes recommendations, suggests a prognosis, and answers questions. We begin with the first of these: the case history.

Written Case History

A written case history is a questionnaire that is completed by the child's caregiver, family member, or by the client if old enough. A *Child Case History Protocol* is available in Chapter 2. The purpose of a case history form is to understand both the past and the present of the child, by gathering information on the child, the disorder for which professional help is being requested, and the family constellation. A detailed case history may also serve as a guide for the clinical interview. A child case history form usually will include questions of various kinds, usually organized into sections whose descriptions follow.

Basic Identifying Information

This section includes the client's name, date of birth, age, address, and phone number. The parent's names, ages, address, and phone number(s) are also reported in this area. The child's physician and his or her contact information may be reported here.

Most printed forms allow the clinician to fill in the identifying information. It is important to have all the needed information because missing pieces of identifying information can be problematic for contacting the child and the family and the referral source.

Referral Source

Documentation of the referral source is important for several reasons. A child who is referred by a physician or another speech-language pathologist is likely to have a medical or clinical history that may need further exploration. The type of physician referral may also provide insight into other deficits or areas of concern. For example, a referral from an otorhinolaryngologist (ENT specialist) may indicate a significant hearing history, a referral from a pediatric neurologist may suggest possible neurologic problems, and a referral from a psychologist may suggest intellectual disabilities or an autism spectrum disorder.

Noting the referral source is also an important part of developing and maintaining professional relationships. If a physician or other rehabilitation professional refers a client, it is often helpful to send a thank you letter, and once the proper release forms are obtained, it may be helpful to provide the referring professional with a brief summary of results and recommendations.

Other Specialists Who Have Seen the Child

Information on other specialists is important in determining if the child's communication difficulties might be part of such other problems, as a hearing loss, physical condition, or neurologic disorder. A clinician may need to obtain background information from one or more of these sources. If the child has been seen by other speech-language pathologists, the clinician needs to follow up with them. The clinician should always obtain the caregiver's permission prior to contacting other specialists or agencies.

In addition, detailed information about previous therapy should be obtained during the interview. The clinician should be aware that if there is a long list of other speech-language pathologists who have evaluated the child, one may be dealing with "searching" parents who are looking for someone to tell them what they want to hear.

Statement of the Problem

The case history form asks the parent or caregiver to describe the problem. This might help the clinician prepare for assessing a specific type of communication disorder or level of severity. The problem statement will also help the clinician determine what the caregivers' primary concerns are, and their level of knowledge regarding the child's communication problem.

    The problem statement should be recorded in the caregivers' own words. During the interview, the clinician may explore the different meanings of this statement and get clarifications to derive a more technical description of the problem.

Developmental History

The case history usually includes an area for the caregiver to report the ages at which the child reached a variety of developmental milestones. This information is helpful in determining if the communicative disorder is part of a larger physical, neurologic, or behavioral disability.

    The clinician should note that the developmental history the caregivers report may be more or less reliable. In some cases, the information may not be available. Careful interview and the use of a prepared inventory will help obtain useful information. To help complete this task, a checklist of developmental milestones of speech, language, and motor skills from 0 to 6 years of age is provided in Chapter 2.

Medical History

The case history includes an area for the caregiver to report any illnesses, accidents, or hospitalizations. The form typically lists several diseases that are of special importance to speech-language development.

    During the interview, the clinician can explore the reported medical conditions further, as needed, to determine whether they are significant to the child's communicative disorder or not. Although communication disorders in some children may not be associated with significant medical conditions, those in others may be, as in the case of children who have genetic syndromes or brain injury.

Family and Social Background

This area is used to collect information on the parents' educational and occupational background, the child's siblings, and the family constellation. It usually includes an area for the parent to comment on how well the child gets along with his or her siblings and peers, as well as the strategies the child uses to communicate at home and in social situations.

    An important piece of information reported in this section concerns the family's language status. It is essential to ascertain whether the child and the family speak a dialect other than the mainstream English dialect and whether the child and the family are bilingual. If they are bilingual, additional information on the two languages the family members speak may be sought during the interview.

Educational Background

It is important to note if the child is attending daycare, preschool, or school. The name of the school and for how long the child has attended it is also important to know. A young child who has attended preschool often separates from the parent and adjusts to the clinical setting more quickly. If the child attends school, it is important to know if the communication problem has interfered with academic performance.

In the case of preschoolers and early elementary-age children, information may also be sought on the home literacy environment. The education of the parents, and the extent to which they read and write at home to provide literacy models may be recorded, or as often the case, explored during the interview.

Although the case history is an economic means for gathering client and family information, it has limitations. The main limitation is variable reliability of information the family members state on the case history forms. Information may vary depending on who completes the form, when it is completed, and whether specific information is even available. For example, a mother might provide different information than a father or grandparent. In the case of an adoption, medical or developmental information may not be known. In addition, the respondent may not understand all the questions, or may have variable abilities for answering them in writing. Some parents may guess more often than others; their guesses may or may not be valid.

Despite such limitations, the case history questionnaire continues to be a valuable tool for collecting client and family information, and is a good starting point for discussion with a parent or caregiver. An extensive interview in which the clinician asks additional questions and gets clarification of information will help mitigate the limitations of information stated on the case history form.

The Initial Clinical Interview

The case history form the caregivers fill out may contain less than the amount of information desired. The information given may be vague or even inaccurate. Therefore, the clinician conducts an *initial interview* with the informants (those who accompany the child to the clinic and provide additional information).

During the initial interview, the clinician goes over the case history form with the informants, typically the parents of the child. The purpose of this verbal exchange, directed mostly by the clinician, is to: (a) get additional details on the child, the family, and the disorder of communication for which help is being sought; (b) obtain clarifications on what the parents have written on the form; and (c) answer any preliminary questions the parents may have about the assessment activities themselves.

This verbal interaction is conducted in a competent and supporting manner, so that the clinician establishes a good professional relationship with the child and the parents, who may begin to trust and feel comfortable working with the clinician. Although not necessarily done during the initial assessment session, additional information or perspective on the child's speech and language skills may be obtained at a later time by interviewing other family members, teachers, daycare providers, or those who have frequent contact with the child.

To begin with, the clinician introduces herself and perhaps engages for a brief duration of small talk (Shipley, 1992). The clinician then gives an overview of what is planned for the session and may ask a series of questions about the child's communication skills and the problems of concern. As the interview proceeds, the clinician adopts a more relaxed and conversational disposition to put the child and the parents at ease. This may encourage the client to talk more freely and ultimately succeed in evoking more detailed information.

The duration of the clinical interview will vary in length depending on the amount and type of information to be exchanged, the completeness of the written case history, and the behavioral dispositions of the people involved, including the clinician. Specific interview questions also will vary, depending on the disorder for which clinical services are being sought. Such disorder-specific questions are included in the *Interview Protocol* provided in the protocols chapters on speech, language, fluency, and voice assessment.

To make clinical interviews efficient and successful, clinicians may follow these guidelines:

1. Be prepared for the interview. If possible, review the written case history ahead of time. Be clear about what you think is the purpose of the interview. Develop a list of questions or key areas you want to cover. A structured, well-planned interview promotes a professional image and reduces clinician anxiety.

2. Always record your interview (audio or video). Do not rely on your memory; take notes on critical information the interviewee offers. However, try not to take excessive written notes, as this tends to take attention away from the client and the informants and may reduce the amount of information they provide. Limit your written notes to a few key points or items you want to explore further at a later point in the interview. You can always review the audio or videotapes for details.

3. Conduct the interview in a physical environment that is comfortable, attractive, and free from distractions.

4. Take your time. Do not rush the informants or limit their responses. Let them speak freely and redirect them only as needed.

5. Avoid too many questions that can be answered with a simple "yes" or "no." Use open-ended questions.

6. Avoid talking too much yourself and do not fall into stereotypical, repetitive responses.

7. Use professional jargon sparingly and define or describe the technical terms in everyday language.

8. Seek information about the client's physical symptoms and etiologic factors by exploring the conditions associated with the onset and development of the disorder.

9. Address the client's and family members' feelings, attitudes, and beliefs regarding the communication problem, its origin, and potential remediation.

10. Ask the same question several different ways during the interview to confirm that you are getting reliable, consistent responses.

11. Be sensitive to cultural differences or language barriers that could interfere with obtaining or sharing information and establishing a positive relationship with the client and the informant.

12. Repeat important points several times during the interview.

13. At the close of the interview, summarize several key points, allowing the informant to rephrase or correct information. Ask if they have any additional questions.

14. Finish the interview by telling them what the next step will be and thanking them.

Hearing Screening

Speech-language pathologists often provide a hearing screening as part of their complete assessment of a child. A hearing screening is typically administered at 20 dB for the frequencies of 500, 1000, 2000, and 4000 Hz. It should be administered in a quiet environment using a well-maintained and calibrated audiometer. *Play audiometry* may need to be used with a young child. A child who fails the hearing screening (does not respond to one or more of the tones presented) should be referred to an audiologist for further evaluation. The form for recording the results of the hearing screening is included as part of the *Orofacial Examination and Hearing Screening Protocol* presented in Chapter 2.

Orofacial Examination

The orofacial examination is an important part of assessment, especially for assessment of speech production. It is designed to evaluate the structural and functional adequacy of the oral mechanism. *Structural adequacy* refers to the normal development of the orofacial structures and their relationship to each other. In addition, the clinician needs to note whether the presence of irregular structures is affecting speech production. *Functional adequacy* refers to how these structures move and perform during speech production (Tomblin, Morris, & Spriestersbach, 2002). During the orofacial examination, the clinician needs to note any irregularities in the strength, range, coordination, and consistency of movements.

The materials needed to complete an orofacial examination include gloves, a flashlight, tongue depressors, a mirror, and a stopwatch or a clock with a second hand. To promote tongue movement while assessing young children, it may be helpful to replace the typical tongue depressor with a lollipop, or to place foods such as peanut butter in locations where tongue placement is desired. A specific and detailed *Orofacial Examination and Hearing Screening Protocol* is provided in Chapter 2. In addition, detailed *Instructions for Conducting the Orofacial Examination: Observations and Implications* are also provided in Chapter 2.

Diadochokinetic Tasks

Diadochokinetic tasks are used to assess a child's production of rapidly alternating speech sounds. It is important to observe the rate, accuracy, and consistency of the child's speech production during these tasks, particularly as single syllables are combined to create longer or more complex utterances. Such an assessment is especially helpful in the differential diagnosis of apraxia of speech. With apraxia of speech, errors are often inconsistent and speech often breaks down as the length and complexity of the utterance increase. The child may correctly produce phonemes in a single syllable, but may fail to produce the same phonemes in a multisyllable production. In addition, sound-syllable transpositions, repetitions, or additions are more likely to occur. Groping and searching behaviors might also be observed if verbal apraxia is present (see *Childhood Apraxia of Speech Assessment Protocol* in Chapter 7). In contrast, if the child's speech errors are the result of faulty learning or muscle weakness, diadochokinetic syllable rates may be slow and speech sound errors are likely to be consistent across trials.

Typically, diadochokinetic syllable tasks consist of having the child produce the following sounds continuously and as quickly as possible: /pʌ/, /tʌ/, /kʌ/, /pʌtə/, and /pʌtəkə/. For young children, the words "buttercup" or "pattycake" are often substituted for /pʌtəkə/.

These phonemes are selected because they require the use of different muscle groups. The phoneme /p/ requires labial activity, /t/ requires elevation of the tongue tip to the front of the oral cavity (alveolar ridge), and /k/ requires posterior tongue elevation to the back of the oral cavity (velum).

Diadochokinetic syllable rates are typically calculated as "repetitions per second," although with young children, the accuracy and consistency of productions may tell us more than just calculating the rate. This is because children's rate of responses from 3 to 5 years may not show significant progressions and by age 4, the vast majority of responses may be both accurate and consistent (Williams & Stackhouse, 1998). In any case, the child's rate of repetitions may be recorded on the *Orofacial Examination and Hearing Screening Protocol*, and compared against Fletcher's (1972) norms provided in the *Diadochokinetic Assessment Protocol*, both available in Chapter 2.

Speech-Language Sample

One goal of any speech-language assessment is to obtain a measure of the child's naturalistic communication behavior. Therefore, the sample should be as representative of the child's "typical" speech and language as possible. This sample can then be used to assess the child's speech, language, fluency, and voice production. Ideally, several speech-language samples should be collected across a number of settings and communication activities. In addition, a representative sample would be based on a spontaneous conversation rather than what is produced in a contrived situation. Unfortunately, most school and clinical environments do not provide the time or opportunities needed to collect multiple and totally naturalistic samples.

The guidelines on taking an adequate speech and language sample are given in Chapter 8 on assessing language skills in children. Speech-language samples, typically recorded on an audiotape, are transcribed for specific kinds of speech or language analysis. A *Language Sample Transcription Protocol* is given in Chapter 9. In addition, a *Speech Sample Analysis Protocol* and a *Language Sample Analysis Protocol* are given in Chapters 7 and 9, respectively. If necessary, the same protocols may be used and attached to a diagnostic report on fluency or voice.

Standardized Assessment Instruments

Standardized tests are commonly used by speech-language pathologists when assessing speech production, receptive and expressive language, and literacy. Typically, standardized tests do not play a major role in the assessment of fluency or voice disorders. Standardized tests help sample speech production skills and language skills to diagnose a speech sound disorder or a language disorder.

Standardized tests make it possible to compare results across various test administrations and examiners. The results of a test may be compared against age-based norms to evaluate a child's standing in relation to his or her peer's skill levels (Anastasi & Urbana, 1997). Standardized tests, however, have significant limitations even when they are administered to children who belong to social and ethnocultural groups that were sampled in the standardization process. The tests are clearly inappropriate for many ethnoculturally diverse children on whom they are not standardized; for such children, many alternative approaches are available. Selected features of alternative approaches, when used in assessing mainstream children, will enhance the reliability and validity of assessment data. Therefore, tests may not be used on all children, and when they are, they should be considered supplemental to more naturalistic assessment procedures, including the language samples, interviews, and alternative procedures.

The characteristics, advantages, and disadvantages of standardized assessment instruments are discussed in Chapter 3. In addition, commonly used standardized tests of speech sound production are listed in Chapter 6, and language tests in Chapter 8.

Alternative and Integrated Assessment Procedures

Many alternative procedures have been developed to mitigate the negative effects of standardized tests that stem from their well-known limitations. One of them, the behavioral assessment is an alternative to the traditional linguistically oriented assessment of communication disorders. It seeks to make a causal analysis of children's verbal behavior (language skills). Other alternative approaches, although typically advocated for assessing children of ethnoculturally diverse or of low income families, offer advantages in assessing all children, including mainstream children. In addition, they all may be especially useful for assessing children who are nonverbal or have extremely limited verbal skills.

Chapter 5 includes a discussion of such alternative approaches as the behavioral (Esch et al., 2010; Lerman et al., 2005), criterion-referenced and client-specific (Hegde, 1998; McCauley, 1996), authentic (Schraeder, Quinn, Stockman, & Miller, 1999; Udvari & Thousand, 1995), dynamic (Gutierrez-Clellen, Peña, & Quinn, 1995), and portfolio (DeFina, 1992). The chapter also presents a comprehensive and integrated approach with a view that it is useful to integrate most beneficial features of alternative approaches with the more traditional approaches.

Assessment of Nonverbal and Minimally Verbal Children

Assessment of children who are nonverbal or minimally verbal, though belonging to a special category, is an important task that clinicians need to master (Beukelman & Mirenda, 2005; Glennen & DeCoste, 1997). Assessment of such children does not follow the basic outline because there are several unique concerns to be addressed. Nonetheless, such basic procedures as the case history, interview, orofacial examination, and hearing screening are relevant to assess children with limited verbal skills.

Beyond the common procedures, the clinician will concentrate on systematically observing and evaluating the nonverbal communication strategies the child exhibits. This is often the starting point of this specialized assessment. Background information on the assessment of children with limited oral language skills is presented in Chapter 14 (resources). The necessary protocols the clinician can use to complete the assessment are provided in Chapter 15.

Subsequent to an assessment of children who are nonverbal or minimally verbal, the clinician will evaluate augmentative and alternative communication (AAC) systems that will be beneficial to the child. Chapter 16 describes the phases of AAC assessment, along with a historical perspective and the currently recommended *participation model*.

Assessment of Literacy Skills

Assessment and management of literacy skills are now within the speech-language pathologist's scope of practice (American Speech-Language-Hearing Association, 2001a). Oral speech-language skills and literacy skills are intertwined. Literacy skills are language-based and adequate language skills promote literacy skills. Children with speech and language disorders experience literacy problems in academic grades (Justice, 2006; Lewis, O'Donnell, Freebrain, & Taylor, 1998). Therefore, it is essential not only to treat speech-language disorders in children, but also to pay attention to strategies that promote literacy skills.

To the extent possible, clinicians can integrate literacy skill assessment into speech and language assessment (Hegde & Maul, 2006). If the literacy assessment needs to be extensive, then additional assessment time will be needed. Chapter 17 presents a primer on literacy assessment, with an emphasis on emergent literacy skills.

Stimulability

Traditionally a part of assessment of any disorder of communication, *stimulability* refers to the child's responsiveness to trial treatment strategies. It is thought that a child's response to stimulability tasks can provide prognostic information and direction for therapy.

Stimulability tasks are different for different diagnostic categories. For example, a child with a speech sound disorder may be asked to correctly produce sounds in error when instructions, modeling, demonstration of phonetic placement, and positive reinforcement for correct responses are provided. A child who stutters may be asked to slow down the rate of speech to see if dysfluency rates go down.

A discussion of stimulability procedures, appropriate to each diagnostic category, is presented in each of the *Resource* chapters of this book. In addition, several of the *Protocol* chapters contain stimulability protocols specific to the diagnostic category.

Postassessment Counseling

After completing the assessment activities, the clinician meets with the parents and the child to: (a) share the results of assessment; (b) suggest whether the child has a communication disorder, and if so, what type of a disorder; (c) provide educational information on the diagnosed communicative disorder; (d) suggest "watchful waiting" and subsequent assessments if appropriate, (e) offer recommendations for treatment, medical follow-up, or both; and (f) respond to caregiver questions regarding the results and recommendations.

The postassessment counseling will address specific issues associated with the particular disorder the child exhibits. Therefore, chapters on speech, language, fluency, and voice protocols describe a specific dialogue between the clinician and the caregivers. Each protocol may be modified or expanded to suit the needs of an individual child and the family members.

A critical feature of postassessment counseling is to tell what the informants have been waiting to hear: Is there a problem, and if there is one, what is the diagnosis; if diagnosed, what is the treatment; if treatment is accepted, what is the prognosis? Therefore, discussing the diagnosis of the disorder, the steps to be taken to remediate the problem, and the prognosis with treatment will be the caregivers' (and older children's) priority. Postassessment counseling in most cases will concentrate on these three concerns of the caregivers and older children.

Related concerns that the clinician needs to address may include factors that contribute to the diagnosed communication problem, as most caregivers ask why their child experiences the problem whereas other children do not. The caregivers also may want to know how severe the child's problem is compared to others who have it. Furthermore, the parents will be concerned about the potential effects of the communication disorder on the academic, social, and eventual occupation life of the child. Addressing these and any other concerns the caregivers may have will be a part of postassessment counseling.

Assessment Report

Following the assessment session, the clinician makes a more complete analysis of results and writes a diagnostic report. Chapter 2 contains an *Assessment Report Outline* to help write a diagnostic report. This outline is appropriate for most diagnostic reports. The outline may be modified as appropriate for a given child and specific disorder. The report may be sent to the parents, and shared with the child's teacher or special education specialist, and with other professionals to whom the child has been referred to.

If the child is scheduled for treatment in the same facility, the clinician may use the assessment results to develop a treatment plan. Before implementing the treatment in the public school setting, the clinician schedules a meeting with the parents or other caregivers to discuss the child's *Individual Family Service Plan* or an *Individual Education Plan*. In other clinics, the clinician may present the written treatment plan to the parents for their approval.

CHAPTER 2

Common Assessment Protocols

- Child Case History Protocol
- Developmental Milestones From 0 to 4 Years of Age
- Instructions for Conducting the Orofacial Examination: Observations and Implications
- Orofacial Examination and Hearing Screening Protocol
- Diadochokinetic Assessment Protocol
- Assessment Report Outline

There are several protocols that are used in the assessment of all children with communicative disorders. These "universal" protocols are common to assessment regardless of the type of communication disorder a child exhibits. All parents who seek clinical services for their children, for example, fill out a standard case history form and respond to questions about the child's developmental milestones; all children clinically assessed for a communication disorder need an orofacial examination, a diadochokinetic test, and a hearing screening. For every child assessed, the clinician is expected to write an assessment report. This chapter provides these standard protocols that are common to all parents and their children seeking clinical services.

In addition to a protocol for completing an orofacial examination, this chapter also provides detailed instructions on making that examination. Furthermore, the instructions also include an explanation of clinical implications of observations made during the orofacial examination.

To make a comprehensive assessment, the common protocols should be combined with a number of specific protocols presented in subsequent chapters. Such a combination helps create an individualized assessment package appropriate for the child being evaluated.

Common Protocol 1
Child Case History

Today's Date _____

Child's Name _____ Date of Birth _____ Gender ___

Address _____ Phone _____

City _____ Zip _____

Mother's Name _____ Age _____

Mother's Occupation _____ Work Phone _____

Mother's Education _____

Father's Name _____ Age _____

Father's Occupation _____ Work Phone _____

Father's Education _____

Does the child live with both parents? _____

If *no*, with whom does the child live? _____

Brothers and Sisters (names and ages) _____

Referred By _____ Phone _____

Address _____

Physician _____ Phone _____

Address _____

Other specialists who have seen the child _____

Address _____ Phone _____

Please attach the most recent report from the physician, agency, or school listed above.

What were the other specialists' conclusions or recommendations? _____

_____

What language(s) does the child speak? _____

If the child is bilingual, which language is dominant? _____

What languages do the parents speak? _____

What language do the parents speak to the child? _____

(continues)

Child Case History (continued)

How does the child usually communicate? (Circle all that apply)

   Gestures   Sign Language   Single Words   Short Phrases   Sentences

Is the child difficult to understand?   Yes   No

If yes, what percentage of speech is intelligible to:

   Parents _____   Other family members _____

   Friends _____   Strangers _____

Describe the child's speech, language, fluency, voice, or hearing problem.

_____

_____

_____

When was the problem first noticed? _____

Who first noticed the problem? _____

What do you think may have caused the problem? _____

_____

Since you first noticed the problem, what changes have you observed in your child's speech, language, fluency, voice, or hearing?

_____

_____

_____

Is the child aware of the problem? _____

What have you done to help your child with the problem? _____

_____

Is there a family history of speech, language, fluency, voice, or hearing problems? If *yes,* who has what problem? Describe the relationship:

_____

_____

Prenatal and Birth History

Describe mother's general health during pregnancy (illness, accidents, prescription and nonprescription medications taken, etc.).

Length of pregnancy _____   Length of Labor _____

Child's general condition at birth _____   Birth weight _____

Circle type of delivery: head first   feet first   breech   cesarean

Describe any unusual conditions associated with the pregnancy or birth. _____

_____

_____

Medical History

Child's general health is: Good   Fair   Poor

If *Fair* or *Poor*, why? _____

Provide the approximate ages at which the child experienced any of the following illnesses or conditions:

Adenoidectomy _____	Asthma _____	Allergies _____
Chicken Pox _____	Colds _____	Convulsions _____
Croup _____	Draining Ear _____	Dizziness _____
Ear Infections _____	Epilepsy _____	Encephalitis _____
German Measles _____	Headaches _____	Hearing Loss _____
Heart Problems _____	High Fever _____	Influenza _____
Measles _____	Mastoiditis _____	Meningitis _____
Mumps _____	Noise Exposure _____	Pneumonia _____
Seizures _____	Sinusitis _____	Tinnitus _____
Tonsillitis _____	Tonsillectomy _____	Visual Problems _____

Vision Problems (Glasses) _____

Other problems _____

List the child's current medications. _____

_____

Describe any major accidents, surgeries, or hospitalizations the child has had.

_____

_____

(continues)

Child Case History (continued)

Developmental History

Write the approximate age when your child began to do the following:

Crawl _____   Sit _____   Stand _____   Walk _____   Feed Self _____

Dress Self _____   Use toilet _____   Use single words _____   Combine words _____

Name simple objects _____   Use simple questions _____   Engage in conversation _____

Does the child have any motor difficulty such as walking, running, or participating in activities that require small or large muscle coordination?

_____

_____

Describe any feeding problems (e.g., problems with sucking, swallowing, drooling, chewing, etc.).

_____

_____

How does the child respond to sounds? _____

Do you suspect any hearing problems? _____

General Behavior

Does the child eat well? _____   Sleep well? _____

How does the child interact with other family members? _____

_____

Is the child: attentive _____   extremely active _____   restless _____

Does the child lose his or her temper? _____

List any problem behaviors noticed _____

_____

Educational History

School or Preschool _____ Grade _____

Teacher(s) _____

How is your child doing in school? _____

Describe the child's difficulties at school _____

_____

Why do you think the child has those problems in the school?

_____

_____

If enrolled for special education services, list main goals of the Individualized Education Plan (IEP) or Individual Family Service Plan (IFSP).

_____

_____

_____

Please add any additional information you feel might be helpful in the evaluation or treatment of the child's problem.

_____

_____

_____

Person completing the form _____

Relationship to the child _____

Signed _____ Date _____

Please attach any report you have from another agency, school, or physician.

Common Protocol 2
Developmental Milestones from 0 to 4 Years of Age

Name _____ DOB _____ Date _____ Clinician _____

Individualize this protocol on the CD and print it for your use.

For a more detailed inventory of language skills in children up to 6 years of age, use the *Normal Language Assessment Protocol* in Chapter 9.

For the behavior exhibited, place a checkmark within the open circle.

SPEECH AND LANGUAGE	MOTOR SKILLS
Birth–3 months ○ startles to loud sounds ○ turns head toward direction of sound ○ quiets or smiles when spoken to ○ seems to recognize parent's voice and quiets if crying ○ makes pleasure sounds (cooing) ○ cries differently for different needs ○ smiles when he or she sees parents	**Birth–3 months** ○ opens hands frequently ○ supports head for more than a moment when held upright ○ raises head and chest when lying on stomach (by the end of the 3rd month). ○ brings hands to mouth ○ takes swipes at dangling objects with hands ○ grasps and shakes hand toys
4–6 months ○ moves eyes in direction of sounds ○ responds to changes in the tone of the speaker's voice ○ pays attention to music and notices toys that make sounds ○ babbles more speech-like sounds with different sounds, including *p*, *b*, and *m* ○ vocalizes excitement and displeasure ○ makes gurgling sounds when left alone or playing with others	**4–6 months** ○ rolls over from front to back and back to front ○ sits while using hands for support ○ reaches for objects with one hand ○ watches own hands ○ tracks visually people and objects
7–12 months ○ enjoys games like peek-a-boo and pat-a-cake ○ turns and looks in the direction of sound ○ listens when spoken to ○ recognizes words for common items (cup, shoe, juice) ○ understands "no" and "hot" ○ begins to respond to such requests as "come here" ○ babbles both long and short groups of sounds ○ babbles with inflection	**7–12 months** ○ sits without assistance ○ crawls forward on belly ○ assumes hands-and-knees position ○ crawls on hands and knees ○ transitions from sitting to crawling to prone position ○ pulls self up to stand ○ walks with assistance or while holding on to furniture ○ stands momentarily without support ○ may walk 2 or 3 steps without support ○ holds own bottle

SPEECH AND LANGUAGE	MOTOR SKILLS
○ produces speech or vocalizations other than crying to get and keep attention ○ imitates different speech sounds ○ produces one or two words (e.g. , "mama," "dada," "bye," "uh oh"); may be unclear	○ drinks from a cup ○ explores objects in different ways (shaking, banging, throwing, dropping) ○ imitates gestures
13–18 months ○ produces at least 3 words ○ uses adultlike intonation patterns ○ combines gestures and vocalization ○ points to a few (1 to 3) body parts when asked ○ points to objects or pictures in a book when named ○ follows simple commands ○ requests "more" of a something	**13–18 months** ○ holds a regular cup or glass without help and drinks without spilling ○ walks without support or help ○ walks across a room without falling ○ takes off shoes without help ○ feeds self
19–24 months ○ follows simple commands and understands such simple questions as "roll the ball," or "where's your shoe?" ○ enjoys listening to stories, songs, and rhymes ○ knows 5 body parts ○ learns to say new words every month ○ has an expressive vocabulary of 50 to 100 words ○ produces some 1–2 word questions (e.g., "what's that ?"or "where mommy?") ○ puts 2 words together ○ begins to use pronouns ○ 25–50% intelligible to strangers	**19–24 months** ○ walks sideways and backward ○ uses pull toys ○ pushes a wheeled toy ○ walks up and down stairs with help ○ climbs and stands on chair ○ seats self in child seat ○ enjoys playing with clay
2–3 years ○ follows simple commands and answers simple questions ○ follows 2-part requests (e.g., "Get the ball and put it in the box.") ○ understands most things said to him or her ○ has an expressive vocabulary of 50–250 or more words; names almost everything in environment ○ understands differences in meaning (e.g., *go-stop, in-on," big-little, up-down,* and *one-all*) ○ 50–75% intelligible ○ verbalizes toilet needs	**2–3 years** ○ carries a large toy or several toys while walking ○ begins to run ○ stands on tiptoe ○ kicks a ball ○ climbs onto and down from furniture unassisted ○ walks up and down stairs holding on to support ○ holds writing utensil and scribbles spontaneously ○ turns over a container to pour out contents ○ builds a tower of 4 blocks or more

(continues)

Developmental Milestones from 0 to 4 Years of Age (continued)

SPEECH AND LANGUAGE	MOTOR SKILLS
2–3 years *(continued)* ○ asks for or directs attention to objects by naming them ○ combines 2 to 3 words ○ produces some prepositions, articles, present progressive verbs, regular plurals, contractions, irregular past tense forms, and auxiliary *is* ○ exhibits multiple grammatical errors	**2–3 years** *(continued)* ○ uses one hand more frequently than the other ○ jumps off floor with both feet ○ balances on one foot for one second ○ undresses self ○ turns pages in a book several at a time
3–4 years ○ follows 2- and 3-part commands ○ understands and asks simple *who, what, where,* and *why* questions ○ understands the concept of "two" ○ understands prepositions *in, on,* and *under* ○ understand expression of *past* and *future* ○ 80% intelligible ○ has an expressive vocabulary of 800– 1500 words or more ○ uses 4-word sentences ○ may use up to 6-word sentences ○ talks about activities at school or at friends' homes ○ says name, age, and gender ○ produces *is, are,* and *am* in sentences ○ produces pronouns (*I, you, me, we,* and *they*) ○ produces some contractions, irregular plurals, future tense verbs, conjunctions, regular plurals, possessives, and simple past tense verbs	**3–4 years** ○ climbs well ○ kicks ball forward ○ runs easily ○ pedals tricycle ○ bends over easily without falling ○ turns pages in a book one at a time ○ builds a tower of more than 6 blocks ○ holds a writing utensil in writing position ○ makes vertical, horizontal, and circular strokes when drawing ○ turns rotating handles ○ screws and unscrews jar lids, and nuts and bolts ○ unbuttons but cannot button ○ uses a spoon well

Source: Adapted from various sources, including the American Speech-Language-Hearing Association (n.d.) (http://www.asha.org/public/speech/development/chart.htm) and the American Academy of Pediatrics (n.d.) http://www.aap.org/pubed .

Instructions for Conducting the Orofacial Examination: Observations and Implications

1. Gather the materials needed to complete the orofacial examination:
   - Gloves
   - Flashlight
   - Tongue depressor
   - Mirror
   - Stopwatch or clock with a second hand
   - Food or drink items (optional)
   - *Orofacial Examination and Hearing Screening Protocol* and optionally, *Childhood Apraxia of Speech Assessment Protocol* or *Dysarthric Speech Assessment Protocol*

2. Position the child so his or her face and mouth are at your eye level.

3. Observe general facial symmetry and the appearance of structures: eyes, nose, mouth, ears, hair/hairline, jaw, eyebrows, forehead, and chin. Note any irregularities or signs of asymmetry.

   Implications
   - Asymmetry, as indicated by drooping of one eye, cheek, or corner of the mouth may indicate neurologic involvement, unilateral facial paresis (weakness), or paralysis.
   - Structures that appear unusual, out of alignment with each other, or asymmetric may indicate craniofacial anomalies or be characteristic of certain syndromes or medical conditions

4. Observe the child's breathing.

   Implications
   - *Clavicular breathing* (characterized by elevation of the shoulders with each breath) may be associated with excess tension in the neck and shoulders and may contribute to hyperfunction in the larynx and consequent voice problems.
   - *Irregular breathing patterns or inadequate respiration* may affect speech prosody or have a negative effect on vocal quality.
   - *Mouth breathing* is often associated with an open mouth posture and forward tongue carriage. If these are observed, the nasal patency should be checked to make sure nasal breathing is possible. If nasal breathing is absent or difficult, and the child's speech is hyponasal, the child should be referred to a medical evaluation to determine why.

5. Observe the child's lips at rest and note any irregularities such as scars or discolorations.

6. Observe labial strength and range of motion on the following tasks:
    *   round/pucker the lip
    *   elongate the lips (smile, showing teeth)
    *   alternate pucker-smile-pucker-smile
    *   open lips wide
    *   close lips tightly and puff up cheeks (sustain intraoral pressure)
    *   bite lower lip as if making an /f/ sound
    *   say "puh-puh-puh"

    Implications
    ○   Labial weakness, as indicated by an inability to round/pucker the lips tightly, elongate the lips symmetrically, or close the lips tightly to sustain intraoral air pressure, may indicate neurologic involvement. If the lips pull to one side during elongation, the pull will be to the stronger side, suggesting a weaker opposite side.
    ○   If the child does not sustain intraoral air pressure because air escapes through the lips, labial weakness is indicated. If air escapes through the nose, along with hypernasality or nasal emission, velopharyngeal insufficiency or incompetence is indicated. Administer the *Resonance and Velopharyngeal Function Assessment Protocol* found in Chapter 13.
    ○   Difficulty producing the /p/ also may indicate labial weakness or incoordination.
    ○   Sequencing or motor programming difficulties, as indicated by searching and groping behaviors, difficulty alternating the pucker-smile, or difficulty coordinating the movements needed to puff up the cheeks or bite the lower lip, may indicate the presence of apraxia.

7. Observe the surface appearance of the child's tongue. Note any irregularities, scars, or discolorations.

8. Observe lingual strength and range of motion as you demonstrate the following movements and ask the child to:
    *   stick the tongue out as far as possible
    *   push against a tongue blade (to assess strength)
    *   elevate the tongue tip as if trying to touch your nose
    *   move the tongue tip down, as if trying to touch the chin
    *   move the tongue tip left
    *   move the tongue tip right
    *   move the tongue to the left, and then to the right sides
    *   put tongue inside cheek on right side and push cheek out (the clinician can push against the cheek to assess strength)
    *   put tongue inside cheek on left side and push cheek out (the clinician can push against the cheek to assess strength)
    *   place tongue tip behind the teeth (alveolar ridge), then slide it back along the roof of your mouth (hard palate)

Implications

- o The following observations indicate lingual weakness or incoordination: An inability to protrude the tongue or push against the tongue blade, difficulty elevating or lowering the tongue tip, difficulty moving the tongue from side-to-side or pushing against the cheek; slow tongue movement, possibly accompanied by tremor; and reduced range of motion. If weakness is on one side (unilateral), then the tongue will deviate to the weak side upon protrusion, and the child will have trouble moving the tongue towards the strong side.

- o Inability to protrude the tongue beyond the lips and a heart-shaped tongue when protruded indicate a short lingual frenulum. This is known as *ankyloglossia* or "tongue tie," which may or may not affect articulation. Have the child attempt to produce several speech sounds requiring tongue elevation (e.g., /t/, /d/, /n/, /k/). The child who cannot make the specific tongue-palate contact to produce these sounds may need to have the frenulum clipped by a physician.

- o Sequencing or motor programming difficulties, as indicated by searching and groping behaviors, difficulty alternating tongue movements, or difficulty coordinating the movements needed to put the tongue in the cheek or draw it back along the hard palate, may indicate the presence of apraxia.

9. Observe the general condition of the teeth and gums. Note any dental appliances or prostheses.

10. Observe the alignment or dental occlusion. Have the child open the mouth wide. Place a tongue blade alongside the teeth on one side and gently pull the cheek out to observe the teeth on that side. Have the child bite down so the upper and lower teeth are together. Compare the alignment of the upper first molar to the lower first molar. Repeat for the other side.

   - *Normal occlusion:* The lower first molar (mandibular) is one-half tooth ahead of the upper first molar (maxillary)
   - *Class I—Neutrocclusion:* The maxilla and mandible are in correct alignment, but individual teeth are misaligned, rotated, or jumbled
   - *Class II—Distocclusion:* The mandible is too far back in comparison to the maxilla (will appear as if jaw is underdeveloped or chin is receding)
   - *Class III—Mesiocclusion:* Mandible is too far forward in relation to the maxilla (midface may appear underdeveloped or jaw may appear overdeveloped)

11. Have the child bite down and observe the dental alignment from the front. Note any irregularities.

   - *Open bite:* While biting down, an open space (vertical space) remains between the upper and lower teeth—may be an anterior open bite or a lateral open bite

- *Overbite:* While biting down, the upper anterior teeth overlap the bottom teeth excessively (more than 1/3 of the lower teeth are covered by the upper teeth)
- *Overjet:* Horizontal projection of the upper incisors in front of the lower incisors ("buck teeth"), commonly associated with a Class II malocclusion
- *Underbite:* The upper incisors rest behind the lower incisors, commonly associated with a Class III malocclusion

Implications

- o Discoloration or cares may be the result of poor dental hygiene, poor nutrition, medications, or other medical conditions.
- o Poorly developed or misshapen teeth may be associated with various medical conditions or syndromes.
- o Poorly aligned or missing teeth can also be associated with various craniofacial anomalies or syndromes.
- o Severe malocclusion or dental alignment problems may interfere with articulation.
- o An open bite or overjet may be associated with a tongue thrust or forward tongue carriage.

12. Observe the general appearance of the hard palate: color, scarring, vault height, and vault width.

Implications

- o Discoloration or scarring may be a sign of a palatal fistula; repaired, unrepaired, or submucosal cleft. The *diagnostic triad for a submucous cleft* is a bifid uvula, a white or bluish line near the border of the hard and soft palate, and a "notch" near the posterior nasal spine that can be felt upon palpation.
- o The shape of the palatal arch varies greatly across children. However, a significantly high, narrow palate or low palate may make articulatory contacts more difficult for some sound productions. Extremely high, narrow palates may be associated with a forward tongue carriage and fronting of speech sounds.
- o *Pronounced rugae* (ridges found near the alveolar ridge) are associated with tongue thrust or forward tongue carriage. They often co-occur with a high, narrow palate, low palate, or large tongue in relation to the palate.

13. Observe the soft palate, uvula, faucial arches, tonsils and pharyngeal area. Assess the velopharyngeal mechanism during the following tasks:

- Have the child sustain "ah" for as long as possible. Observe the symmetric elevation of the uvula and medial movement of the faucial arches upon phonation.
- Have the child say "ah-ah-ah" forcefully. See the uvula move up and down symmetrically with phonation.

- Have the child sustain /u/ while you alternately occlude and open the nostrils (pinch and release the nose gently). This is called the *alternate nose holding technique.* The quality of voice should not change as you occlude and releases the nose. Any change in quality is an indication of hypernasality. A protocol for a more detailed evaluation of velopharyngeal function is presented in the voice protocols, Chapter 13.

Implications

- A bifid uvula (incomplete cleft of the soft palate) may be associated with a submucous cleft or velopharyngeal insufficiency (VPI). See the *diagnostic triad for submucous cleft palate,* described earlier.

- Asymmetry of the faucial arches or deviation of the uvula to one side may indicate neurologic involvement. The arches will tend to "droop" on the weak side, and the uvula will deviate to the strong side upon elevation.

- A change of vocal quality (hypernasality) during the alternate nose holding technique (above) may indicate VPI. Administer the *Resonance and Velopharyngeal Function Assessment Protocol* found in Chapter 13.

- Enlarged tonsils are often observed in children and they usually have no adverse affect on a child's speech. At times, however, enlarged tonsils are associated with general health, resonance, and hearing problems, and forward tongue carriage. These, in turn, could affect speech production.

- A weak or absent *gag reflex* may be associated with velopharyngeal weakness or neurologic impairment. For some children, however, lack of a gag reflex is normal.

- A hyperactive gag reflex may be associated with hypersensitivity requiring the clinician to try desensitizing the child, or may prohibit use of a tongue blade in the mouth.

- Children with oral hypersensitivity may also have trouble using a toothbrush, or may be extremely picky about what foods they will eat.

Common Protocol 3
Orofacial Examination and Hearing Screening Protocol

Child's Name: _____ DOB: _____

Examiner: _____ Date of Exam: _____

☐ Facial Symmetry at Rest
Comments:

☐ Breathing
Comments:

SCORING KEY
+ within normal limits
− deviation noted
W weakness noted
NR No Response

Lips
☐ Appearance at Rest
☐ Round Lips (pucker)
☐ Draw Corners Back (smile)
☐ Close Lips and Puff Cheeks
☐ Bite Lower Lip

Describe Lip Deviations or Indications of Weakness:

Tongue
☐ Surface Appearance at Rest   Describe:
☐ Lingual Frenum
☐ Stick Out as Far as You Can   ☐ Push Against Tongue Blade to Assess Strength
☐ Tip Up   ☐ Tip Down
☐ Tip Right   ☐ Tip Left   ☐ Alternate Left to Right
☐ Push Against Inside of Each Cheek or Tongue Blade on Each Side to Assess Strength
☐ Place Tip on Alveolar Ridge   ☐ Draw Tip Back along Hard Palate

Describe Tongue Deviations or Indications of Weakness:

Dentition and Occlusion
☐ General Condition of Teeth   ☐ Describe:
☐ **Occlusion** Based on Lateral View of First Molars (Check below, as appropriate)
  o Normal occlusion: mandibular first molar is one-half tooth ahead of maxillary first molar
  o Class I, Neutrocclusion (maxilla and mandible are in correct occlusion, but individual teeth are misaligned, rotated or jumbled)
  o Class II, Distocclusion (mandible is too far back in relation to maxilla)
  o Class III, Mesiocclusion (mandible is too far forward in relation to maxilla)

☐ Alignment (Check below, as appropriate)
    o Open bite   o Overbite   o Overjet   o Underbite

Hard Palate

☐ General Appearance   ☐ Vault Height   ☐ Vault Width

Comments:

Soft Palate and Pharynx

☐ Appearance and Symmetry of Soft Palate at Rest
☐ Appearance of the Uvula   ☐ Bifid Uvula
☐ Appearance of Faucial Arches at Rest   ☐ Palatine Tonsils

Describe any deviations of the soft palate or faucial arches, at rest:

Velopharyngeal Mechanism

Assess the velopharyngeal mechanism during the tasks described below:

Have the client sustain "ah" for as long as possible.
Have the client say "ah – ah – ah."

☐ Vertical movement of the velum (up and back)   ☐ Symmetry of movement
☐ Medial movement of the lateral pharyngeal walls   ☐ Symmetry of movement

Have the client sustain /u/ while you alternate occluding and opening the nostrils.

Was there a change in vocal quality?   YES   NO
Was hypernasality present?   YES   NO

Comments:

Diadochokinetic rates

Task	Repetitions	Seconds	Repetitions per Second
/pʌ/	_____	_____	_____
/tʌ/	_____	_____	_____
/kʌ/	_____	_____	_____
/pʌtə/	_____	_____	_____
/pʌtəkə/	_____	_____	_____

Comments on the rate, accuracy, and consistency of productions during diadochokinetic tasks:

(continues)

Orofacial Examination and Hearing Screening Protocol (continued)

Hearing Screening

	500 Hz	1000 Hz	2000 Hz	4000 Hz
Right Ear	_____	_____	_____	_____
Left Ear	_____	_____	_____	_____

Completed at _____ dB (loudness level)

○ Passed.   ○ Failed the hearing screening—audiologic evaluation recommended.

○ Hearing Screening not completed. Why?

Comments on the Hearing Screening:

Common Protocol 4
Diadochokinetic Assessment Protocol

To obtain results that represent the child's best attempt at the task, give clear instruction to the child and provide an opportunity for the child to practice. Ask the child to take a deep breath and say /pʌpʌpʌ . . . / as quickly as possible, for as long as the child can. Record the number of repetitions and the number of seconds. Repeat for /tʌtʌtʌ . . . /, /kʌkʌkʌ . . . /, /pʌtəpʌtəpʌtə . . . /, and /pʌtəkəpʌtəkəpʌtəkə . . . /. Calculate repetitions per second.

/pʌ/ _____ ÷ _____ = _____
      # of repetitions   # of seconds   repetitions per second

/tʌ/ _____ ÷ _____ = _____
      # of repetitions   # of seconds   repetitions per second

/kʌ/ _____ ÷ _____ = _____
      # of repetitions   # of seconds   repetitions per second

/pʌtə/ _____ ÷ _____ = _____
      # of repetitions   # of seconds   repetitions per second

/pʌtəkə/ _____ ÷ _____ = _____
      # of repetitions   # of seconds   repetitions per second

Comment on the accuracy and consistency of the child's productions:

Typical diadochokinetic rates (repetitions per second) for Children, 6 to 13 years old. Adapted from Fletcher (1972). The data presented in this table can be used as a guideline for "normalcy;" however, it is important to note that with young children the accuracy and consistency of their productions may tell us more than just calculating the rate.

Age in years	/pʌ/	/tʌ/	/kʌ/	/pʌtə/	/pʌtəkə/
6	4.1	4.0	3.6	2.0	.97
7	4.1	4.0	3.7	2.9	1.0
8	4.7	4.5	4.1	2.4	1.2
9	5.0	4.8	4.3	2.5	1.3
10	5.4	5.2	4.6	2.7	1.4
11	5.5	5.5	5.0	3.1	1.5
12	5.9	5.7	5.1	3.1	1.5
13	6.0	6.0	5.4	3.5	1.7

Common Protocol 5
Assessment Report Outline

Identifying Information

CLIENT: DATE OF BIRTH:

ADDRESS: DIAGNOSIS:

CITY/STATE/ZIP: REFERRED BY:

PHONE NUMBER: CLINICIAN:

DATE OF REPORT:

Background and Presenting Complaint

This information will be extracted from the Case History Form and the Interview.

Include in the first paragraph:

- The name, age, and gender of the client
- The place where the evaluation was completed
- The date of the evaluation
- Who accompanied the child and who served as the primary informant for the assessment
- The caregiver's presenting complaint or primary concern
- Information on any prior speech-language services

History

Onset and Development of the Disorder

This information will be extracted from the Case History Form and the Interview.

- Describe the time and conditions of the onset of the disorder for which help is being sought
- Describe how the disorder has changed over time
- Describe the parental reactions to the disorder and the steps they took to help the child
- Describe the child's reaction to his or her communication problem
- Describe previous professional evaluation and treatment and the effects of previous clinical services
- Describe services received from other professionals
- Describe the effect of the disorder on the child's social, academic, and personal life
- Take note of any associated clinical conditions

Pregnancy, Birth, and Developmental History

This information will be extracted from the Case History Form and the Interview.

This section may be more or less detailed, depending on the age of the child.

- Describe whether the pregnancy was full term and whether the pregnant mother had any significant illnesses that affect the embryonic and fetal growth (e.g., anemia, infectious diseases, alcoholism)
- Describe whether the delivery was normal or was associated with complications
- Describe the health of the newborn; take note of any congenital clinical conditions
- Describe the early growth and development, including any feeding problems; concentrate on speech, language, and general behavioral development

Medical History

This information will be extracted from the Case History Form and the Interview.

This section may be more or less detailed, depending on the presence or absence of medical complications.

- Describe the child's illnesses, allergies, sensory deficits (e.g., hearing loss or visual problems), neuromotor problems (e.g., cerebral palsy), and craniofacial anomalies including the clefts of the lips and palates
- Describe medical or surgical treatments the child may have received and the consequences of such treatments
- Describe the child's current health

Family, Social, and Educational History

This information will be extracted from the Case History Form and the Interview.

This section should be as detailed as possible to understand the family constellation that influences treatment outcome.

- Describe the members of the family with whom the child lives
- Take note of the parental education and occupation
- Describe the language or languages spoken by parents, other family members, and the child; pay special attention to the child's bilingual status; ascertain the child's proficiency in the primary and secondary language
- Describe the family literacy environment and support for literacy activities at home
- Describe the child's social environment, play activities, and playmates at home and in the neighborhood
- Give an overview of the child's educational activities, strengths and weaknesses, and the effects of the communication disorder on the child's academic achievement; include any comments from the child's teacher

(continues)

Assessment Report Outline (continued)

Observations and Assessment Results

Hearing Screening

Results will have been recorded on the Orofacial Examination and Hearing Screening Protocol included in Chapter 2.

- State whether the child passed or failed the hearing screening test
- If the child failed the hearing screening test, note the need for a complete audiologic evaluation

Orofacial Examination and Diadochokinetic Tasks

Results will have been recorded on the Orofacial Examination and Hearing Screening Protocol included in Chapter 2.

- Summarize your findings of the orofacial examination
- State whether the orofacial structures are adequate for speech production
- Summarize any deviations that might affect speech production
- Suggest needed additional referrals (e.g., a genetic counselor, an orthodontist, a neurologist, an audiologist)

Speech Sound Production

Results will have been recorded on protocols included in Chapter 7.

See also, Chapter 6.

Note that this section will be detailed as outlined if the child has been assessed for a speech sound disorder (an articulation or a phonological disorder); if not, general comments about the child's production of speech sounds may be made in the report.

- Summarize the results of any standardized tests
  - include an inventory of phoneme errors
  - list phonological process
  - report any standardized scores
- Summarize the results of your speech sample analysis
  - list phoneme errors and phonological processes observed
  - compare the results of standardized test results and speech sample analysis
  - state the percent intelligibility of speech
  - discuss factors contributing to intelligibility
  - comment on prosody, voice, and fluency as observed during spontaneous speech
- Summarize the results of any alternative assessment procedures used
  - specify the procedures (e.g., child-specific, authentic, dynamic, portfolio)
  - summarize the findings and compare them against the findings of other measures used, including standardized tests and speech samples

- Write a summative statement about the existing and missing speech production skills that integrates observations based on standardized tests, language sample, and alternative procedures used

Language

Results will have been recorded on protocols included in Chapter 9.

See also, Chapter 8.

Note that this section will be detailed as outlined if the child has been assessed for a language disorder; if not, general comments about the child's language skills may be made in the report.

- Summarize results of standardized language tests
  - comment on the child's vocabulary (estimated size, variety)
  - list morphologic features correctly produced and those that are missing or incorrectly produced
  - comment on the syntactic structures produced and syntactic errors noted
  - describe the pragmatic or conversational skills observed and those that are judged inappropriate or missing
- Summarize the results of your language sample analysis
  - Describe the observed semantic, morphologic, syntactic, and pragmatic language skills the child produced during the language sampling
  - List the expected language skills the child did not produce
  - Compare the results of language sample analysis with those of standardized tests
  - Comment on the child's language comprehension as noted throughout the assessment session
- Summarize the results of any alternative assessment procedures used
  - specify the procedures (e.g., child-specific, authentic, dynamic, portfolio)
  - summarize the findings and compare them against the findings of other measures used, including standardized tests and speech samples
- Write a summative statement about the existing and missing language skills that integrates observations based on standardized tests, language sample, and alternative procedures used

Fluency

Results will have been recorded on protocols included in Chapter 11.

See also, Chapter 10.

Note that this section will be detailed as outlined if the child has been assessed for a fluency disorder; if not, general comments about fluency may be made in the report.

- Summarize the results of the speech sample analysis; state the percent dysfluency rate

(continues)

Assessment Report Outline (continued)

- Describe the types of dysfluencies the child produced during assessment
- Describe the child's avoidance reactions: speech situations and words the child typically avoids
- Describe the child's negative emotional reactions as assessed through interviews or standardized assessment batteries
- Describe in general terms the motor behaviors (e.g., eye blinks, hand and feet movements, facial grimaces) that are associated with dysfluencies

Voice

Results will have been recorded on protocols included in Chapter 13.

See also Chapter 12.

Note that this section will be detailed as outlined if the child has been assessed for a voice disorder; if not, general comments about the child's voice may be made in the report.

- Summarize the results of clinical observations and results of specific assessment tasks presented to the child
- Summarize the results of instrumental assessment of vocal parameters
- Describe the voice disorders that have been observed and measured during assessment
- Describe the resonance disorders that have been observed and measured during assessment
- Comment on potential and suspected laryngeal pathologies associated with the noted voice problems
- Describe the vocally abusive behaviors, if relevant
- Summarize the laryngologist's report, if one is available

Associated Clinical Conditions

Information on any associated clinical conditions will be extracted from the case history, interview, and any report received from other professionals (e.g., psychologists, psychiatrists, genetic counselors, physicians, and audiologists).

See Chapter 8 for some associated clinical conditions.

Note that this section may be omitted if associated clinical conditions are absent.

- Describe any associated clinical conditions and the observed behavioral characteristics, including:
  - hearing loss
  - intellectual disabilities
  - autism spectrum disorders

- ○ craniofacial anomalies and genetic syndromes
- ○ neuromotor deficits, including traumatic brain injury and cerebral palsy
- ○ psychiatric or behavioral problems, including attention deficit and hyperactivity disorders
- ○ myofunctional disorders
- ○ physical growth problems
- ○ any other clinical condition noted or reported
- • Summarize the reports of relevant specialists, if available

Diagnostic Summary and Prognosis

Write a section on diagnostic summary and prognosis in which you:

- • Summarize your major findings
- • State your diagnosis, if appropriate
- • Estimate a level of severity
- • Discuss strengths and weaknesses of the child
- • Give a prognostic statement based on your observation, judged motivation, family support, response to any previous treatment, and results of your stimulability test:
  - ○ prognosis with treatment, if recommended
  - ○ prognosis without treatment
  - ○ conditions under which a good prognosis may be obtained (e.g., regular treatment, follow-up by parents, completion of assigned work at home)

Recommendations

Cover the following in making your recommendations:

- • State whether you recommend speech, language, voice, or fluency therapy
- • Estimate the frequency and duration of treatment
- • Make needed referrals to other professionals, including an audiologist if the child failed the hearing screening test
- • Discuss areas where additional data need to be collected (i.e., additional assessment, a home speech sample, or diagnostic therapy)
- • Describe recommended treatment goals

To practice writing assessment reports, see *A Coursebook on Scientific and Professional Writing for Speech-Language Pathology* (4th ed.) by Hegde (2010). Clifton Park, NY: Delmar, Cengage Learning.

CHAPTER 3

Standardized Assessment

- Standardized and Norm-Referenced Tests
- Test Construction
- Reliability
- Validity
- Questionnaires and Developmental Inventories
- Strengths of Standardized Tests
- Limitations of Standardized Tests
- Prudent Use of Standardized Tests
- Assessment in a Multicultural Society

Standardized testing of human behavior or skills has a long history in psychology. The term "mental tests" dates back to 1890, when the American psychologist James McKeen Cattell used it for the first time (Anastasi & Urbina, 1997). The testing movement is the result of a need to determine the intellectual, sensory, and behavioral ("personality") characteristics in individuals. The educational need to classify children with limited intellectual abilities has been an important force in the development of psychological tests. The European experimental psychologists of the 19th century had discovered that to measure sensory discrimination and reaction time of human participants, the conditions and instructions must be standardized; such standardization was incorporated into measuring any kind of human performance, including psychological tests. By the end of the 19th century, people attending scientific or industrial expositions were taking various tests that assessed their sensory and motor skills, the result of which were compared against norms (Anastasi & Urbina, 1997).

Formal and systematic measurement of intelligence, begun with the French psychologists Binet and Simon at the beginning of the 20th century, heralded the modern era of psychological testing. In subsequent years, tests to measure aptitude, personality, and educational achievement were developed. The need to assess various abilities of a large number of army recruits at the beginning of World War I in 1917 gave a significant boost to psychological testing.

Speech-language pathology has borrowed and accepted the tradition of assessing communication skills through standardized tests. Clinicians now commonly use them to diagnose disorders of communication and to qualify children for intervention in public schools. In this chapter, we describe the essential features of standardized tests as a means to assess communication skills and diagnose communication disorders. We take note of the strengths and limitations of standardized tests. In the next chapter, we will discuss assessment of children of ethnocultural minority groups for whom many available standardized tests are inappropriate. In Chapter 5, we describe alternatives to standardized assessment, along with an integrated and comprehensive approach that may be appropriate to all children.

Standardized and Norm-Referenced Tests

Standardization is a research process that includes careful selection of test items, administration of the items to a representative sample drawn from a defined population, statistical analysis of results, establishment of age-based norms, and development of instructions and response scoring procedures. A standardized test should be self-contained in that all needed stimulus materials and recording forms should be included in it. The instrument should allow for uniform administration and scoring of responses by different examiners in varied settings to minimize any influence examiners and settings may have on the skills being measured.

Most standardized tests also are *norm-referenced*. Norm referenced tests are always standardized. Norm-referenced tests help compare a client's performance to the performance of another group of individuals called the *normative group*. A *norm* is the performance measure of a normative group on a tested skill. The normative group is usually a representative sample of individuals of the same age and possibly the same sex as the client.

A norm-referenced test should provide detailed information on the normative sample, including:

- The size of the sample; the American Psychological Association (1999) states that it should not be less than 100; meeting only this minimum requirement of a sample size, however, will result in a test of extremely limited applicability.

- The ethnocultural and socioeconomic levels of the individuals selected for standardization; the greater the variety of these variables and the more adequate the different subsamples selected, the higher the applicability of the test.

- The geographic distribution of selected participants for standardization; once again, the more varied the geographic distribution of the samples, the wider the applicability of the test.

- Other relevant variables, including the IQ or medical status of the sample; when children are the participants, the manual should also specify the range of education and occupation of the parents.

- Descriptive statistics; the manual should include means and standard deviations for all groups on whom the test items have been administered; additional statistical transformation of the raw scores (e.g., percentiles) also may be specified.

The test developers carefully select test items that they believe represent the skill the test seeks to measure. The test items are then administered to the normative group. The results are analyzed to establish the *normal distribution of scores*. This normal distribution is often represented by a bell-shaped curve with the range of scores or values measured on the horizontal access and the number of participants receiving a particular score on the vertical access. The bell-shape results because there will be a concentration of people in the middle (median or mean score) with a rapid decrease in the number of people as one moves away from the middle in either direction (see Table 3–1.) In other words, most people's scores will center around the mean, and progressively fewer people's scores will deviate from the mean to the progressively greater extent. The peak of the bell-shaped curve will represent the mean or median score, the average performance on the test. This would also be the 50th percentile.

Because the mean represents a statistical average of individual performance, the score of an individual may not exactly correspond to the mean; it may deviate, or be different from, the mean. The extent to which an individual's score deviates away from the mean is called the *standard deviation*. In a normal curve:

- 68.26% of all scores will fall within 1 standard deviation of the mean (34.13% above and 34.13% below the mean)

- 95.44% of all scores will fall within 2 standard deviations of the mean (47.5% above and 47.5% below the mean)

- 99.72% of all scores will fall within 3 standard deviations of the mean (49.85% above and 49.85% below the mean)

A given individual's score on a test may be understood in terms of standard deviation from the mean. The distribution within which a score falls is indicative of the extent to which the score deviates from the average score for the standardization sample.

The *raw score* of an individual is the initial score given based on his or her correct responses to test items. Typically, the raw scores of different individuals on most standardized tests are not meaningfully compared with each other. Therefore, most standardized test scores are statistically transformed into other kinds of scores, collectively known as *derived scores* or *scales*. Such derived (transformed) scores of different individuals may be compared to determine their relative strengths and limitations. Percentiles, standard scores (*z*), and stanines are among the more frequently encountered transformed scores in standardized test manuals (Anastasi & Urbina, 1997; Van Ornum, Dunlap, & Shore, 2008).

Percentiles

Percentiles, also called *percentile scales*, represent the percentage of individuals in the standardization sample scoring at or below a given raw score. The 50th percentile would represent the mean or median score. Therefore, those who score above the 50th percentile are "above average" and those who score below the 50th percentile are "below average" in the tested skill. Percentiles are a ranking system except that the lower the percentile, the lower the skill level and the higher the percentile, the higher the skill level.

A person whose score represents the 30th percentile is thought to have performed lower than 70% of those in the normative sample: a significantly below average performance. On the other hand, a person whose score represents the 95th percentile will have scored better than 94% of individuals on whom the test was standardized: a very high score because only 5% of the sample did better than that person. The highest raw score in the standardized sample would have a percentile rank of 100, although it does not mean a perfect raw score on the test. The lowest raw score of an individual in the standardized samplewould have a percentile rank of zero, although once again, it does not mean a zero raw score.

Percentages of correct responses and percentiles refer to different measures. Percentage of correct responses is calculated on the basis of the number of correct and incorrect *responses* out of the total number of test items. The percentile, on the other hand, is based on the number of *individuals* who score below or above a particular raw score.

Percentile ranks are commonly used in comparing individuals on a skill being assessed. They are available for most standardized tests. A limitation of percentile ranks is that they can tell that two individuals are apart on a skill (one with a higher level than the other), but the scores cannot tell *how much apart*. Generally, scores around the mean are clustered and, hence, are close to each other. Scores that are at the extremes are fewer and also farther apart than those that are clustered around the mean. The distance between a score of 90 and 99, away from the mean, may be much bigger (larger differences between the individuals) than the distance between the scores 40, 50, and 60 (around the mean, with smaller differences in skills measured).

Standard Scores (*Z* and *T* Scores)

The *standard scores* represent the degree to which a child's score deviates from the mean. Deviation from the mean is expressed in terms of a *standard deviation* (SD); it is a measure of the distance between the group mean and an individual score. There are two common types of standard scores: the *Z score* and the *T score*.

The *z* scores are linearly derived standard scores. *Z* scores are based on the assumption that the mean is zero and the *SD* is 1. *Z* scores retain the original relationship between the raw scores. To calculate a *z* score, the clinician needs to know the score of an individual (X1), the mean for the standardization group (M), and the *SD* of the normative sample. The formula for calculating the *z* score is as follows:

$$z = \frac{X - M}{SD}$$

If a child's score is 70, the mean for the standardization sample is 60, and the *SD* for that sample is 5, then the child's *z* score is 2 (70 minus 60, divided by 5). This means that the child's score fell 2 *SD* above the mean. If another child's score is 60, but the mean is 70, and the *SD* is the same 5, then the child's *z* score will be –2 (60 minus 70, divided by 5). This means that the child's score fell 2 *SD* below the mean. As these examples show, if a child's score deviates to the negative side of the mean, then the *z* score value will be negative; if it deviates to the positive side of the mean, the *z* score value will be positive. The *z* score for a child who scores the same as the sample mean will be zero (no deviation from the mean). Note that it is clinically much more meaningful to know that the child performed at, below, or above the mean for the standardization group than to say that the child scored 60 or 70 on a test.

The T scores are technically *normalized standard scores* because the distribution of scores of the standardization sample will have been transformed to fit a normal probability (bell-shaped) curve (Anastasi & Urbina, 1997). The T scores are based on the assumption that the mean is 50 and the *SD* is 10. Consequently, on a T score scale, a child who scores 60 is judged to be 1 *SD* above the mean and a child who scores 30 is 2 *SD* below the mean.

Most test manuals provide a table of *z* scores or T scores to readily interpret a child's raw score on the test. Clinicians then can make diagnostic and intervention decisions based on the interpretation.

Stanine

Developed by the U.S. Air Force, a *stanine* is a statistical product of World War II. It is based on a nine-unit scale with a mean of 5 (representing the average performance) and an *SD* that approximates 2. The term stanine is created out of *standard* and *nine*. Because the scores range only from 1 to 9, all raw scores are converted to one of the single digits within that range. Percentages under the normal curve are used to assign stanine to a distribution of test scores. The same percentages are then assigned to each stanine, as shown in Table 3–1.

According to the table, the lowest scoring 4% of the individuals tested will get a stanine of 1 whereas the highest scoring 4% of individuals tested will get a stanine of 9. Stanine scores of 2, 3, and 4, respectively, represent 7, 12, and 17% of the tested individuals. Note

Table 3–1. Percentages Under the Normal Curve and Stanine Score Assignment

Percentage	4	7	12	17	20	17	12	7	4
Stanine	1	2	3	4	5	6	7	8	9

that the mean is 5 with the largest percentage of individuals; the other percentages are roughly evenly distributed on either side of the mean. Scores 6, 7, 8, and 9 represent the corresponding percentages of individuals with above-average performance.

Equivalent Scores

Unlike the scales described so far which compare an individual's scores to the normal distribution, equivalent scores suggest that a given score is representative of a particular age group or educational grade. For example, a 7-year-old could obtain a raw score of 70 on a standardized test. The test manual then may suggest that a raw score of 70 on the test was typically obtained by 6-year-old children in the standardization sample. This is interpreted to mean that the 7-year-old child's tested skills match that of a 6-year-old and that the tested child's skills are *more like those of a child who is 1 year younger*. These types of age- or grade-equivalent scores are not standard psychometric measures, although they are popular in educational assessment. Parents and teachers alike find age- or grade-equivalent scores easy to understand; tested children may be classified as performing at, below, or above their age or grade levels. Many tests provide such equivalency scores and most clinicians, especially in educational settings, use them in reporting test results.

Clinicians, however, should be aware of serious limitations of equivalent scores. Such scores do not take into account variations in performance that might be common or expected in a particular age group. For example, we know that the 7-year-old child in the previous example scored similar to a typical 6-year-old, but we do not know how unusual this is. That score could be within the 40th percentile indicating that it is not that unusual for a child of that age, or it could be more than 2 standard deviations below the mean, indicating that it is unusual or *below normal limits* for that age. This example shows that age- or grade-equivalency scores are not accurate indicators of impairment (McCauley & Swisher, 1984a, 1984b). In fact, age- or grade-equivalent scores may be "the least useful or most dangerous scores to be obtained from standardized tests because they lead to gross misinterpretations of a client's performance" (Haynes & Pindzola, 2004, p. 63). Clinicians should prefer one of the standard scores to equivalent scores.

Test manuals should provide instructions for interpreting raw scores using the various scales. It is important for the clinician to review this information prior to interpreting test results. In general, however, any score that falls in the bottom 5% of the normal distribution, or approximately −1.5 to −2.0 standard deviations below the mean is cause for concern (Haynes & Pindzola, 2004).

Basal and Ceiling Levels

Many standardized tests, particularly language and intelligence tests, require the examiner to establish a *basal level* and a *ceiling level*. Tests will define both the levels in terms of correct and incorrect scores. A basal score is the entry level and the ceiling score is the test-terminating score.

In many relatively long tests, testing may begin at some arbitrary level judged appropriate for the child, instead of at the very beginning of the test. This will help save test administration time. If the judged entry level proves wrong, the clinician may move down to find the basal level. In a given test, for example, a basal score might be defined as 5 consecutively correct responses. If at the initial level of testing, a child scored only 2 out of 5 responses correctly, the judged entry level would have been too high; the examiner then moves down the test items to find the first 5 consecutively correct responses. Once a basal is established, all test items prior to it are considered *correct* and the testing continues forward.

A ceiling in a given test might be defined as 6 out of 8 consecutively incorrect responses. In this example, the examiner continues to present the test items until the child gives 6 incorrect responses on 8 consecutive test items. The ceiling represents the highest number or level of test items administered or the point at which the test administration is stopped because the remaining higher level items are all considered *failed*. A test may require that a basal and ceiling be established to calculate a raw score.

Test Construction

Clinicians who select and administer standardized tests to assess and diagnose disorders of communication should have a basic knowledge of how they are constructed. Such knowledge is helpful in carefully evaluating available tests and selecting the most appropriate ones to assess a given set of skills.

Test developers generally consider the following principles in constructing and standardizing assessment tests. However, some test developers may be more successful than others in adhering to the principles of test construction.

Test Purpose. Tests are designed for different purposes, some limited and others more ambitious. Therefore, the experts designing a test must clearly state the purpose for which a test was created so that the practitioners do not misuse them. The authors should also present evidence that the test measures what it purports to measure. This is a matter of *validity*, which is addressed in a later section.

Stimulus Items. Stimulus items should be carefully selected to meet the purposes of the test. Simply put, stimulus items should help assess the targeted skills. These stimulus items may include verbal instructions, photographs, drawings, objects, and written information. These test items should also be assessed for their relevance, validity, and reliability. The selected photographs and drawing should be attractive, clear, and unambiguous. All stimuli should be culturally appropriate for the intended population of children.

Test Administration and Scoring Procedures. These procedures are predetermined and specified in the manual so that different administrators stimulate and score the responses in a uniform manner, thus minimizing the influence of individual examiners. To maximize consistency in test administration and scoring, written directions must outline exactly what the examiner does and says to give test instructions and administer the test. Specific rules for scoring client responses must be developed, along with accompanying resources (e.g., conversion tables for raw scores, percentiles, standard scores, stanines, means, and standard deviations).

Normative Sample. Norm-referenced tests are expected to assess skills that are representative of the children in the relevant population (e.g., children in the age range of 2 to 7 years or children belonging to certain ethnocultural groups). Because the test cannot be standardized on the entire relevant population, which is typically very large, the test developers select a much smaller **normative sample** that is expected to represent that population.

Although the normative sample is smaller than the population it represents, it cannot be too small to be biased. Test developers select a sample of participants they believe represents the relevant population. According to the *Standards for Educational and Psychological Tests* compiled by the American Psychological Association (1999), the number of participants in each group should not be less than 100. For most nationally or even regionally used tests, one probably needs a much larger sample than 100 participants. The sample should adequately represent the various educational, socioeconomic, and occupational levels of the families from which the participants are sampled. Proportionate sampling of children who belong to different racial and ethnic groups and those who live in different geographic regions (e.g., rural, urban, and suburban) is also important. Standardized tests that are considered inadequate often will not have sampled the participants adequately to achieve the stated test purpose.

Statistical Analysis. The test developers should provide the range of raw scores as well as derived scores. Various statistical analyses of the normative data may be made to give derived scores of the kind described previously. The analysis should include means and standard deviations for all groups in the normative sample. Confidence intervals and information on the standard error of measurement also should be included.

Validity and Reliability. It is important to establish that the test measures what it purports to measures and that it does it consistently. These are matters of validity and reliability, respectively. The test manual should include information on the kinds of validity the authors established. Minimally, the manual should report construct validity. Test-retest, interjudge, and internal consistency types of reliability should also be reported (Hutchinson, 1996). Other kinds of reliability and validity, if reported, will enhance the usefulness of a test. Because of their technical nature and importance to test selection, the concepts and procedures of reliability and validity are discussed in some detail in the next section.

Test Manual. A comprehensive test manual is essential to properly administer a test and to make correct interpretation of the results. Hutchinson (1996) states that the manual should include detailed information on the following: the rationale for the test; a description of how the test was developed; the purpose of the test; examiner qualifications; detailed instructions for the administration, scoring, and interpretation of the test; reliability and validity indexes; information on the normative sample; and descriptive statistics. The manual should be written in a clear and concise language while giving all essential information. Informative tables and attractive graphs will help understand the procedures of analysis and facilitate interpretation of results.

Reliability

Reliability is consistency across repeated measures of the same phenomenon with the same instrument. That a standardized test is reliable means that the results obtained for the same individuals are replicable and that different examiners report similar scores for the same individuals. Consistency of measures is critical for both standardized and naturalistic measures. A test will not be trustworthy if it cannot provide consistent results when administered to the same individuals by different examiners or when the same examiners administer it to the same individuals on different occasions.

Typically, reliability, much like its twin concept of validity to be described in the next section, is expressed as a correlation coefficient (Hegde, 2001, 2003; Salvia & Ysseldyke, 1981). Standardized tests often report such reliability correlation coefficients. It is preferable for tests to have correlation coefficients of .90 or above. The closer a coefficient of reliability is to 1.0, the more reliable is the test.

Reliable measurement of communicative behaviors is a difficult and often neglected issue in speech-language pathology. The difficulty is common to both standardized tests and naturalistic observations (e.g., speech and language samples). It is not always evident that clinicians can reliably measure the frequency of stuttering or make reliable judgments about various voice qualities.

Some factors facilitate acceptable reliability of measures whereas others impede it. To achieve improved reliability, it is necessary to:

- Define the behavior being assessed in operational (measurable) terms; poorly defined or broadly conceptualized skills are hard to measure in the first place, let alone reliably.

- Describe the administration and scoring procedures in clear and precise language; standardized tests that do not give clear instructions on test administration and response scoring cannot lead to good reliability of scores; similarly, clear and precise description of speech-language sampling procedures and scoring methods will facilitate reliable measures.

- Train test administrators or observers of naturally occurring behaviors (as in obtaining a speech-language sample or judging voice deviations) to follow standard procedures; poorly trained test administrators or observers cannot be expected to get consistent measures on the same individuals even with the same tests or methods of observation.

- Simplify the behavior to be assessed or observed; although oversimplification of a complex skill will not serve any purpose, the more complex or abstract the behavior being assessed, the more difficult it is to achieve reliable measures; breaking a complex behavior into more easily observable components might be helpful.

- Record the observational or testing session; although not commonly done, beginning clinicians may audio-record a testing session until they become proficient in test administration; naturalistic observations (e.g., language sampling) is typically audio-recorded for later analysis.

- Take note of the natural variability of the behavior or skill being measured; some behaviors, not matter how well the observers are trained and how carefully the measurement procedures are developed, may fluctuate across time and situations; stuttering is known to vary in this manner; some voice characteristics also may naturally vary; the only available solution to this natural variability of a phenomenon being measured is to control the conditions under which it is observed and repeat observations until the behavior stabilizes and its measures are consistent.

A concept central to reliability is *error of measurement* (Hegde, 2003). When a phenomenon is measured repeatedly, the measured values will be unlikely to be identical, even if the phenomenon is stable; very few phenomena, if any, are stable over time. Furthermore, some behaviors are more stable than others. Speech-language production and comprehension skills may be relatively more stable than frequency of stuttering or the "mood" of a person. Consequently, some fluctuations in scores across repeated measurements is unavoidable because the behavior being measured may change over time, combined with errors in measurement. Therefore, variability in repeated scores obtained for the same individuals may have two sources: a true difference (variability) in the behavior being measured, and an *error variance* that is due to common and unavoidable errors in measurement. A reliable test minimizes the error variance.

Reliability is established in different ways, giving rise to different kinds of reliability. Each type captures a different aspect of reliability, and addresses different kinds of measurement concerns.

Interobserver Reliability

Interobserver reliability, also known as *interjudge reliability*, is consistency of test scores recorded by two or more examiners administering the same test to the same individuals. In the context of language samples or other naturalistic (nonstandardized) measures, interobserver reliability refers to consistency of measured values across observers who measure the same phenomenon in the same individuals. Whether it is a standardized or more naturalistic measure, reliability is a basic requirement that all observations and measurements must fulfill.

Interobserver reliability is higher if two or more observers are trained strictly according to the manual of a test or trained the same way to make naturalistic observations. But the critical issue here is whether the test itself allows for acceptable interobserver reliability. If two well-trained test administrators cannot get similar scores on the same individual, for the same and relatively stable behavior, then perhaps there is a reliability problem with the test itself.

Intraobserver or Test-Retest Reliability

Also known as *intrajudge reliability*, **intraobserver reliability** is the consistency of scores the same individuals obtain when the same examiner readministers the test or repeats a naturalistic observation. In the context of standardized tests, intraobserver reliability is typically described as *test-retest reliability* because the main method of establishing this type of reliability is to repeat the test on the same individuals. In the context of nonstandardized naturalistic measurement of skills (e.g., speech-language sampling, baserating, probing during or after treatment), the term *intraobserver reliability* is more appropriate than *test-retest* reliability. Obviously, if repeated administrations of a test or naturalistic observations of a behavior yield divergent scores, the clinician cannot make diagnostic or treatment decisions.

The test-retest method is probably one of the easiest methods of establishing reliability of standardized tests. The examiner then correlates the two sets of scores of the same persons. An obvious question for the test constructor is the optimum time duration between the two administrations of the same test to the same individuals. If the duration is too short, the individuals tested may simply recall their responses from the first administration; this will inflate the reliability correlation coefficient. If the duration between the two administrations is too long, the behavior being measured may change, thus yielding a low reliability correlation coefficient. Generally, the same individuals are retested within a month, perhaps in two weeks. Tests standardized for children usually have shorter durations between retests than those developed for adults because of more rapid changes in skills in the former, as against the latter, populations. Even for adults, however, the interval should not exceed 6 months unless there is some special reason to extend it (Anastasi & Urbina, 1997).

Another question that needs to be answered about the usefulness of retest reliability is whether the skill being measured will change, often improve, because of the testing itself. Motor dexterity test scores may improve because of practice the individuals gain during the test. Speech sound productions may improve with repeated practice. The problem, however, is more acute in measuring opinions and attitudes than relatively stable speech-language skills. We return to this problem in a later section on inventories and questionnaires.

To facilitate an understanding and evaluation of a test, its manual should specify not only the test-retest correlation coefficient, but also the interval between the two administrations. The manual should further specify any changes that may have occurred in the life of the individuals who were retested (e.g., illness, counseling, or treatment during the interval). If the retest reliability of a test is good, but an individual clinician does not get consistent scores on the same individuals, it is possible that the clinician needs training in the administration and scoring of the test.

Alternate- or Parallel-Form Reliability

Alternate-form reliability refers to the consistency of measures when two forms of the same test are administered to the same person or group of people. Obviously, it requires two versions of the same test (Hegde, 2001). This type of reliability minimizes some of the problems inherent to retest reliability. For instance, alternate forms of the same test may reduce the chances of recall of responses from the previous administration because the test items that sample the same behaviors may be different on the two forms. When there is an appropriate temporal interval between the two administrations, alternative form reliability indicates both the degree of temporal stability of responses and the consistency of test items.

The main difficulty in establishing parallel-form reliability is the construction of two versions of the same test that include items comparable in difficulty. If one form is easier than the other, or if one form contains items more familiar to certain individuals than to others, then the scores on the two forms may not reflect its true reliability. If the two forms are administered about the same time in quick succession, the resulting acceptable reliability coefficient will only indicate consistency across forms, not temporal stability. Such a coefficient may also partly reflect some degree of practice effect. The test manual should, therefore, specify the time interval between the two parallel-form administrations. Furthermore, because of the need to construct two parallel forms of the same test, a two-fold effort is needed to standardize a test and establish this type of reliability.

Split-Half Reliability

Split-half reliability is a measure of internal consistency of a test. To establish this type of reliability, an examiner correlates the scores from one-half of the test with those from the other half of the test. Another method of calculating split-half reliability is to correlate responses given to odd-numbered items with those given to even-numbered items. The correlation calculated with the split-half method is sometimes described as *coefficient of internal consistency*. Such a coefficient does not suggest stability of scores across time because there is only a single administration of the test.

To establish split-half reliability, both halves of a test should be equivalent in the content and difficulty level; the entire test should measure the same skill. Split-half reliability is desired for some tests, but may be inappropriate for a test whose items are in a hierarchical order. For example, some tests begin with easier items and progress toward increasingly difficult items. Splitting such a test into equivalent halves will yield low reliability coefficients. A solution to this problem is to correlate the responses on odd-even items; this method samples items throughout the test to create two halves. Therefore, responses given to both the easier and more difficult items are sampled for correlation.

A test that reliably measures something may not measure something specific. In other words, what a test measures reliably may not be what the examiner wants to measure in given individuals. Therefore, having decided that a test reliably measures something, the clinician needs to evaluate whether what is measured is what was intended to be measured. This is the matter of validity.

Validity

Validity is the extent to which a test measures what it is constructed to measure. It reflects the *truthfulness* of the measure. For example, if a test claims to measure a child's expressive vocabulary, it should adequately measure that skill. If it measures something else, it is invalid for the purpose of measuring expressive vocabulary, although it may measure some other skill quite validly (as well as reliably). Therefore, note that validity of a test is always judged against what it is *purported* to measure.

Validity of a test is also judged against an examiner's intended use. Many tests may be used for different purposes, some not suggested by the original test developers. For example, a test of speech sound production in longer sentences may later be used to assess the maximum speed with which syllables are produced without losing intelligibility. In such contexts, it is the test user who should judge whether the test is valid for the new purpose for which it will be administered. In a general sense, validity is "the extent to which interpretations of the test scores are meaningful and acceptable" (Hegde & Maul, 2006, p. 96). Communication is a complex process that involves many kinds of skills, so it is important that the test actually measures what the test developer intended it to measure and what an examiner uses it to measure.

There are different kinds of validity, but the kinds are simply a result of different ways in which a test's validity can be established. Some types of validity are based on expert's careful judgment whereas other kinds require statistical analyses of additional data gathered to demonstrate a new test's validity. It is a common misconception that a test is fully valid if it contains *any one* of the several types. A truly valid test, however, should demonstrate all major kinds of validity, a description of which follows.

Content Validity

Content validity is demonstrated by expert judgment that the test indeed includes items that are relevant to assess the purported skill. To validate a test through this method, one should have a thorough knowledge of the skill being measured. If the experts find that a test of English morphologic features contains items to sample the production of English morphologic features, then the test is claimed to have content validity.

Three major criteria guide the content-validation of a test under construction (Salvia & Ysseldyke, 1981):

- Appropriateness of the items included: The test should contain only those items that help sample the purported skill and it should not contain items that are judged irrelevant to the skill being measured; most carefully designed tests meet this criterion.

- Completeness of the items sampled: The number of items included in the test should be sufficient to make a comprehensive assessment of the skill being measured; unfortunately, many standardized tests fail to meet this criterion because they assess a skill with a single or few items.

- Way in which the test items assess the content: The manner of assessment should fit the skill; for example, speech sounds need to be evoked in words and in three word-positions (initial, medial, and final); morphologic features should be evoked with specific kinds of questions, whereas certain conversational skills (e.g., topic maintenance) should be assessed through narrative speech.

Content-validation of a test requires that the entire skill range to be tested is described beforehand, not after the fact. The test items should be appropriately balanced across subskills; they should not be overloaded on skills for which it is easier to write objective test items. Content validity is not achieved by a superficial examination of resemblance of the test items to the skill being measured; such an examination may suggest what is known as *face validity*, which is unsatisfactory. Content validation requires an expert's critical examination of each item's relevance and ability to sample the behavior under observation.

Mere content validity, though reported to be satisfactory, is not a sufficient justification to use a test. The test must have other kinds of validity as well, although all other kinds begin with content validity. A test that includes irrelevant items, an inadequate number of relevant items, or empirically invalid evoking procedures for assessing a skill is unlikely to have other kinds of validity.

Construct Validity

Construct validity is the degree to which a test measures a predetermined theoretical construct. A *construct* is a theoretical statement supported by prior empirical observations or experimental data on a behavior or skill being measured. In essence, a test, to have construct validity, should produce test scores that reflect a theoretical statement known to be valid about the behavior being measured. For example, observational studies on language acquisition in children have supported the theoretical statement that expressive vocabulary improves with age. Therefore, a test of expressive vocabulary in children should yield scores that show progressive improvement with age. Similarly, tests of speech sound production should reflect positive changes across the age levels, a theoretical construct supported by empirical evidence. Another construct a speech or language test may use in demonstrating its validity is the difference in scores of children within the normal range of intelligence and those with significantly below-normal IQs.

Construct validity is expressed in terms of a correlation coefficient: according to the examples given, age levels and the test scores should be positively correlated. Most speech and language tests have the potential to meet the requirements of construct validity because of known developmental changes in communication skills across progressively higher age groups. A test that does not reflect such changes may be judged invalid.

Construct validity may be demonstrated not only by positive correlation with some variables, but also by low or negative correlation with other variables. For instance, a test of oral reading skills is expected to correlate poorly with arithmetic reasoning skills because they are theoretically unrelated skills. The validity of a test of oral reading skills that correlates highly with a test of arithmetic reasoning skills may be extremely suspect. When low or negative correlation with other variables is used as the theoretical construct, the resulting validity is sometimes described as *discriminant validation,* still a variety of construct validation (Anastasi & Urbina, 1997).

Another kind of construct validity, especially relevant for clinical disciplines, is based on experimental findings (Anastasi & Urbina, 1997). For instance, if prior experimental research has confirmed that a particular treatment procedure effects significant changes in certain language skills, a relevant language test given before and after that treatment should yield different scores. If the pre- and posttest scores of that language tests do not show improvement in children who have received that effective treatment, then perhaps the test is not valid. In such instances, the clinician, of course, will have measured language skills through other means (e.g., language samples or systematic probes) and will have documented improvement in those skills.

Construct validity, especially when based on well-established empirical and experimental findings, can be a strong indicator that the new test measures what it purports to measure. When combined with good content validity, acceptable construct validity may inspire confidence in the use of a standardized test.

Construct validity is as good as the theoretical construct on which it is based. Clinicians cannot always assume that the constructs themselves have strong empirical support. Even the widely held assumption that language skills improve across age levels may be more true for younger children than for older students and adults. Some generally believed theoretical constructs may be invalid. Moreover, just because the test scores correlate well with a theoretical construct does not mean that it is valid. For instance, a child language test may correlate well with height in children (both increase), but the relation is spurious. The theoretical construct and the skill being measured should be meaningfully related.

Criterion Validity

Criterion validity is the assurance that the test measures what it purports to measure because it is correlated with another meaningful variable. Unlike both content and construct validity that are inherent to the test itself, criterion validity requires some external variable to validate a new test.

Several types of external variables may serve as criteria for establishing the validity of a new test. We consider the two most common forms relevant for speech-language tests: concurrent validity and predicative validity.

Concurrent Validity. Concurrent validity refers to the degree to which a new test correlates with an established test that is already regarded as valid for measuring the same skill or behavior. For example, the scores on a new test of articulation may be correlated with those of an established test whose acceptable validity has been demonstrated. The new test is judged valid if the scores on it positively correlate with those of the older, reliable test designed to assess the same skill. On a given individual, the new and the old test should lead to similar decisions: the same or similar skill level or the same or similar deficiency level, suggesting the same diagnosis.

An important consideration is that the two tests should lead to same decisions on a given individual, but the two test scores should not correlate too high. Only a moderate correlation between the scores of the two tests is desirable; too high a correlation means the two tests are very similar. Perhaps the new test is an unnecessary duplication. A moderate correlation, although ensuring concurrent validity, will suggest that the new test helps assess aspects of the same skill untouched by the older test.

Predictive Validity. The degree to which a test predicts future performance on a related task is called **predictive validity**. Unlike content, construct, and concurrent validity, predictive validity takes time to establish; it may not be reported in the first edition of the test. As the test gains acceptance, the scores made by individuals may be checked against some other criterion of performance. For example, the scores of children on a language competence test, accumulated over a period of time, may be correlated with grade-point average or other indexes of academic performance as they become available (Hegde, 2001). If children who scored relatively high on the language test also scored relatively high grade-point averages (and vice versa), then the test accurately predicts the future academic performance, which is the criterion predicted.

Several other criteria may be used in establishing predictive validity of new tests. A single test may be validated against multiple criteria, provided that the test is designed for multiple use. Each use of a test may be validated against its own predictive criterion. For example, a phonological skills test may be validated against (correlated with) spelling skills or oral reading skills, two related but distinctly different domains, measured years later. Scores on a morphologic language test designed for preschool children may be correlated in the future when the same children's scores on writing sills become available. Similarly, the scores on a test of oral narrative skills may later be correlated with written language skills.

Most college students know that the admission officers believe their admission tests (including the Graduate Record Examination-GRE) are valid because the scores predict performance in future college courses. A real estate salesmanship test may be eventually validated against the number of homes the agents sell.

Like other kinds of validity, the criterion validity has its limitations. As noted, it may not be available at the time a test is first published. Unless other kinds of acceptable validity are reported for it, an invalid test may become entrenched before it is shown to be incapable of predicting relevant future performance. In some cases, there may be what is known as *criterion contamination* (Anastasi & Urbina, 1997). For instance, classroom teachers who know their students' scores on a language test may give better grades to those who scored better on the (language) test, and lower grades to those who scored lower on the test. The resulting high criterion validity for the language test may be specious.

As Anastasi and Urbina (1997) point out, different types of validities may be interrelated, in that the construct validity is a more inclusive term. For instance, predictive validity—that the scores of a test accurately predict some future performance—may be considered a theoretical construct the test meets. Similarly, the assumption that one valid test should correlate moderately but not too highly with another valid test, also may be considered a theoretical construct similar to the well-recognized theoretical construct that speech-language skills in children increase with chronologic age. It is also evident from the previous discussion that validity of a test may evolve over time. Evidence of predictive validity of a test is especially likely to accumulate in the years following its initial publication.

A broader understanding of validity and reliability of tests and limitations of different kinds of validation and reliability procedures will help clinicians select the most suitable tests in assessing their clients. Clinicians also need to appreciate the basic strengths and limitations of all standardized tests, including those that report acceptable reliability and validity. We address these issues in a later section in this chapter; we describe commonly used standardized tests in Chapters 6 (speech sound production tests) and 8 (language tests).

Questionnaires and Developmental Inventories

In addition to standardized tests, speech-language pathologists often rely on questionnaires and developmental inventories to seek information about the children's speech and language skills from their parents or caregivers. This information may be particularly helpful when trying to evaluate young or difficult-to-test children, or as a supplement to other information obtained during the assessment. Parents may be asked to respond to questionnaires and inventories that itemize and organize various behaviors into a developmental or observational list.

There are several advantages to using inventories or developmental questionnaires to obtain information from parents regarding their child's speech, language, and general development. For instance, parent-reported information may:

1. Provide a way to tap into a parents' unique knowledge of how their child communicates on a day-to-day basis in a variety of settings and situations.

2. Offer information on changes in the child's skill over an extended period of time; this kind of information can be obtained only through parental input.

3. Give insight into the parental actions and reactions to any limitations or deficiencies they note in their child's speech and language skills.

4. Help assess young children's (under age 3) communication skills without the use of costly and structured tests that require time, training, and child cooperation.

5. Represent an infant's or toddler's communication skills better than a language sample collected in a clinical setting; the results of the former source may be less influenced by factors such as setting, content, and examiner unfamiliarity.

6. Assist in planning for the assessment session because it can be obtained prior to actually seeing the child; such information may be helpful in selecting child-specific tools and procedures needed to complete the evaluation.

7. Offer an adjunct to supplement the clinician's observations.

8. Help establish rapport and create a "therapeutic alliance" between the parents and the clinician because of the clinician's request that the parents take part in assessment.

9. Eliminate the need for expensive stimulus items.

10. Afford a cost-effective and time-efficient means for a general evaluation or screening of a child's language.

11. Provide a valid and efficient means of assessing a child's naturalistic communication skills.

12. Offer a means of checking the reliability of information obtained in the clinic.

The reliability and validity of parent/caregiver-reported information is a concern to professionals. Parents or caregivers may not provide completely accurate information. Some parents or caregivers may miss subtle language behaviors that a trained clinician would note and others might overestimate their child's speech and language skills. Generally, any recalled information is subject to memory problems. Also, the older the child on whom the parents recall early developmental information, the greater the chances of memory distortions. Despite these concerns, several studies have shown that parents and primary caregivers can be excellent informants and that there is a strong relationship between parent-reported information and clinician-measured data (Boudreau, 2005; Conti-Ramsden, Simkin, & Pickles, 2006; Dale, 1991; Dale, Bates, Reznick, & Morisset, 1989; Fenson et al., 1993; Meisels, 1991; Miller, Manhal, & Lee, 1991; Squires & Bricker, 1991).

Strengths of Standardized Tests

Standardized tests are commonly used mostly for historic, regulatory, and practical reasons. A variety of historical trends, actual strengths, educational policies, training of clinicians, and commonly offered arguments justify the use of standardized tests:

- The history of standardized assessment in the United States is longer than that of alternative approaches; many standardized tests are readily available.

- Standardized tests have been historically promoted as "objective" in the sense that the examiner's biases would not influence the results. Other kinds of assessment, are often dubbed as "informal," implying subjective.

- Many clinicians tend to receive little or no systematic training in using alternative procedures; therefore, they continue to use what they are trained in.

- Some school districts may have a policy of qualifying children for services based only on the results of standardized tests, although the federal special education laws do not require that the decisions be based on the results of standardized tests.

- The concept that deviation from a statistical norm suggests a disorder in need of remediation is entrenched in the U.S. educational and clinical establishment. Most people seem to more easily grasp that concept than such alternative views as skill deficiency or mastery levels that do not match the social and academic demands the child faces.

- The tests are convenient and easier to administer. Once learned to administer, standardized test administration is more routine and easier than designing a child- and family-specific speech-language assessment procedure.

- It is much easier to analyze and interpret the results of standardized tests than the results of alternative assessment procedures.

- Standardized tests are conveniently packaged. All stimulus materials, acceptable and unacceptable response characteristics, response scoring procedures, and interpretations are ready-made for the clinician. Most alternative procedures require extensive preparation, often special preparation for individual clients.

- Clinicians believe that standardized tests are efficient even if they inadequately sample communicative behaviors. A variety of speech and language skills may be sampled in a relatively short duration, even if each behavior is only sampled superficially.

- Tests permit comparison of results across various test administrations and examiners. More flexible alternative assessment results do not easily lend themselves to such comparisons.

- Although many alternative approaches are available to assess communication, none have replaced the standardized tests.

- Clinicians may believe that many standardized tests, although inappropriate to assess children who belong to ethnocultural minority groups, are quite appropriate to assess mainstream children on whom the tests may have been standardized. The strong possibility that the tests may provide only limited information even on children who belong to the standardization group is often unappreciated.

- Some who favor standardized testing believe that tests are indeed more capable of avoiding bias in assessing all people, including minority cultural groups, than clinicians who make judgments without objective test scores. Used appropriately, test results may "provide a safeguard against favoritism and arbitrary and capricious decisions" (Anastasi & Urbina, 1997, p. 549). This may be especially true when the tests are appropriately standardized on specific target groups (various cultural minorities) with test items that are unique to the specific groups.

- At least certain kinds of biases are not a property of the test itself, but a matter of faulty interpretations of results. Tests do not say why a child behaved in a certain manner during testing; the clinician will have to find out the answer. For instance, a language test might reveal that a child belonging to a certain cultural minority does not maintain eye contact during conversation. The test cannot be faulted for discovering this fact. No test makes inappropriate cultural or clinical decisions because "tests couldn't see whether the youngster is in rags or tweeds, and they couldn't hear the accents of the slum" (Gardner, 1961, pp. 48–49). If anything goes wrong with the finding in our example, it is the clinician's interpretation that the child who did not maintain eye contact or the one with a dialect (accent) has a language disorder.

- An additional argument in favor of prudent use of standardized tests in assessing cultural minorities is that it is indeed both fair and essential to know what negative effects unfavorable social conditions have on the skills of people so that appropriate remedial actions can be taken. Using procedures that are insensitive to the negative consequences of unfavorable socioeconomic conditions does a disservice to people who experience such consequences (Anastasi & Urbina, 1997).

- Test constructors now follow widely accepted ethical guidelines in standardizing tests. Authors of tests have been making and continue to make systematic efforts to eliminate biased stimuli, culturally loaded instructions, stereotypic characterization of diverse people, and so forth. Test developers are making significant efforts to sample ethnoculturally diverse populations.

- Standardized tests, like any kind of assessment instruments, may be misused. It is the clinician's responsibility to use them properly. This argument correctly puts the responsibility on those who train clinicians in assessment procedures and their fair and objective interpretations that lead to beneficial consequences to those who take tests.

Reasons and arguments such as these have made the administration of standardized tests the main task of assessment in speech-language pathology, psychology, and education. However, a prudent use of standardized tests requires that the clinicians understand their limitations as well.

Limitations of Standardized Tests

Limitations of standardized tests and objections to their widespread use began to surface in late 1950s and early 1960s. Various legal challenges to the fairness of intelligence testing and passage of civil rights laws in the 1960s forced attention to the limitations or inappropriateness of standardized tests in assessing people from cultural minority groups. Critics contend that some practical advantages of standardized tests have overridden their serious and multiple disadvantages. Indeed, even the strongest advocates of standardized testing are fully aware of its limitations and offer thoughtful discussions (e.g., see Anastasi & Urbina, 1997, a classic, still a current, and highly respected, book in psychological testing). Over the decades, the validity of standardized tests as a means of assessing communication and its disorders also became a matter of serious concern. Due to extensive discussions in psychological, educational, and communication disorders literature, the limitations of standardized tests are now well recognized (Adler, 1990; Haynes & Pindzola, 2004; Hegde, 1998; Hegde & Maul, 2006; Laing & Kamhi, 2003; Owens, 2004; Washington & Craig, 1992; Wetherby & Prizant, 1992). Currently, a variety of weaknesses, reasons, and arguments question the use of standardized tests, especially in the context of assessing communication and its disorders:

- The highly structured and standardized formality of most standardized tests do not allow for a sampling of natural social interactions inherent to communication and what is sampled may not represent the client's functional communication skills in social situations.

- Most standardized tests provide limited opportunity for the child to initiate interaction. Test items evoke responses, but do not allow for much spontaneous communication.

- Many tests artificially isolate individual aspects of communication (e.g., expressive syntactic skills or receptive vocabulary). Test items do not help assess language skills that are integrative of different structural aspects.

- Speech and language tests generally are less efficient in assessing and scoring more global conversational skills and abstract language production than they are in assessing the production of discrete words and grammatic morphemes.

- Most standardized tests sample verbal language and overlook preverbal or nonverbal communication.

- The standardized formats and protocols allow for little individual variation in communication across children.

- Most standardized tests limit the role of family members in the assessment process and intervention planning.

- Few standardized tests of early language skills have good predictability of language and communication skills expressed at a later age.

- Norm-referenced standardized tests of speech and language are based on the assumption that all children learn communication skills in a certain invariable sequence. This assumption, however, is highly questionable and individual differences in learning language are well documented.

- Comparing a child's performance with the norms is one of the most troublesome, even if cherished, aspects of standardized tests. A child that does not demonstrate a particular speech or language skill by a certain age may be labeled *disordered*; this may be valid only if individual differences in language acquisition were insignificant.

- Standardized tests typically do not include children with language disorders or those with other clinical conditions that may affect language skills in their normative sample. Therefore, the *norms* do not accurately reflect the general population, which includes children with limited language skills.

- The interaction style of many young children may not match the type of interaction required on a given test. In fact, there is little interaction except for giving responses to preselected test items.

- Standardized tests do not sample behaviors adequately. Although most test constructors pay attention to the sample size (the number of children tested), they ignore the problem of inadequate sampling of skills (Hegde, 1998). Most tests contain only one or a few stimulus items for any particular skill; the results may not be an accurate representation of the child's behavior in social settings.

- Standardized tests are designed only to determine whether or not a problem exists compared with a sample of the general population. Therefore, they may not identify a child's overall strengths and weaknesses.

- Standardized test items can be subjectively scored. Even though they are constructed to be objective, it is nearly impossible for the examiner to completely eliminate some subjective scoring. This may skew the scores a client receives on a given test.

- Standardized tests assume that the average performance for an age level on a certain task sets the age norm for that behavior. This is not always the case because of individual differences that exist within the range of normalcy (Hegde, 1998). Therefore, clinicians should be wary of using age-equivalency scores to describe a child's level of functioning.

- Results from standardized tests do not always translate into specific treatment goals. Additional measurements, including language samples and baserates, are often necessary to specify treatment goals.

- Standardized tests, at best, help make a structural assessment of communicative behaviors; they do not allow for a functional analysis of skills. A behavioral *functional assessment*, designed to find out what variables maintain the current behaviors, better suggests effective treatment options than a mere structural assessment. See Chapters 1, 5, and 8 for more information on functional assessment.

- The stimulus items or procedures of some standardized tests may be discriminatory or inappropriate for children of diverse cultural or socioeconomic backgrounds. Lack of responses to such items may not suggest skill deficiency.

- The participant sampling may be biased against children from low income, minority, or rural families. Although sampling of minority children in test standardization is on the increase, many historically standardized tests have included, for the most part, children from the mainstream social strata.

- Most tests are standardized on local, not national, samples. Although efforts are being made to draw larger and nationally more representative samples, many tests are not designed to be used nationally; nonetheless, they are used nationally.

- Children of some ethnocultural minority groups may react differently to unfamiliar examiners. Children from different cultural backgrounds may communicate better in their own social and cultural situations than in formal and unfamiliar testing situations.

It is unlikely that the use of standardized tests, regardless of their increasingly appreciated limitations, will decline significantly because of some of the historic views, current training of clinicians, and educational policies. Therefore, it is important to limit the negative consequences of tests by using them prudently.

Prudent Use of Standardized Tests

Probably the best way of limiting the negative consequences of standardized tests is to develop and use a new approach to assessment that integrates the strengths of various alternative assessment procedures, including functional (behavioral) assessment, as well as those of standardized assessment. In Chapter 5, we not only review alternative assessment approaches, but also describe a new integrated approach.

Prudent use of standardized tests that help minimize their negative consequences requires that the clinicians consider: (a) the ethical issues in standardized assessment, (b) criteria for selection of standardized tests, (c) fair and valid interpretation of test results, and (d) assigning a valid role to standardized tests in assessment. Among several sources the clinicians should regularly consult are the Standards for Educational and Psychological Testing, which is a set of guidelines jointly developed and published by the American Educational Research Association (http://www.aera.org), American Psychological Association (http://www.apa.org), and the National Council on the Measurement in Education (http://www.ncme.org). The current standards were published in 1999; revised standards are expected to be published in 2013 (to check on the progress, visit http://teststandards. net or http://www.ncme.org). In addition, speech-language pathologists should consult the relevant position papers and other publications of the American Speech-Language-Hearing Association.

Ethical Issues in Standardized Assessment

Ethically responsible use of standardized tests is based mostly on the codes of conduct that professionals adhere to. For instance, before administering a test, clinicians should get themselves trained in its administration and scoring. This is part of the ethical code of most professionals, who are required to provide only those services they are qualified to offer (American Speech-Language-Hearing Association, 2003; Anastasi & Urbina, 1997).

An ethical principle that authors should adhere to is to avoid publishing or releasing in other ways, tests that are not adequately standardized. A test should be made available for general use only when it has been standardized with acceptable reliability and validity. Diagnostic tests of various kinds should not be made available in popular media.

All clinicians are expected to protect the privacy of their clients, and this applies to the results of standardized tests as well. Clinicians should always seek to test skills that are relevant to making a valid diagnosis, designing an intervention plan, and providing other kinds of services. All test takers should be informed of the purpose of testing, the general testing format, and how the results will be used. The results of the tests and other assessment procedures should be held with strict confidentiality.

Test publishers, too, have certain ethical responsibilities in selling standardized tests. Publishers limit the sale of tests to qualified (usually a master's degree in a relevant discipline), and perhaps also licensed, professionals. Tests should not be sold to those who do not meet such qualifications, nor should such persons seek to purchase standardized tests.

Criteria for Selection of Standardized Tests

Selecting the most appropriate test for a given child or situation can be a daunting task. What follows is a brief description of major criteria that can be helpful in selecting a test that is appropriate for the child being assessed.

Select a test that has a detailed and comprehensive test manual. The test manual should contain specific instructions on administration of the test and scoring and interpretation of the results. The manual should contain detailed information on the size and make-up of the normative sample, the sampling method used, test reliability, and validity. Tests that come with poorly written manuals with missing information should be avoided.

Select a test that is based on a large and diverse normative sample. Tests that have sampled too few participants or have not included sufficient number of participants from diverse cultural, linguistic, and socioeconomic groups are generally inappropriate. If a test had sampled subgroups, the number of participants in each should be 100 or more.

Select a test that samples the skills adequately. Tests that give multiple opportunities to produce a skill (e.g., a given phoneme or grammatic morpheme) should be preferred to those that give only one or two production opportunities.

Select a test that has been recently revised and thus provides current normative data. Tests should be updated on a regular basis to keep the normative data current. Racial and cultural composition of societies and educational and economic status of people change over time and the test norms should reflect such changes. Avoid dated tests, and regularly check for revised editions of tests you use.

Select a test that has strong reliability and validity. Tests that offer different kinds of reliability and validity should be preferred over those that report only one kind or a weaker kind. Tests that offer strong and extensive evidence of reliability and validity data should be preferred over those that offer only limited or weak data.

Select a test that has appropriate stimulus items. Tests that contain dated stimuli and stimuli that are socially and culturally inappropriate to the child being assessed should be avoided.

Select a test that you are well trained to administer. A clinician who is not trained in the administration and scoring of a new or better test that becomes available should first get the training.

Select a test that will yield useful diagnostic information and help design treatment goals or procedures. Some tests may provide solid assessment results that are not easily translated into treatment goals and methods. Tests that generate both solid diagnostic information and treatment suggestions should be preferred. If no such test is available, consider alternative assessment procedures, especially functional assessment, described in Chapter 5.

The clinician would not base selection of a test only on one or two criteria just summarized. To be selected, a test should meet multiple criteria. The greater the number of criteria a given test meets, the more useful it is in making reliable and valid clinical judgments.

Fair and Valid Interpretation of Test Results

It is generally believed that test results are strictly interpreted according to the test manual. Although all clinicians strive to make justified interpretations of test results, it is not uncommon for them to face dilemmas in finding the meaning of the results. The manual itself may be unhelpful, ambiguous, or unclear about interpretations.

Fair and valid interpretation of test results has been a particular concern in assessing children and adults who belong to ethnocultural minority groups on whom the tests administered have not been standardized. Potential misinterpretation of results in cases of such children (as well as adults) is now well recognized. The best solution is not to administer tests that are standardized only on mainstream children to children of ethnocultural diversity. Unfortunately, in certain situations (as in a school district that requires standard test scores to qualify a child for services), clinicians may be forced to use an available test. In such cases, it is the clinician's responsibility to interpret the test results in light of the child's ethnocultural and linguistic background. Rigid adherence to the manual may lead to faulty interpretations of results. This issue is further addressed in the next section.

The need for fair and valid interpretation may require some flexibility even in the case of children of the kind who were included in the standardization sample. For instance, positive or negative results of an articulation test that gives only one opportunity to test a speech sound may have to be checked against the results of a speech sample before concluding that the child does or does not produce the sound. If the clinician observes that the child was somewhat puzzled by a speech or language stimulus item and gave a wrong response, the clinician may hold judgment until other kinds of evidence emerges to make a better judgment.

Although the results of a test should be generally interpreted according to the manual, the clinician should not ignore signs that the test, for whatever the reason, may not have sampled the child's behavior adequately or fairly. Not heeding such signs, because of the assumption that the manual is inviolable, may do more harm than good to the child tested.

The Role of Standardized Tests in Assessment

Finally, prudent use of standardized tests requires that the clinician assign a proper role to them in the larger context of assessment. Clinicians who believe that the standardized tests are the only or the main means of assessment of communication skills will give them an exaggerated status and, consequently, run the risk of drawing invalid conclusions. Such clinicians fail to assign a proper role to standardized tests in assessment.

Attention to all ethical issues, careful selection of tests, and fair and valid interpretations will be productive strategies if the tests are seen as one of several sources of information on the child's communication skills. Tests need not be a primary source; it should never be the sole source. We have noted earlier that a detailed case history, a carefully done interview, an adequate language sample taken in the clinic and home, and reports from other professionals provide information that tests cannot provide. Furthermore, we will see in Chapter 5 that various alternative approaches, including client-specific and criterion-referenced, authentic, portfolio, and functional assessment offer valuable information and mitigate the negative consequences of standardized tests.

A proper role for standardized tests is that they are one potentially useful source of information. No strong advocate of standardized tests has considered their results infallible (Anastasi & Urbina, 1997). It is often said and written that case history, interview, and language samples *supplement standardized tests.* Assigning a proper role to tests, one might say that *standardized tests supplement* other procedures that adequately sample social communication in more naturalistic contexts.

Assessment in a Multicultural Society

As noted in earlier sections of this chapter, a significant issue with the use of standardized tests is their appropriateness in assessing children who belong to various ethnocultural minority groups. In fact, the limitations of standardized tests are often discussed in the context of assessment in an ethnoculturally diverse society.

Tests standardized on mainstream American children are especially not useful in assessing varied ethnocultural groups. Children who speak a dialect other than Standard American English either because of African American culture or because of bilingual status of the family are a case in point. Because of special concerns in assessment of children belonging to various ethnocultural groups, we have devoted Chapter 4 to this topic.

CHAPTER 4

Assessment of Ethnoculturally Diverse Children

- Assessment in Ethnoculturally Diverse Societies
- Can Speech-Language Assessment Be Culture-Free?
- Limitations of Standardized Tests in Assessing Ethnoculturally Diverse Children
- Assessment of African American Children
- Assessment of Bilingual Children
- Traditional and Alternative Assessment Approaches

We have noted in the previous chapter that standardized tests have multiple limitations, most of which are relevant to assessing children of all backgrounds, including the mainstream children on whom the tests are standardized. Those limitations get magnified when tests are used in assessing children of ethnocultural diversity. Therefore, the practice of assessing ethnoculturally diverse children with standardized tests has come under serious scrutiny from educators, psychologists, and speech-language pathologists.

Clinicians need to gain a significant body of knowledge about fair and valid assessment of children coming from ethnocultural backgrounds that vary from the American mainstream culture, language, and dialects. This chapter gives an overview of a growing body of scientific and professional literature on multicultural and bilingual issues in speech-language pathology (Brice, 2002; Brice & Brice, 2009; Goldstein, 2004; Kamhi, Pollock, & Harris, 1996; Kayser, 1995; Roseberry-McKibbin, 1994, 2002; Seymour, 2004; van Keulen, Weddington, & DeBose, 1998).

Assessment in Ethnoculturally Diverse Societies

In recent decades, the demographic profiles of countries that permit immigration have changed significantly. For instance, United States population has become more racially, ethnically, and linguistically diverse in recent decades. Consequently, children attending many U.S. schools come from varied ethnocultural backgrounds. Those children speak a variety of languages and English dialectal variations at home. Communication disorders in such children may be evident in their first language, second language, or both.

According to the 2010 U.S. Census (http://www.census.gov), of the total population of 311 million (2011 estimate) 63.7% are White (non-Hispanic), 12.6% are African American, 4.8% are Asian American, 0.9% are American Indian and Alaska Native, 0.2% are Native Hawaiian or Pacific Islander, and 16.3% are Hispanic or Latino.

The states of California, Texas, and Florida are home to more than half of all Hispanic people living in the United States. Children of Hispanic background speak different varieties of Spanish and those of Asian backgrounds speak different languages. Speech-language pathologists are especially concerned with diagnosing communication disorders in bilingual and bicultural children whose English proficiency is limited. According to the National Center for Educational Statistics (http://nces.ed.gov/fastfacts), the number of school-age children (5 to 17 years) who spoke a language other than English at home increased from 4.7 million (10% of the population) in 1980 to 11.2 million (21%) in 2009. It is projected that in 20 years, children from diverse cultural backgrounds will be in the majority in the U.S. public schools. Most children who have limited English proficiency are of Hispanic or Latino background with Spanish as their first language. Over the past decade, the number of school-age children with limited English language skills with other primary languages spoken at home has more than doubled (http://nces.ed.gov/fastfacts). African American (AA) children, on the other hand, are not bilingual in the usual sense. Many, however, may speak African American English (AAE) when they enter school (Stockman, 2010). Due to such changing demographic factors, speech-language pathologists, whatever their background, are likely to have a significant number of clients that come from a culture different from their own.

Assessment of children coming from diverse cultural backgrounds poses special challenges. Commonly used standardized tests are inappropriate for children of minority culture, language, or dialect. Many standardized tests of intelligence, personality, interests and aptitudes, and speech-language skills routinely used in the United States and other western countries have historically been standardized on samples drawn from monolingual, native, and standard English-speaking people of majority. Children with limited English proficiency or children who are bilingual but their English is influenced by their first language have not been included in the normative sample in sufficient numbers to represent them. But more importantly, even those tests that do include children of minority language or culture in their standardization samples do not sample their language characteristics; most if not all test items pertain to standard English. Also, native minorities who speak a dialectal variation of English (e.g., the African Americans in the United States) have neither been sampled adequately nor are their language characteristics included in the test content.

Ethnocultural factors affect the appropriateness, fairness, and validity not only of standardized tests, but also of methods of interviewing parents and collecting a naturalistic language sample. Cultural barriers or differences in communication styles can restrict the value of information received. Some people may be uncomfortable sharing certain information with a stranger, and this may be intensified when the interviewer is from a different race or culture. People of certain cultural backgrounds may find it more difficult to share personal information with strangers. Finally, a language barrier may interfere with effective communication.

Children from diverse language backgrounds tend to score lower on standardized tests, and are often inappropriately placed in special education programs (Haynes & Pindzola, 2004; Kamhi, Pollock, & Harris, 1996; Taylor & Payne, 1983). Therefore, it is now accepted that the accurate assessment of speech and language skills in culturally diverse children should not depend solely on the use of standardized, norm-referenced, test procedures (Craig & Washington, 2000; Hegde & Maul, 2006; Laing & Kamhi, 2003; Taylor & Payne, 1983; Washington, 1996; Wyatt, 1995). It is doubtful if standardized tests should be used at all in some cases. Similarly, using nonverbal tasks or testing the children in their native language may not be adequate or practical solutions (Tomblin, Morris, & Spriestersbach, 2002). Nonverbal tasks may not fully represent the verbal skills the children are capable of or need to learn to meet social and academic demands. Clinicians may have no expertise in the child's native language to make an assessment in that language. Finally, a fair assessment of English language skills in ethnoculturally diverse U.S. children is needed because of educational demands placed on them; such demands, even with a push for bilingual education, will have to be met only with English proficiency.

Can Speech-Language Assessment Be Culture-Free?

Speech-language pathologists are among the most recent professionals to face the challenge of assessing culturally diverse children and adults with what they traditionally had: standardized tests. But the challenge is not new. It has been recognized as early as 1910 that the tests standardized on one cultural group or a single socioeconomic stratum within a single culture may not be appropriate for assessing members of other cultures or socioeconomic strata. That assessment issues and migration of people are intertwined is historically illustrated. Testing intelligence of new immigrants arriving at Ellis Island in the United States in the first decades of the 20th century required what eventually came to be known as *culture-free* or *cross-cultural* tests that could be administered to individuals who came from varied cultural backgrounds and spoke different languages (Knox, 1914). It is the same old immigration issue that challenges speech-language pathologists in the 21st century.

Psychologists and sociologists have devised various kinds of assessment instruments that are relatively free from cultural restraints or experiential factors. Nonverbal tests of intelligence that avoid even verbal instructions have been in existence at least since the 1920s. For example, the Goodenough Draw-A-Man test, a nonverbal test of intelligence, was originally published in 1926 (Goodenough, 1949). The Leiter International Performance Scale (Roid & Miller, 1997), another nonverbal test of intelligence, was first published in 1940. Both the tests claim to have eliminated *biases due to culture and language*. These and other nonverbal tests have been used to assess intelligence of people living in different countries and cultures for well over half a century.

The main strategy in developing culture-free psychological tests that could be administered to individuals of varied ethnocultural groups was to eliminate variables related to cultural influence. The most powerful variable that is firmly rooted in an individual's culture is *language* which psychologists could eliminate by designing nonverbal tests of intelligence and other abilities that required no verbal interaction between the examiner and the test taker. It is not a controversial statement that a person who does not speak a particular language can still be intellectually exceptional, not just average. However, attempts at eliminating the influence of culture and language in understanding and assessing people's behaviors and skills may prompt a philosophical debate and pose a practical dilemma; to understand behaviors, is it not necessary to understand the cultural conditions under which people behave? The problem is more acute for speech-language pathologists who need to assess language in all its naturalistic cultural context. Any attempt at eliminating the culture in assessing communication and its disorders will create empty assessment strategies. Because for speech-language pathologists, eliminating the influence of culture and language in assessing communication leaves little else to assess, they need to squarely face the problem of assessing language skills in the context of the client's culture.

Some speech-language pathologists have proposed that biases in assessing ethnoculturally diverse children may be reduced or eliminated by using processing-independent skills that minimize dependence on language (Campbell, Dollaghan, Needleman, & Janosky, 1997; Laing & Kamhi, 2003). Various memory and perceptual tasks are thought to represent skills *underlying* language but not directly influenced by language. But assessing such tasks is similar to assessing nonverbal skills in an effort to avoid language skills, but still seeking to assess language, but only indirectly. There is no assurance that memory and perceptual skills and other nonverbal skills validly represent social communication skills. How does one measure comprehension or production of speech sounds, grammatic features, turn-taking in conversations, topic maintenance, and understanding of proverbs through such nonverbal skills as digit-span memory? A strategy that requires the clinician to abandon the assessment of language skills to avoid bias in assessing language skills offers no solution to the problem at hand.

Language assessment is culturally based, because as Skinner (1957) stated, verbal behavior is shaped and maintained by a verbal community. The important principle to adhere to is that verbal communities differ in their cultural practices, and therefore, assessment procedures cannot be culture free, but they should be culture-specific, and as Craig and Washington (2000) put it, culture-fair.

Limitations of Standardized Tests in Assessing Ethnoculturally Diverse Children

Most of the problems in using standardized tests to assess ethnoculturally diverse children center around a mismatch between the children and the assessment instrument (Cole & Taylor, 1990; Craig & Washington, 2000; Fagundes, Haynes, Haak, & Moran, 1998; Kohnert, 2007; Laing & Kamhi, 2003; Stockman, 2000; Tomblin, Morris & Spriestersbach, 2002; Washington, 1996; Wyatt, 1995). As an example, Cole and Taylor (1990) showed that some of the commonly used tests of speech sound production may misclassify AA children who speak the African American English dialect as having a speech sound disorder if the features of that dialect are not taken into account. Their analysis revealed that 19% of the test items of the Arizona Articulation Proficiency Scale (Fudula, 1974), 21% of the Templin-Darley Test of Articulation (Templin & Darley, 1969), and 14% of the Photo Articulation Test (Pendergast, Dickey, Selman, & Sorder, 1974) are subject to misinterpretation when administered to AA children. Cole and Taylor's study showed that when normally speaking AA children were tested and scored according to the standard English scoring criteria, seven children on the AAPS-R, six on the Templin-Darley, and three on the PAT were falsely identified as having a speech sound disorder. It should be noted that a subsequent study by Washington and Craig (1992) suggested that AA children in the U.S. southern and northern states may speak different varieties of African American English and that these varieties should be considered in scoring the articulation and language tests.

Several factors affect the reliability and validity of tests administered to children. Among these are the language or languages spoken at home, general cultural environment in which the child is raised, the family communication patterns or the verbal environment, values and orientations affecting diseases and disorders, the child's experience in taking tests, and lack of familiarity of tests and the examiners (Roseberry-McKibbin, 2002). In addition, several properties of the test and the way the examiner interacts with the child also may create problems in evaluating communication skills of children from diverse backgrounds. Finally, interpretation of results obtained from tests administered to ethnoculturally diverse children may pose special problems.

Variables Related to the Child and the Family

Standardized test-taking, though spreading around the world, is an American and perhaps Western European phenomenon. Many children in Asian and African countries, and those of minority cultural groups in the United States, may only have limited experience in taking standardized tests. These children may misinterpret the directions or may not fully grasp all the instructions given them. They may not ask questions or request that the directions be repeated. Learning in the child's culture may be more dependent on modeling and manual guidance than detailed verbal instructions.

Some children may find the formal testing situation threatening because of a potential negative evaluation that may follow. Tests may mean different things to different children; prior failure or negative educational placement or consequences that may have followed earlier testing may add to the child's misgiving about the test and the testing situation. The child's performance under these circumstances may not reflect true skill levels. Other children, again because of their lack of experience with test-taking, may not be highly motivated to do well. They may fail to understand the significance of testing, may be unaware of the consequences of failure, and thus may not perform as well as they possibly could.

Timed tests may be especially troublesome to children of certain minority cultural groups partly because of the different cultural value placed on time. Many children may not be used to taking tests that allot only a specified amount of time for completion. The child may have been conditioned to complete a task well at one's own pace, rather than trying to finish it as quickly as possible under time pressure.

The child's culture may place an emphasis on quiet performance, rather than competitive display of skills. Individual achievement may be less valued than cooperative group performance; trying to appear better than others may have been discouraged by parents or caregivers. A child with this kind of upbringing may not perform well on a test not because of lack of skills, but because of the alien nature of the task demand.

Cultural values and orientation toward disabilities and their remediation differ across societies. Mainstream American culture considers speech, language, and hearing problems to be significant disabilities that may require medical or therapeutic intervention. Other cultures may not place such a high value on verbal communication, and even if they do, the people in it may not be used to the concept of treating communication problems. Therefore, people may tend to be more accepting of verbal skill deficiencies. The parents may encourage compensatory skills from the beginning, instead of seeking formal intervention.

Variables Related to the Test and the Examiner

Tests of mainstream American English standardized on mainstream children will sample language, communication styles, and particular aspects of social communication that are not especially relevant to the minority children and their cultural background. Standardized tests may be based on the assumption that all children have been exposed to the same or similar vocabulary, concepts, and life experiences. Children from culturally diverse backgrounds may not perform well on a test because their life experiences and exposure to vocabulary may have been different from those of mainstream children (Laing & Kamhi, 2003). Children from different social strata within the same general culture also may have vastly different language experiences. Even children within the same social stratum within the same culture but living in different home environments may have different life and language experiences.

Stimulus materials, especially pictures or drawings, may fail to evoke correct responses from a child because of their unfamiliarity. Such stimulus items may not have been a part of the child's home and general social environment. Stories or topics used to assess conversational or narrative skills may be unfamiliar to, or inappropriate for, children of diverse cultural backgrounds, resulting in poor performance. If stories and topics are selected from the child's cultural background, better narrative skills may be observed. Similarly, tests that do not emphasize speed may better sample the skill.

It is clear that if the standardization sample did not include children of different ethnocultural groups in proportions to represent the population, the norms established by the test will *not* be relevant to many specific cultural groups. In an effort to remediate this problem, test developers now attempt to include more representative proportions of diverse populations in their sample. Merely including a correct proportion of minority groups in the standardization sample, however, is not enough to make the test norms applicable to the included minority groups. For instance, including a correct national proportion of AA children in standardizing a mainstream (standard) American English language or speech test is not sufficient to make the test relevant to assessing children who speak African American English. It is not just the adequate sampling of the participants that makes a test relevant to the sampled group; in addition to appropriate sampling, the *nature* of the test items and how the responses are scored, also are important in generating norms that apply to varied groups. For example, to do justice to children who speak the African American English, the test should contain African American English dialectal variations of speech and language features, evoked through culture-specific stimulus materials, and the responses scored according to the rules of that language. The same requirements will apply to tests designed to assess Hispanic American, Asian American, or Native American children. There is now evidence that refined and more representative sampling technique does not necessarily eliminate overidentification or underidentification of communication problems in minority children (Washington & Craig, 1992, 1999).

During testing, clinicians or test examiners may interact with the child in unfamiliar ways. Both verbal and nonverbal behavior of the clinician may be unfamiliar to the child. There may be dialectal differences between the child's speech and the clinician's speech. The test items may not sample the child's dialectal differences, and the test (and the examiner) may require responses that are not in the child's dialectal repertoire. In such contexts, poor performance on a test may reflect a language difference rather than a language impairment. If these differences are scored as "errors" on a test it may lead to overidentification of a disorder. On the other hand, a child who actually has a language impairment may be missed because it is mistakenly interpreted as a language difference. This can lead to underidentification.

Valid Interpretation of Test Results

Misinterpretation of test results is a major concern when standardized tests are administered to children of ethnocultural minority. Most misinterpretations arise because of a lack of understanding of the child's cultural background and accepted communication patterns within that culture. As noted before, a test may simply indicate that a particular response or skill is either produced or not produced; this is a factual observation and the test is neither to be applauded nor faulted for that. How to interpret this presence or absence of a skill is a matter of judgment when the child tested belongs to an ethnocultural minority group. For example, lack of a child's eye contact during conversation may be a negative finding in the American mainstream culture, but it may be normal in some cultures (e.g., Asian or Native American culture), especially when the child interacts with an adult. A child may omit certain phonemes or substitute others. This, too, may be due to the child's dialect or bilingual status.

As described in later sections of this chapter, there are two distinct ethnoculturally diverse groups that require a somewhat different approach to assessing and interpreting test results. One group of children are bilingual and the other group, though monolingual, speak a different dialect of English.

Some Suggested Ways of Using or Improving Standardized Tests

Over the years, speech-language pathologists have researched or suggested several strategies in an effort to overcome the various types of biases and drawbacks of administering standardized tests on children of ethnocultural diversity (see, for example, Cole & Taylor, 1990; Kayser, 1989; Rhyner, Kelly, Bramtley, & Kruger, 1999; Taylor & Payne, 1983; Washington & Craig, 1992; Westby, 2002). Unfortunately, suggested ways do not always and fully eliminate the problems they address; nonetheless, the following may be considered:

- Translating the standardized text into the child's primary language. However, a mere translation of a test is not equivalent to standardizing it on a minority group; translated items may not be valid or appropriate for the child and they may not sample the dialectal variations.

- Standardizing an existing test on minority populations. This is probably the best solution if new test items that are relevant to the minority populations are created anew; if not, it is not likely to sample the unique speech and language features of minority children. This strategy requires extensive efforts and resources, and perhaps for this reason, very few tests are standardized entirely on minority groups.

- Using tests that include a small percentage of minorities in the standardization sample. As noted, sampling children of different ethnocultural groups without changing the test content is insufficient; the test content should be selected such that they are relevant to the communication patterns of specific groups: a difficult proposition when the items have to be relevant to a vast majority of children.

- Developing local norms that are more representative of the population being served. Apparently a practical solution, but this means a test needs to be standardized in many different locations or regions of the country. Another potential problem is that tests, once published, tend to get used nationally, despite their local standardization.

- Modifying existing tests to make them more appropriate for children from diverse cultures. These may include such changes as:
  - removing particularly difficult or biased test items so that they are not counted in the calculation of the final score; however, such modifications may negatively affect the interpretation of the overall test scores and reliability and validity of the test results;

- ○ changing stimuli to parallel forms that are more appropriate for a particular cultural and linguistic group; this will create a shadow of a standardized test without the benefits of standardization on the relevant cultural group; reliability and validity of such procedures are not clear;
  - ○ changing the scoring to permit dialectical variations to be considered correct; another, apparently practical solution, but it is less efficient than directly sampling the dialect of the child and analyzing the results in the context of the child's culture and communication patterns.

- Adopting alternative assessment approaches. This is an attractive suggestion but it does not improve the application of standardized tests in assessing cultural minority groups. Most alternative approaches, as described in Chapter 5, avoid, but do not seek to improve, standardized tests.

The problems associated with standardized test assessment of children from ethnocultural diversity are complex and numerous. Modification of the content, administration procedures, stimulus items, instructions, adjusted scoring systems, and interpretation of standardized tests risks questionable reliability and validity of the test administered while also not sampling the relevant, culture-specific skills of minority children. In any case, if the results of a test do not apply to a given child, interpretation should be tentative, cautious, withheld, or entirely abandoned.

The identification of a communicative disorder and subsequent development of an effective treatment plan for any child require adequate assessment. To date, however, there are no widely accepted procedures for evaluating children from culturally diverse backgrounds. In Chapter 5 we consider alternative approaches that avoid standardized tests or greatly minimize their role; these, too, unfortunately, have not gained widespread acceptance.

Assessment of African American Children

A variation of English associated with the African American culture is preferably called African American English (Seymour, 2004; van Keulen, Weddington, & DeBose, 1998), but it is also called *Black English (BE)* (Dillard, 1972), *Black English Vernacular (BEV)*, or *African American Vernacular English (AAVE)* (Laing, 2003; Vaughn-Cooke, 1987). Phonological and language characteristics of African American English (AAE) have often been compared with those of Mainstream American English (MAE), which is also known as Standard American English (SAE) or General American English (GAE). Such comparative studies of the two forms of English are made to understand the differences and similarities from a scientific point of view and to understand fully the nature of AAE.

Linguistic scholars (Dillard, 1972; Green, 2002; Labov, 1972), speech-language pathologists (Kamhi, Pollock, & Harris, 1996; Stockman, 2010; Taylor, 1983), and the American Speech-Language-Hearing Association (1983) view AAE as a variety of English in its own right, that is, a product of the African American culture. Because there are actually more similarities than differences between the MAE and AAE, it is debatable whether it is a unique form of language; it certainly has its unique phonological, morphologic, syntactic, and pragmatic features not found in MAE. Such unique features have prompted some scholars to believe that AAE is a separate language (van Keulen et al., 1998).

AAE is colorful and eloquent. Its distinct rhythm and communication style is a product of the rich African American cultural heritage. AAE is characterized by a greater degree of emotional and gestural expression than MAE. Verbal behavior of some African Americans may be more intense than what is typically found in other ethnocultural groups. Touching and physical contacts are a part of the African American communication pattern, but eye contact between an adult and a child may be less common than in the mainstream American culture.

African American communities value family relationships, support for family members, and a general loyalty to family. African American elderly are held with respect. Common good of the group is more valued than individual achievement, especially if the latter is detrimental to the former. A broader concept of the family may include unrelated persons. Children are especially valued, loved, and supported but they may be reared more authoritatively than in other cultural groups.

For the speech-language pathologists, excellent sources are now available on AAE (Craig & Washington, 2000; Craig et al., 2003; Dillard, 1972; Hecht, Collier, & Ribeau, 1993; Kamhi, Pollock, & Harris, 1996; Pearson, Velleman, Bryant, & Charko, 2009; Roseberry-McKibbin, 2002; Stockman, 2010; van Keulen et al., 1988; Willis, 1992; Wolfram, 1994). An increasing number of research studies on AAE learning in children and on assessing communication disorders in them is being published in the journals of the American-Speech-Language-Hearing Association (Stockman, 2010). To make a valid assessment of speech-language skills of AA children, clinicians should consult these and other sources and keep abreast of research to better understand the African American culture, family, and social communication style.

Both phonological and language characteristics of AAE should be understood to make a fair assessment of communication skills of children who speak AAE. A majority of phonological, semantic, and grammatic characteristics of AAE are similar to those of MAE. Therefore, a thorough analysis of an African American child's pattern of communication should take into consideration the features MAE and AAE share. As a next step, it is essential to identify the unique speech and language features of AAE that suggest only a difference, not a disorder. Without such an analysis, the child may be mistakenly diagnosed as having a speech sound or language disorder (Craig et al., 2003).

In assessing phonological and language properties of an African American child, the clinician first should establish that the child indeed is an AAE speaker, although most preschoolers and those who enter grade school speak AAE. African American adults, on the other hand, may or may not speak AAE, and if they do, they may code-switch between the two forms of English. Some African American adults may not speak AAE at all. Furthermore, a few rural southern Whites, especially from the lower socioeconomic strata, may produce specific expressions that are typical of AAE. For instance, /f/ for /θ/ substitution and some final cluster reductions (e.g., *rd, ld, st, ts,* and *ks*) that characterize AAE, may be heard in Southern English dialect, even if infrequently or inconsistently (Fasold, 1981; Washington & Craig, 1992; Wolfram, 1986). Whether and to what extent a child's speech will contain AAE characteristics may depend on the family's socioeconomic and educational status (Wolfram, 1986; Washington & Craig, 1992). AA children from upper socioeconomic status and children whose parents have higher education may use fewer features of AAE than those from lower socioeconomic strata and limited family education. Almost all of African American preschool children (94% to 100%) from low-income families living in such urban centers as Detroit may be AAE speakers, possibly because of their lack of exposure to MAE (Craig & Washington, 2002; Washington & Craig, 1992). Children from all socioeconomic and educational strata may use a few features, though with varying frequency. For example, a child from an upper socioeconomic and educational status may still omit the postvocalic *r* in such words as *sister*, (pronounced as *sistə*), but may not substitute /f/ for /θ/ in such words as *bath* (pronounced as *baf in AAE)*; children from middle and lower socioeconomic classes are likely to produce both variations. Therefore, a child who does not substitute /f/ for /θ/ may still be an AAE speaker, even if occasionally, who belongs to an upper class.

Not only the socioeconomic class, but also the geographic regions of the United States may affect the production and pattern of AAE among African American speakers. This is true of MAE as well, as no dialect of any language is free from the influence of geographic variations. For instance, a study by Washington and Craig (1992) pointed out that AAE features of the AA children in the northern states of the country (e.g., Michigan) may be different from the pattern found in the children living in the southern states (e.g., Mississippi). Their study found that the Arizona Articulation Proficiency Scale-Second Edition (Fudala & Reynolds, 1986) did not require adjustment for AAE dialect (scoring modifications) when administered to children in the Detroit area, whereas this and other tests of articulation did require adjustments when administered to AAE speaking children in Mississippi, as reported by Cole and Taylor (1990).

Tasks used in assessment also may evoke to a greater or lesser extent features of AAE in children who speak that dialect. For instance, Washington, Craig, and Kushmaul (1998) found that picture description evokes more AAE features than free-play speech. Connor and Craig (2006) reported that sentence imitation tasks may not evoke AAE features; when the expectation is the production of MAE, many AA children who can code-switch are likely to produce MAE instead of AAE.

Generally, age and the grade in which the child is studying may be important to consider in judging whether an African American child is an AAE speaker. Although most preschool children may be AAE speakers, children in the upper grades may be both AAE and MAE speakers as the medium of instruction in the schools is MAE (Pearson, Velleman, Bryant, & Charko, 2009). As they move through the elementary grades, AA children gain progressively greater proficiency in MAE and learn to code-switch.

It is important to note that there is no clinical concern when children or adults speak AAE all the time, speak it some of the time, or include only some of its features some of the time, or even all the time. It is clinically relevant only when it risks a misdiagnosis of a communication disorder. It is this risk that speech-language pathologists should avoid by understanding the AAE features and excluding those as the bases for diagnosing a disorder.

Speech Characteristics of AAE

AAE and the MAE share the same set of consonants (Green, 2002; Pearson et al., 2009; Stockman, 2006). One particular consonant, /ð/ of the MAE, may be virtually absent in some AAE speakers as it is typically replaced by /d/, however. All MAE vowels are present in AAE, although some diphthongs may be reduced to single vowels. The pattern of MAE sound production by African Americans who speak AAE may differ, however. Differences between AAE and MAE may be more pronounced in consonant than vowel productions and in syllable and word structures (Pearson et al., 2009). The clinician, while noting the production of common (shared) sounds and syllables, should pay special attention to features that contrast (different in AAE, compared to MAE), as summarized from the various research literature (Bailey & Thomas, 1998; Cole & Taylor, 1990; Craig, Thompson, Washington, & Potter, 2003; Laing, 2003; Pearson et al., 2009; Rickford, 1999; Stockman, 1996a, 2010; Wolfram, 1994; examples are from these and other sources):

Vowel changes include the following;

- Reduction of the diphthong /aʊ/ to single vowel in some contexts (e.g., "at" for *out*)
- Reduction of /ɔɪ/ to single vowel in some contexts (e.g., "all" for *oil*)
- Reduction of /aɪ/ to single vowel in some contexts (e.g., "ass" for *ice*)

Omission or weak production of consonants is a characteristics of AAE:

- *Variable omission* of several *final consonants* is a significant aspects of AAE; it should be noted that all sounds listed here may not be omitted by all AAE speakers; the same sound omitted in the final word-positions may be produced correctly in the initial or medial positions
- Omission (or lessening) of the word-final /l/ (e.g., "too" for *tool)* and the medial /l/ (e.g., "a'ways" for *always*)
- Omissions of the word-final /d/ (e.g., "ba" for *bad* and "goo" for *good)*
- Omission (or lessening) of the word-final /r/ (e.g., "doah" for *door* or "mudah" for *mother*)
- Omission of the word-final /m/ (e.g., "hæ for *ham*)
- Omission of the final nasal sound or an oral stop. Whether the following word begins with a consonant or a vowel may have an effect on the production of sounds in the previous word. For instance, the /t/ in *best buy* is more likely to be omitted than the /t/ in *right on*. A consonant that is also an English morphological feature may be omitted in redundant contexts (e.g., the omission of the plural *s* in such expressions as *two cup*; the lexical quantifier *two* makes the plural morpheme redundant).
- Omission of final *g* (e.g., "I am goin'" for *I am going)*

To a variable extent, other word-final consonants that may also be omitted include /b/, /p/, /k/, /n/, and /v/ (Craig et al., 2003; Stockman, 1996a).

Substitution of consonants also is a feature of AAE:

- /d/ may replace /ð/ in the word-initial positions (e.g., "dis" for *this*)
- /d/ may replace /ð/ in the word-medial positions (e.g., "broder" for *brother*).
- /v/ may replace /ð/ in word-final positions (e.g., "smoov" for *smooth*)
- /t/ or /f/ may replace the /θ/ (e.g., "tin" for *thin* or "teef" for *teeth*).

- /b/ may replace /v/ (e.g. "balentine" for *valentine)*
- /n/ may replace the word-final /ŋ/ in unstressed syllables (e.g., "son" for *song)*
- /s/ may replace a /z/ as a devoicing feature (e.g., "his" for *hiz)*

Consonant cluster reduction, especially in the word-final positions, is another significant feature of AAE (Craig et al., 2003; Stockman, 1996a):

- -sk may be reduced to /s/ (e.g., "des" for *desk)*
- -ft may be reduced to /f/ (e.g., "lef" for *left)*
- -st may be reduced to /s/ (e.g., "tes" for *test)*
- -kst may be reduced to *ks* (e.g., "neks" for *next)*
- -ʃr may be reduced to a non-English cluster *sr* (e.g., "srink" for *shrink)*
- -ɵr may be reduced to /ɵ/ (e.g., "thow" for *throw)*
- -nɵ may be reduced to either *nf* or *nt* (e.g., "tenf" or "tent" for *tenth)*
- -mf may be reduced to *mp* (e.g., "triump" for *triumph)*
- -nd may be reduced to /n/ (e.g., "lan" for *land)*
- -ls may be reduced to /s/ (e.g., "fas" for *false)*

Many other clusters also may be reduced to a single consonant. For example, such clusters as -lm, -lp, -ld, -lt, -lk, -nd, -kt, -sp, among others, may be reduced to single consonants (Stockman, 1996a). Any cluster reduction in an African American child should be carefully considered as a potential feature of AAE.

Unstressed syllable reduction or deletion, is another significant feature of AAE:

- Deletion of an unstressed single vowel forming the syllable shape (e.g., "way" for *away* or "bout" for *about)*
- Deletion of an unstressed vowel with the preceding word ending in a vowel (e.g., "go'way" for *go away)*
- Deletion of an unstressed syllable in word that is a preposition or conjunction (e.g., "hind" for *behind* or "cause" for *because)*

The unstressed syllable is *retained* in other contexts:

- The unstressed syllable is produced when the word is a noun, adjective, or verb (e.g., the initial syllable is produced in *begin* but may be deleted in *before)*
- The unstressed syllable is produced when the word has three syllables (e.g., the initial syllable is produced in *depression,* but may be deleted in *divorce* (Stockman, 1996a).

Other Features that characterize the speech of AAE speakers include:

- Sound reversal (e.g., "aks" for *ask)*
- Stressing the initial syllable in a word that may be unstressed in MAE (e.g., "**po**lice" instead of *police* or "**De**troit" for *Detroit)*

- Lower fundamental frequency of voice than found in MAE speakers
- Higher variations in pitch than found in MAE speakers
- Rising pitch contours
- Falling pitch contours on questions

During assessment, the clinician is likely to find that the phonetic inventory of a child who speaks AAE is more similar to the inventory found in other children. The same MAE phonemes are found in AAE, but the pattern of production may be different. Sounds correctly produced in other contexts may be omitted or substituted in certain word medial and final positions. Therefore, such omissions and substitutions are not disorders of articulation. It is this different pattern of phoneme production that gives AAE its most characteristic feature. Similarly, persons who speak English as a second language also omit or substitute phonemes.

Language Characteristics of AAE

Assessment of children who speak AAE should also take into consideration the **patterns of language features** (mostly morphologic and syntactic differences). Unique rules of morphologic and syntactic productions may be extracted from AAE. Various features of MAE may be omitted, substituted, or modified. Distinctions that are not made in MAE may be made in AAE. Language features of AAE to be considered in assessing a child who speaks it include the following, although not all features may be found in all speakers and some may be variable within the speaker (Craig et al., 2003; Mufwene, Rickford, Bailey, & Baugh, 1998; Stockman, 2010; Washington & Craig, 2002; several examples are from these and other sources):

Omission of several MAE grammatic features is a significant aspect of AAE. For example, AAE speakers may:

- Omit noun possessives (e.g., "it Kaneesha house" for *It's Kaneesha's house*)
- Omit the plural morpheme (e.g., "she got five pencil" for *she has five pencils*)
- Omit third person singular (e.g., "he work downtown" for *he works downtown)*
- Omit the copula (e.g., "he a nice man" for *he is a nice man*)
- Omit the verbal auxiliary *(e.g.,* "they going on a vacation" for *they are going on a vacation*)
- Omit the present tense form of auxiliary *have* (e.g., "I been here for two hours" for *I have been here for two hours*)
- Omit the past tense form of *have* (e.g., "he done it again" for *he has done it again*)
- Omit the regular past tense *ed* (e.g., "he kick me" for *he kicked me*)
- Omit the present tense morpheme (e.g., "he live in Africa" for *he lives in Africa*)
- Omit the auxiliary *is* when the described action is not permanent, but only temporary (e.g., "he working" to suggest that an unemployed man is working

temporarily; contrasted with "he be working" to suggest that a man with a permanent employment is also working presently)

- Omit the present progressive *ing* (e.g., "what are you lay___ in the sun for?" for *what are you laying in the sun for?*)

- Omit the infinitive marker *to* (e.g., "I don't know how ___ do it" for *I don't know how to do it)*

- Omit the definitive article *the* (e.g., "now ___ food is ready" for *now the food is ready)*

- Omit the preposition (e.g., "hey, get out the way" for *hey, get out of the way)*

Replacement of certain MAE features with other features is also a feature of AAE speakers:

- Auxiliary *is* may replace the auxiliary *are* (e.g., or "they is doing fine!" for *they are doing fine*)

- Copula *is* may replace the copula *are* (e.g., "you is not bad!" for *you are not bad)*

- Past tense *was* may replace its plural form (e.g., "they was doing well" for *they were doing well* or "you was nice to me" for *you were nice to me)*

- *None* may replace *any* (e.g., "he don't need none" for *he doesn't need any)*

- *Them* may replace *those* (e.g., "them houses, they be old" for *those houses are old* or "Where do you get them shoes?" for *where do you get those shoes?)*

- *Gonna* may replace future tense *is* and *are* auxiliary forms (e.g., "He gonna do it" for *he is going to do it* or "they gonna be fine" for *they are going to be fine)*

- *Does* may replace *do* (e.g., "he do cook well" for *he does cook well* or "It do make sense" for *it does make sense)*

- Auxiliary *be* may replace the auxiliary *is,* as noted, to suggest a permanent as well as a current condition (e.g., "he be working" to suggest that the man has a permanent job and is working today)

- Indefinite article *a* may replace *an* (e.g., "I see a elephant" for *I see an elephant)*

- Present tense form may replace an irregular past term (e.g., "Then they all fall" for *then they all fell")*

- *Hisself* may replace *himself* (e.g., "he lives by hisself" for *he lives by himself)*

- Pronoun replacements (e.g., "them not goin' to do" for *they are not going to do it)*

- *It* may replace *there* ("it seems it's a lot more here" for *it seems there is a lot more here)*

Addition of certain features that are not found in MAE is a feature of AAE speakers:

- Add *at* at the end of *where* questions (e.g., "where is the cat *at?*" for *where is the cat?)*

- Add a second auxiliary (e.g., "I might could have done it" for *I could have done it)*

- Add a double negatives for emphasis (e.g., "I don't never want no cake" for *I don't want any cake* or "I have not seen no one" for *I have not seen anyone)*

- Add *been* to emphasize past events or actions (e.g., "I been had an accident when I was 20" for *I had an accident when I was 20* or "I been known that" for *I have known that*)
- Add *done* to a past tense construction (e.g., "he done painted the house" for *he painted the house*)
- Add an implied pronoun to restate the subject (e.g., "my mother, *she* cannot make it" for *my mother cannot make it*)
- Add the regular plural morpheme to irregular plurals (e.g., "you have all these mens here" for *you have all these men here)*
- Add a possessive when not needed (e.g., "this one is mines" for *this one is mine)*
- Adding *done* to emphasize something just done (e.g., "done wash(ed) the car" for *I just finished the car wash*)

Several other unique features also characterize AAE language production:

- Subject-verb agreement variation (e.g., "I gets too hot" for *I get too hot* or "I knew you was going to do it" for *I knew you were going to do it*)
- Noninverted question (e.g., "what we can do about it?" for *what can we do about it)*
- Production of a pronoun and a noun (e.g., "Jane she cooks good" for *Jane cooks good)*
- Production of *ain't* as a negative auxiliary (e.g., "you ain't seen that yet" for *you have not seen it yet)*
- Abbreviation of *about* (e.g., "he is bouta fall of " for *he is about to fall of)*
- Reduction of an unstressed syllable (e.g., "kem" for *became)*
- Multiple agreement markers for regular nouns and verbs ("he tries to kills him" for *he tries to kill him)*
- Overcorrection of irregular terms (e.g., "they felled" for *they fell)*

Studies have revealed that five AAE grammatic features offer the greatest contrast with MAE in both children and adults from low and middle socioeconomic levels: (1) *deletion of the copula,* (2) *deletion of the verbal auxiliary,* (3) *subject-verb variation* (lack of agreement), (4) o*mission of the past tense morpheme,* and (5) *multiple negation* (Oetting & Pruitt, 2005; Stockman, 2010; Washington & Craig, 2003). The *noninverted question* form may be less frequent in children than in adults. It should also be noted that AAE phonological patterns interact with morphosyntactic features, creating combined patterns (Craig et al., 2003; Washington & Craig, 2002). For instance:

- Consonant cluster reductions and regular plural omissions may be responsible for such expressions as "their boot(s)" (missing *s*)
- Consonant cluster reductions and lack of subject-verb agreement may result in such expressions as "he work(s) in the yard" (missing *s*)
- Postvocalic consonant reduction and missing past tense may result in such expressions as "she show(ed) him how to do it" (*ed* missing)

- Post vocalic consonant reduction and omission of the possessive morpheme may result in such expressions as "my mother'(s) hat" (*s* missing)

In assessing an African American child's speech and language skills, the clinician should take into consideration these described features of AAE. No diagnosis of a communication disorder will be made on the basis of features that are characteristics of AAE.

AAE Speech and Language Learning Patterns

AA children in the United States learn two dialects. Many children, especially from lower socioeconomic backgrounds, may acquire AAE as their first dialect at home and learn the MAE dialect of their geographic region when they enter school (Pearson et al., 2009). Much of the research has been concerned with the differences between the two dialects; very few studies have been done on the learning patterns in typically developing children (Pearson et al., 2009; see Stockman, 2010 for a review of studies).

We summarize here the AAE and MAE learning patterns found in AA children (Bland-Stewart, 2003; Cole & Taylor, 1990; Craig & Washington, 2002; Craig, Washington, & Thomson, 2005; Kamhi, Pollock, & Harris, 1996; Pearson et al., 2009; Pruitt & Oetting, 2009; Stockman, 1996, 2008, 2010; Stockman, Karasinski & Guillory, 2008, among others), while recommending clinicians to keep abreast of expanding research:

- AA children's pattern of **speech sound learning** is similar to those of MAE learners; speech sound mastery advances with increasing age levels
    - By age 2, AA children produce single consonant and clusters in conversational speech; they produce all of the 15 most frequently occurring English consonants: /m/, /n/, /p/, /b/, /t/, /d/, /k/, /g/, /w/, /j/, /f/, /s/, /h/, /l/, and /r/. Stockman (2006a, 2008) includes these 15 consonants in her *minimal articulatory competence* of 3-year old AA children; if an AA child does not produce some of these sounds by age 3, then there is reason for clinical concern.
    - By age 3, AA children produce 8 to 9 word initial consonant clusters, especially those involving obstruents plus sonorants (e.g., *br, pr, dr, tr, gr, kr, tw, sl, sm, sn,* and so forth)
    - By ages 5 and 6, such later learned fricatives as /z/, /ʃ/, and /tʃ/ may be evident in some word positions; at least 75% of children may produce the initial /l/ and /s/ blends
    - Consistent with AAE, word final consonants may be variably absent; however, such other phonologic patterns as fricative stopping, velar fronting, liquid gliding, and voicing assimilation are comparable to those found in MAE children
    - At age 3;4 to 3;11, 81 to 82% of consonants may be judged correct, in reference to AAE phonological patterns; at age 3;7 to 6;1, 95 to 98% of consonants may be correct in single-word productions
    - Except for the final stop omissions, consonant production and mastery patters are similar across AAE- and MAE-speaking children; there are a few notable exceptions, however; AAE children master /ð/ much later, but they master /r/

in prevocalic positions and /rs/ final clusters, /s/ in initial and final positions, and /z/ in final positions sooner, than MAE-speaking children

- Generally, AA children achieve their **oral language mastery** by age 6, similar to other children
  - AA children learn to produce the various grammatic features in a pattern and sequence similar to those learning MAE
  - The number and variety of words learned increase as expected during the early years, although some effect of socioeconomic status may be evident; all semantic categories (e.g., action, state, location) found in other children also are found in AA children
  - AA children combine words by 18 months; as expected, their mean length of utterance (MLU) increases with each higher age level (e.g., an MLU of 1.3 at 18 months increases to 3.39 at age 3 to 4; and then to 6.61 to 7.42 at age 4 and 6 years
  - By age 3, AA children produce declarative, imperative, interrogative, and negative sentence types; they also produce complex sentences at this age and show consistent increases in subsequent years; the most complex syntax may be found in children with highest density of AAE
  - AA children learn the grammatic morphemes in a manner similar to other children except for a few that contrast between AAE and MAE; for instance, possessive –s, third person singular –s, past tense -ed, contractible copula, and auxiliary may be variably absent at age 3 or higher
  - Pragmatic language skills of AAE speakers are roughly comparable to those of MAE speakers
  - AA children begin to exhibit narrative-like talk between 2 and 3 years of age; older children effectively code-switch during their narration from AAE to MAE
  - AA children's speech contains conversational structures at age 3 and 4; they take appropriate conversational turns at age 4.
  - AAE speakers use the same types of conversational repair strategies as the MAE speakers

Strategies for Assessing African American Children

The basic procedures and approaches of assessment of AA children do not differ from those of other children. A case history, orofacial examination, and hearing screening needs to be completed. The family interview will include standard questions as well as those that are specific to understanding the culture and communication patterns of the African American family. Although most standardized tests are not appropriate for assessing AA children, a few acceptable tests may be a part of this assessment.

Washington and Craig (1992) report that the Arizona Articulation Proficiency Scale-Second Edition (Fudala & Reynolds, 1986) may be acceptable for assessing AA children, even without a scoring adjustment for AAE. The authors caution, however, that this may be true only for AA children in such northern states as Michigan, but not for AA children in such southern states as Mississippi unless adjusted for AAE dialect, as demonstrated by

Cole and Taylor (1990). Most other tests of articulation also may require scoring adjustment: a questionable practice that raises issues of reliability and validity. Instead of administering an inappropriate test and changing the scoring method, clinicians should use language samples, child-specific criterion-based procedures, and other alternative procedures described in the next chapter to asses speech sound productions; the results may be accurately analyzed in light of AAE.

The Expressive Vocabulary Test (Williams, 1997) also may be acceptable for assessing AA children (Thomas-Tate, Washington, Craig, & Packard, 2006). On the other hand, a commonly used test of vocabulary, the Peabody Picture Vocabulary Test (Dunn & Dunn, 1981, 1997) is deemed unsuitable for AA children (Stockman, 2000; Washington & Craig, 1992), although it may have a place in a comprehensive alternative assessment package. The Preschool Language Scale (Zimmerman, Steiner, & Pond, 1992) may penalize AA children for their use of double negatives and omissions of possessives, third person singular, copula, and auxiliary, and therefore, may overdiagnose language disorders (Qi et al., 2006).

Laing (2003) describes an *alternate response mode* (ARM) procedure in which the child is tested in the manner of McDonald's (1964) *Deep Test of Articulation*. In this procedure, Laing had AA children produce target words for testing combined with a single, constant word (e.g., tru*ck*-eyes, wat*ch*-eyes, va*se*-eyes, etc.) to assess the production of the italicized sounds in the examples. The method was effective in reducing final consonant deletions that are typical of AAE, thus minimizing the risk of overdiagnosing a speech disorder in AA children.

Stockman (2006, 2008) has researched the concept of minimal competency core as a way of assessing AAE-appropriate speech sound production. Stockman suggests the previously listed 15 word-initial consonants as the minimum number of speech sounds to be assessed in AA children. This is one of the alternative methods of assessing AA children, and we discuss this further in the next chapter.

Clinicians may choose one of the few assessment instruments especially designed for AAE, listed in Table 4–1. The norm-referenced Diagnostic Evaluation of Language Variation has a screening and a full version (Seymour, Roeper, & de Villiers, 2003, 2005). Both the versions help distinguish language difference from a language disorder.

The other two instruments listed in Table 4–1 by Washington and Craig (2004) and Craig and Washington (2000) are not standardized published tests; useful nonetheless because they are AAE-specific and are based on research data. Both use child-centered free play language samples and specific language tasks that offer criterion-referenced method to screen or assess language skills of AA children in urban settings. The language screening protocol (Washington & Craig, 2004) includes the number of different words in a language sample, the Kaufman Assessment Battery for Children (Kaufman, & Kaufman, 1983), and a nonword repetition task that help identify AA children with language disorders. Washington and Craig point out that these measures are not affected by the AAE features. In their study on an assessment battery, Craig and Washington (2000) demonstrated that the average length of communication units (MLCU) measured in words or morphemes, frequencies of complex syntax, and number of different words are valid language production tasks that can help distinguish AA children with language disorders from typically developing AA children. In addition, responses to *Wh*-questions and responses to probes of active and passive sentences can help assess language comprehension in children

Table 4–1. Assessment Instruments for African American English

Assessment Instrument	Age Range	Skills Assessed
A language screening protocol for use with young African American children in urban settings. (Washington & Craig, 2004)	3 years to 5 years (study participants)	Not a standardized test, but a researched screening protocol; helps assess number of different words, nonword repetition, Wh-question comprehension, and picture description.
An assessment battery for identifying language impairments in African American children. (Craig & Washington, 2000)	4 years to 11 years (study participants)	Not a standardized test, but a researched assessment battery to evaluate the length of communication units, frequencies of complex syntax, number of different words, and language comprehension.
Diagnostic Evaluation of Language Variation-Screening Test (DELV-Screening Test) (Seymour, Roeper, & de Villiers, 2003)	4 years to 12 years	Mainstream American English and language variation due to regional and cultural language differences; helps distinguish language differences from disorders.
Diagnostic Evaluation of Language Variation-(DELV)-Norm-Referenced (Seymour, Roeper, & de Villiers, 2005)	4 through 9 years	Noncontrastive, shared elements of language variations; helps assess language disorders by ruling out several American English dialectal features.

with language disorders. Lower sores on these tasks may suggest a language disorder in AA children.

A comprehensive and valid assessment of AA children will need an integrated approach that incorporates the best features of alternative approaches and the essential elements of the traditional approach. We describe such a model in the next chapter. In addition, we provide assessment protocols in Chapter 7 (Speech Production) and Chapter 9 (Language Skills) to make a proper ethnocultural analysis of AA children's speech sounds or language skills and disorders.

Assessment of Bilingual Children

Bilingual children may exhibit various levels of proficiency in English that they are trying to master as a second language. Such children are described as either children with limited English proficiency (LEP) or English Language Learners (ELL). Although the first and the home language of a significant number of ELL is Spanish, there are children in U.S. schools who speak languages from all corners of the world, including Asia, Eastern Europe, Russia, Africa, the Caribbean islands, and Central and South America.

Diagnosis of communication disorders in ELL with limited English proficiency because of their bilingual status requires evidence that a disorder exists in both languages (Brice, 2002; Goldstein, 2004; Hamayan & Damico, 1991; Kayser, 2002; Long, 1994; Roseberry-McKibbin, 1994, 2002). Results of tests administered in English to bilingual children should be interpreted cautiously. If a language disorder exists, it is likely to manifest itself in both languages the child speaks, although with varying proficiency. Therefore, assessment needs to be done in both languages. If the results of an assessment show that there is only a problem in the second language (English), then it is possible that the child does not have a speech or language disorder, but has not yet mastered the second language to the extent expected. What this child needs is an educational program that includes an intensive English language instruction, not clinical intervention for a communication disorder.

Bilingual Learning Patterns

Assessing a bilingual child requires knowledge of a dual-language learning process (Brice, 2002; Brice & Brice, 2009; Goldstein, 2004; Kayser, 1995; Kohnert, 2007; Roseberry-McKibbin, 1994, 2002). A simple search of any aggregate database will reveal an increasing number of research papers being published over the years on dual language acquisition and assessment issues related to bilingual children with communication disorders. Without a critical knowledge of this ever increasing database, several normal features of bilingualism can be misinterpreted as a sign of a communication disorder. For instance, grammatical mistakes or speech sound substitutions bilingual children make during the time they are learning English should not be a basis to diagnose a language or speech disorder.

Research on bilingual language (and speech) learning has been expanding in recent years. The main trends and principles of bilingual learning summarized here, though coming from Spanish-English bilingual research, may be applicable to other children whose first language is Asian or American Indian. Therefore, to assess all bilingual children, clinicians should critically evaluate the studies on bilingualism (Brice & Brice, 2009; Dollaghan & Horner, 2010; Fabian-Smith & Goldstein, 2010a, 2010b; Gutierrez-Clellen & Simon-Cereijido, 2007; Gutierrez-Clellen, Simon-Cereijido, & Sweet, 2012; Kohnert, 2007; Paradis & Genesee, 1996). One difficulty clinicians need to overcome is the bilingual (or monolingual) literature's heavy theoretical and mentalistic-linguistic speculations. Speech-language pathologists need to rephrase the bilingualism's concept into empirical terms that are better aligned with treatment procedures which are based mostly on empirical learning principles.

From a descriptive standpoint, bilingual learning may be simultaneous or sequential. In *simultaneous bilingualism*, children are exposed to two languages at the same time and master them even if somewhat unevenly. In *sequential bilingualism*, the child will have mastered one language substantially before learning another language. If the parents speak two different languages at home, the child is likely to be in a simultaneous bilingual situation from the very start of speech-language acquisition. Learning a second language, if that is more reinforcing to the child, may result in the functional loss of the first language, sometimes called *subtractive bilingualism* or *L1 attrition*. In other cases, a second language may be learned while preserving the first language, described as *additive bilingualism* (Lambert, 1977). From a learning standpoint, it is doubtful whether children engage in language addition and subtraction. In a bilingual situation, teachers and parents may reinforce the verbal behaviors of a particular language, and withhold their reinforcement for the same kind of behaviors of another language. In such cases, reinforced behaviors (of one language) will be strengthened while those of the unreinforced will decline.

Verbal behaviors of the first language (e.g., Spanish, Mandarin, or Punjabi) may decline when parents who do not speak English well are urged to switch to English at home, on the assumption that children's English learning will then accelerate (Wong-Fillmore, 1991). In such cases, children may not show normal gains in their first language behaviors, and the poor English to which they are exposed to at home may fail to advance their English skills. This often happens with children in elementary school who begin to spend more time in an all English-speaking classroom. According to some studies, it takes approximately 2 to 3 years to achieve proficiency in social language skills in the second language and 5 to 7 years to achieve academic language proficiency (Collier, 1987; Cummins, 1984). Children examined during this phase of bilingualism may appear to have inadequate communication skills in both the languages (Anderson, 2004). But such children may not be diagnosed with a language disorder, yet they need to be reassessed at a later time.

Another feature that may complicate assessment of bilingual children is code switching or code mixing, both referring to alternation of two languages in the same conversational episode. A full sentence spoken in one language and the next sentence spoken in a different language is *code switching,* and including words from different languages within a sentence is *code mixing*, and both forms may be observed in most bilingual children and adults (Brice, 2002; Brice & Brice, 2009). Neither code switching nor mixing is an indication of a language disorder; most speakers who are competent in two or more languages code switch or code mix when the audience is appropriate (i.e., in the presence of others who do the same). Many bilingual Asians or Hispanics who speak English well constantly switch and mix English words and sentences with their native languages in informal conversations. This behavior seems to be strictly under the audience-stimulus control, because it is present in the presence of some conversational partners and absent in the presence of other partners.

In some cases, children and adults who have mastered the two languages may exhibit a phenomenon described as *fossilization*, an unfortunate term that gives no indication of its learning history while evoking a geological process to explain an aspect of verbal behavior. In fossilization, some unusual expressions or grammatic errors in the second language become fixated, resulting in idiosyncratic errors. Roseberry-McKibbin (2002) gives the example of a Spanish speaker with excellent mastery of English who may say "the news are that . . . " Similarly, an English native speaker who has learned Spanish well may routinely use the word *reducio* instead of the correct *redujo* to mean *reduced* (Brice, 2002). Such persistent errors of grammar and usage are common in fist language speakers, although not requiring any special term (such as *fossilization)*; for instance, agreement problems like "the clinician . . . . and they . . . " in which *they* refers to the singular noun, are now quite common among native speakers and writers of English. Although not an indication of a language disorder, fossilized expressions are thought to be resistant to change; however, their persistence is likely due to them being reinforced over the years. Clinicians might think that it is possible to change them by reinforcing correct alternatives.

A more complete understanding of variables related to simultaneously learning of two languages needs much more research; research is especially sparse on Asian American children and American Indian children learning English. Bilingual learning is complex because of the potential mutual influence of the two languages and their interactions. All kinds of possible influences and interactions have been hypothesized; many hypotheses seem to suggest some autonomous processes, instead of learning variables. More evidence is needed to fully validate the current crop of linguistic and cognitive hypotheses. Among the several hypotheses, language transfer has special clinical implications (Brice & Brice, 2009; Paradis & Genesee, 1996).

The language transfer hypothesis includes both positive and negative transfer. *Positive transfer* is the facilitative effect of one language over the other. Generally, positive transfer is said to occur when the two languages a child learns share common features (often described as linguistic rules). For instance, the regular plural -*s* occurs in both Spanish and English; therefore, a child who has learned the plural inflection in one of the two languages is likely to learn the same inflection in the other language with much less difficulty (Goldstein, 2004). Similarly, a speech sound that is present in one language may promote positive transfer to the same sound present in the other language. In learning terms, positive transfer is acceptable generalization, something that clinicians observe in treatment sessions.

In negative transfer, also described as *interference*, a feature of one language may have a negative effect on the acquisition of some aspects of the other language. Speech sounds that are missing in the first language but present in the second may be acquired with difficulty or may be omitted while speaking in the second language. For instance, a Spanish speaker may pronounce the English word *Julie* as *Yulie* because of the absent /dʒ/ in Spanish. A European or an Asian speaker of English whose first language does not contain contrastive /v/ and /w/ may substitute one for the other. Similarly, grammatic features missing in the first language also may be omitted in the second; a correct word order of one language may be used incorrectly in the other. For example, a Spanish speaker might say, "The boy bicycle," omitting the possessive morpheme. An Asian language speaker might say, "You are going now?" (a wrong English word order generalized from the verbal behavior of the first language). Negative transfer also is generalization in learning terms, only unacceptable in the new or different verbal community.

Studies have shown that *reduced language learning opportunities* may be associated with poverty (Edwards, 1989; Gilliam & de Mesquita, 2000, Qi, Kaiser, Milan, & Hancock, 2006; Roseberry-McKibbin, 2008). Therefore, socioeconomic conditions are an important variable to consider, especially with children of minority background because of the relatively high rate of poverty among minority and bilingual families. Both monolingual English-speaking and bilingual children who come from impoverished backgrounds often perform poorly on standardized language measures (Edwards, 1989). To negatively affect language learning, environmental and cultural deprivation has to be severe, because families in lower socioeconomic strata can still provide the minimum environmental support for language learning (Hart & Risley, 1995, 1999). Even those children, who come from low socioeconomic strata, but meet the normative expectations, may be unfamiliar with certain words, phrases, situations depicted, and stimuli shown on standardize tests. Therefore, alternative assessment strategies are important in assessing children from lower socioeconomic strata, including those who may be bilingual.

Primary Language and Secondary English Dialects

A pervasive effect of the first language on the production of the second is described as *foreign accent*. Whereas accent refers primarily to the phonologic effect of the first language on the second, a *dialect* is a variation in speech, language, and prosodic features; being a more comprehensive term than *accent*, dialect is a varied form of a language and is not necessarily restricted to the influence of a fist language (Westby, 2002).

Dialects of a language are a product of a geocultural history of groups of individuals, and are not always due to bilingualism. English, being the language of international commerce and spoken around the world in different countries, exists in many forms. The authoritative Oxford Advanced Learner's Dictionary (2005) states that, "English is not just one standard language, but can be thought of as a 'family' which includes many different varieties" (p. R91). To indicate words that are integrated into British or American English from a variety of global "Englishes," the dictionary uses abbreviations for Australian, Canadian, Indian, Southeast Asian, South African, East African, and West African English. Within each of those major regions, English varies. British English has the Irish, Scottish, and other several regional dialects. The various American English dialects (e.g., the Eastern, Central Midland, North Central, Southern, Northwestern, and Southwestern) are well known to students of phonetics. Many native English dialects of the United States, Canada, United Kingdom, Australia, New Zealand, and South Africa are a product of geocultural factors, not bilingualism.

On the other hand, many dialects heard in a specific geographic region may be due to the influence of a second language. A child's second language English dialect may be due to the child's first language, Spanish or Russian, for instance. Another child's English dialect may be a product of an Asian, African, or Middle Eastern primary language.

Based on a speaker's dialect, people sometimes may make negative judgments that speech-language pathologists avoid. The American Speech-Language-Hearing Association (ASHA) (1983, 1985) has a long-standing position on social dialects: Dialects are normal variations in language and are not disorders of speech or language. It is ASHA's position that:

1. No social dialect of English is a communicative disorder. These dialects are a legitimate variety of English used for communication and social solidarity.

2. A person speaking a dialect of English may also manifest a clinically significant communicative disorder that is unrelated to the dialect.

3. The speech-language pathologist should distinguish between communicative disorders and dialectical differences.

4. Speech-language pathologists must be familiar with procedures for culturally unbiased testing.

Speech-language pathologists have an ethical responsibility to familiarize themselves with the various English dialects, especially those that are spoken in their service area. To minimize cultural bias, these dialectical differences should be taken into account when selecting assessment procedures, diagnosing a disorder, and planning treatment.

General Strategies for Assessing Bilingual Children

There are general as well as specific strategies for evaluating speech and language skills of bilingual children. General strategies apply to all bilingual children whereas specific strategies apply to children of particular primary language that influences English as their second language. The main theme of the general strategies is to consider both languages in assessing communication skills of a bilingual child.

Determining Language Dominance

Very few bilingual children in need of clinical services are equally proficient in their primary language as well as English. It is often the case that the child will have one dominant language and one somewhat weaker language. During preschool years and the earlier elementary grades, their first language may be dominant in many children who are just beginning to learn English. Soon, as the bilingual child's social milieu expands to include more English-speaking peers and academic demands in English increase, the child's English proficiency may also increase. The first language may show loss or attrition and English may eventually become the dominant language. Assessment is likely to pose significant challenges when the child is learning both languages, and when the shift to English as the dominant language has just begun, but the process is not completed. Once English becomes the child's dominant language and exclusive medium of instruction in school, most clinicians will conduct the assessment in English. The clinician would still analyze the results in light of the child's first language characteristics, however. This is necessary to differentially determine a language difference versus a language disorder because the influence of the first language on English cannot be ruled out.

In most cases, the situation may not be clear cut; the dominant language may not be apparent; proficiency in each may vary across topics or partners of conversation as well as contexts of communication. For example, a child from an English-Spanish speaking bilingual family may talk to the parents in English about his or her school experiences, but may talk in Spanish about family matters. Therefore, the clinician needs to interview the parents as well as teachers to gauge the amount of each language produced at home to determine language dominance.

Determining Language Proficiency

Beyond language dominance, the clinician needs to assess *language proficiency*. A child may lack desired proficiency even in his or her dominant language. Language proficiency testing is generally done by a specialist in English as a Second Language (ESL). Information provided by parents and teachers may also be taken into account. Determination of language proficiency should include consideration of the child's communication competence for daily activities, auditory and verbal skills, reading, and writing. Speech-language pathologists can make important contributions to the academic success of the child by making a comprehensive assessment of speech and language skills that help determine language proficiency.

Finally, as noted earlier, no disorder is diagnosed solely on the basis of a dialectal variation of English. The influencing factors that created the dialect may be noted, however. The client or the family may want to minimize the dialectal variation; in such cases, without diagnosing a disorder, the clinician may offer requested treatment services.

Getting Help from Interpreters

Assessment of bilingual children may require the help of an interpreter. Interpreters are beneficial or even necessary when assessing a child in his or her primary language or when interviewing family members with limited English proficiency. To get reliable and valid information through an interpreter, the clinician should take several steps. Hegde and Maul (2006), Lynch and Hanson (1992), and Westby (2002) provide several suggestions for the successful partnership with an interpreter. Individuals selected as interpreters should meet certain requirements:

1. Interpreters must be proficient in both the languages targeted for assessment; they typically involve the clinician's and the family members' language or languages.

2. Interpreters must understand and appreciate the cultural differences of both parties. Interpreters who do not understand the values, beliefs, and patterns of interaction associated with a particular culture may not help communicate effectively and may generate misinformation about the child and the family.

3. Interpreters should receive training specific to the assessment being done. They should be familiar with professional or unfamiliar vocabulary that might be used, the purpose of the evaluation, standardized test administration procedures, the interview format, and paperwork requirements.

4. Interpreters should have a basic knowledge of the process of speech and language acquisition and second language acquisition.

5. Interpreters should follow professional ethical principles and understand their role in the assessment process.

6. Family members, neighbors, or the child should not serve as interpreters. Lacking in training, they may not play the role of a professional interpreter. They may induce data distortions by faulty translations or interpretations.

During assessment, the clinician should modify his or her style of interaction; for instance:

1. The clinician should speak directly to the child or family members, not to the interpreter.

2. The clinician should avoid professional or technical jargon and figurative language that might be difficult to translate or lead to misunderstanding.

3. The clinician should check the client's or informant's understanding of information and exchange of information throughout the assessment.

4. The clinician should review the information and "debrief the interpreter" (Lynch & Hanson, 1992). A debriefing session is a brief meeting, following the

assessment, in which the interpreter and clinician can review the information collected and discuss any problems with the interpreting process. This is also an opportunity for the interpreter to share his or her impressions regarding the family's emotions or reactions during the session. Although subjective, these impressions might provide valuable insight regarding the family's acceptance of the problem and their understanding of the clinical process.

Developing Databases on Languages Spoken in the Service Area

Clinicians cannot be expected to know all the different languages their potential clients may speak. In some school districts, children may speak a dozen or more foreign languages. Even a proficiently bilingual clinician only can directly and with little external support serve children who speak the same two languages as herself or himself. Therefore, it is essential to develop a database of languages spoken in the clinician's service area.

Many local school districts and area speech-language-hearing clinics have been developing systematic information on the minority languages their students speak. Speech and language characteristics of minority languages may be described and listed. Cultural dispositions to communication and its disabilities may be documented through interviews of parents and research studies. Clinicians may use such databases to make valid decisions about normal communication patterns within the culture of a child and potential communication disorders.

A combination of strategies described so far will help assess a bilingual child fairly and accurately. Unfortunately, there are no substitutes or shortcuts to a clear understanding of the child and the family's culture and communication patterns. A native knowledge of the child's primary as well as secondary languages offers the best chance for evaluating communication skills in both the languages. It is, however, impractical to expect clinicians to know multiple languages well enough to make valid assessment of varied bilingual children. Therefore, clinicians need multiple approaches, as well as such resources as well-qualified interpreters and local databases on language differences.

Specific Strategies for Assessing Bilingual Children

Because bilingual children are a varied group, assessment strategies have to consider the particular primary language the child and the family members speak. Each primary language has its own unique effects on how a bilingual child produces English speech sounds and language features. Therefore, in the following sections, we describe assessment strategies for Asian, American Indian, and Hispanic bilingual children. In the next chapter, we review various alternative assessment models and describe a comprehensive and integrated approach to assessing all children, including those who are bilingual or bidialectal.

Assessment of Asian American Children

Assessment of children of Asian background possibly poses the greatest challenge to clinicians because of the linguistic diversity found in Asia and countries within the continent.

Asia is home to many languages and dialectal variations of those languages. Furthermore, Asian languages belong to different language families. Therefore, any single characterization of the influence of "Asian languages" on English should be suspect. An Asian American child's speech characteristics should be analyzed in relation to his or her specific primary language, although what is generally available to clinicians is a general description of *some* Asian speech characteristic.

Just the two Asian countries, China and India, have several hundred languages. China alone has more than 80 languages and countless dialectal variations; India has more than 20 official languages and over 400 spoken languages with many dialects of each. Similarly, the Southeast Asian countries have numerous languages and dialects. An additional complicating factor is that Asia is home to languages that belong to different language families including: (1) Sino-Tibetan (e.g., Thai, Yao, Mandarin, Cantonese); (2) Indo-Aryan, Indo-European, or Indic (e.g., Hindi, Bengali, Marathi and others spoken in India); (3) Dravidian (e.g., Kannada, Tamil, Telugu, and Malayalam spoken in India); (4) Astro-Asiatic (e.g., Khmer, Vietnamese, Hmong); (5) Tibeto-Burman (e.g., Tibetan and Burmese); (6) Malayo-Polynesian or Astronesian (e.g., Chamorro, Ilocano, Tagalog); (7) Papuan (e.g., New Guinean); (8) Altaic (e.g., Japanese, and Korean), and (9) Arabic and Persian (spoken in the Gulf countries and Iran, respectively).

Research on the acquisition of English as a second language in Asian American children living in the United States is extremely limited. Possibly, most of the research findings summarized earlier on bilingualism would also apply to Asian American children learning English. Therefore, clinicians should keep in perspective research on bilingualism in assessing Asian American children's communication disorders.

Much of the available descriptions of Asian languages apply mostly to Chinese Han language with two dominant dialects, Mandarin and Cantonese (Cheng, 1991). These characteristics may or may not apply to other Asian speakers. Some general characteristics of Asian American speakers that variably apply to speakers of different first languages are available (Roseberry-McKibbin, 2002). In using these characteristics in assessment, clinician should not overgeneralize them; the assessment strategy should be specific to the child's family background and the particular Asian language.

Speech Characteristics of Some Asian American Speakers

Omission or deletion of sounds:

- Omission of final consonants because many Asian languages are open-syllable languages in which more words tend to end in vowels rather than consonants (e.g., "sha" for *shop* or "ha" for *hot*)
- Deletion of /r/ (e.g., "gull" for *girl* or "tone" for *torn*)

Substitution of sounds for sounds that do not exist in the primary Asian language:

- /l/ may replace /r/ (e.g., "lize" for *rise*)
- /r/ may replace /l/ (e.g., "raundy" for *laundry*)
- /ʃ/ may replace /tʃ/ (e.g., "sheep" for *cheap*)
- /b/ may replace /v/ (e.g., "base" for *vase*)

- /v/ may replace /w/ (e.g., "vater" for *water*)
- /p/ may replace /f/ (e.g., "pall" for *fall*)
- /a/ may replace /æ/ (e.g., "block" for *black*)
- Voiceless cognates may substitute voiced sounds (e.g., "Fresno" for *Frezno*)
- /d/ may replace /ð/ (e.g., "dose" for *those*)
- /t/ may replace /θ/ (e.g., "tin" for *thin*)

A few **vowel errors** noted include the following:

- Deletion of syllables in polysyllabic words (e.g., "Ephant" for *elephant*)
- Reduction of vowel length (causing choppiness of speech)

For some basic information on other Asian languages (e.g., Arabic, Vietnamese, Hmong, Korean, Japanese, and a few others), see Peña-Brooks and Hegde (2007).

Language Characteristics of Asian American Speakers

Omission of certain grammatic forms may characterize certain Asian American children or adults who speak English as their second language:

- Regular plural morphemes (e.g., "I see two sheet of paper" or "give me five book")
- Verbal auxiliaries (e.g., "he walking fast" or "they eating a lot")
- Verbal copula (e.g., "she very nice" or "they very big")
- Possessive morphemes (e.g., "that is Dad hat" or "this is Mom dress")
- Regular past tense morphemes (e.g., "he work hard last year" or "they talk all day yesterday")
- Articles (e.g., "give me book" or "cat is here")
- Conjunctions (e.g., "John ___ Jane are coming")
- Forms of have (e.g., "we ___ been to the store")

Addition of grammatical markings may be observed in some bilingual Asian American children and adults:

- Past tense double marking (e.g., "he didn't went with his friends")
- Double negative (e.g., "they don't have no food to eat")

Misuse or incorrect use of grammatical forms may be heard in the speech of some bilingual Asian American children and adults:

- Pronouns (e.g., "her wife is here")
- Prepositions (e.g., "she is in home")

- Comparatives (e.g., "this is gooder than that" or "this is good than that")
- Lack of inflection on auxiliary *do* (e.g., "he do not have enough")
- Incorrect word order in interrogatives (e.g., "you are going now?")

Strategies for Assessing Asian American Children

In assessing Asian American children's English language skills, it is first necessary to determine if: (a) the child is bilingual, and if so, (b) to what extent, and (c) the socioeconomic and educational status of the family. Many Asian American children come from college-educated parents, both of whom speak English at home. In such cases, the child may have acquired English with only a negligible influence of the parents' native language. Where there is an influence of the child's primary language, it is essential to find out the characteristics of the particular Asian language the family speaks.

There are no standardized, norm-referenced tests of speech and language skills to assess Asian American children. Therefore, clinicians should take an extended language sample and analyze it in light of the child's first language characteristics. Clinicians can design child-specific tasks to sample grammatic morphemes and syntactic structures. Conversational speech may be the main vehicle to assess pragmatic language skills. If the child is monolingual English speaker or has acquired English as the first language, then more commonly used procedures may be useful. Chapter 7 (Speech Production) and Chapter 9 (Language Skills) offer protocols to assess features of Asian-influenced English speech and language.

Assessment of Hispanic Children

Assessment of communication skills of Hispanic children in the United States is also complicated by the many varieties of Spanish that influence their English language production. Although a majority of children of Hispanic background speak the Mexican variety of Spanish, there are children in particular states or regions who speak other varieties. For instance, in parts of Florida and other Eastern United States, bilingual Hispanic children may speak the Caribbean variety, including the Cuban and the Puerto Rican Spanish. Bilingual Hispanic children in various other parts of the country may speak Spanish of Spain or Spanish varieties of South and Central American countries. Therefore, it is essential to understand the particular variety of Spanish that influences a Hispanic bilingual child's English.

There are a variety of sources on language acquisition in bilingual children in general and English-Spanish bilingual children in particular (Brice, 2002; Brice & Brice, 2009; Goldstein, 2004; Kayser, 1995; Kohnert, 2007; Peña-Brooks & Hegde, 2007; Roseberry-McKibbin, 2002). These and other sources help clinicians understand the cultural and linguistic diversity of Hispanic children in the United States.

Compared to English, Spanish has a simpler phonological system. Spanish has only 5 vowels: /i/, /e/, /u/, /o/, and /a/ compared to 15 in English. The English consonants /v/, /θ/, /ð/, /z/, /dʒ/, and /ʒ/ as well as the nasal /ŋ/ and the liquid /j/ are absent in Spanish. To the contrary, the Spanish consonants /ŋ/, /ʎ/, /ɣ/, /χ/, /r̃/, and /β/ are absent in English. Spanish and English share the following phonemes: stops (/p/, /b/, /t/, /d/, /k/, and /g/;

nasals /m/ and /n/; fricatives /f/, /s/, and /ð/; affricate /tʃ/; liquid /l/; glides /w/ and /j/; and vowels /i/, /e/, /u/, and /o/.

Some Spanish consonants that are similar to certain consonants in English, may be produced differently; for example, the Spanish /s/ may be produced more frontally, giving the impression of a lisp. Spanish consonantal clusters are fewer and simpler; the /s/ cluster, the most common in English, does not occur in Spanish; final clusters are rare in Spanish. Spanish has only a few consonants in word final positions (only /s/, /n/, /r/, /l/, and /d/). Finally, Spanish vowels a, e, i, o, u may also be found in word-final positions.

What follows is a general description of Spanish-influenced English features to be considered in assessing Hispanic children.

Speech Characteristics of Spanish-Influenced English

Substitutions of sounds that may characterize Spanish-influenced English include:

- /i/ may replace /ɪ/ because of fewer vowels in Spanish (e.g., "Peen" for *pin* or "Cheeldren" for *children*)
- /ɛ/ may replace /æ/ (e.g., "Met" for *mat*)
- *ah* may replace /æ/ (e.g., "Cahn" for *can*)
- /b/ may replace /v/ (e.g., "Boice" for *voice*)
- /tʃ/ may replace /ʃ/ (e.g., "Cheep" for *sheep*)
- /d/ may replace /ð/ (e.g., "Dose" for *those*)
- /z/ may replace /ð/ (e.g., "Zat" for *that*)
- /t/ may replace /θ/ (e.g., "Tin" for *thin*)
- Voiceless final consonants may replace voiced final consonants (e.g., "Mase" for *maze*)
- /j/ may replace /dʒ/ (e.g., "Yune" for *June*)
- /ŋ/ may replace /n/ (e.g., "Tang" for *tan*)

Omission of sounds include the following:

- Many final sounds may be omitted (except for /a/, /e/, /i/, /o/, /u/, /l/, /r/, /n/, /s/, and /d/ that end words in Spanish, hence produced)
- /h/ may be omitted in the word initial positions (e.g., "Ouse" for *house*)

Different manner of productions of certain English sounds include the following:

- More frontal production of /s/ (leading to an impression of a lisp)
- Dentalized production of /t/, /d/, and /n/ (produced with the tip of the tongue positioned against the back of the central incisors)
- Deaspiration of stop sounds (resulting in weak production of aspirated stops, giving the impression of omission)
- Trilled production of /r/

Addition of sound include the following:

- A schwa may be inserted at the beginning of initial consonant clusters (e.g., "ʌschool" for *school*)

- /r/ may be trapped (as in the English word *butter*) or trilled

- /h/ may be silent in word-initial positions (e.g., *old* for *hold* or *it* for *hit*)

Language Characteristics of Spanish-Influenced English

Differences in word order include:

- A noun may precede an adjective (e.g., "The pencil red" for *The red pencil.*)

- The verb may precede an adverb (e.g., "He drives very fast his motorcycle" for *He drives his motorcycle very fast.*)

Omission of grammatic morphemes include:

- Regular plural allomorphs may be omitted (e.g., "I see two book" for *I see two books.*)

- Regular possessive allomorphs may be omitted (e.g., "The boy bicycle" for *The boy's bicycle.*)

- Regular past tense allomorphs may be omitted (e.g., "They talk yesterday" for *They talked yesterday* or "We paint last month" for *We painted last month.*)

Different patterns of grammatical productions include:

- Double negatives (e.g., "I don't want no more" for *I don't want any more.*)

- Production of the word *more* instead of a comparative (e.g., "This house is more small" for *This house is smaller.*)

Varied prosodic features include:

- Spanish stress patterns superimposed on English productions (e.g., "baking" with an emphasis on the final syllable)

- Speech with reduced pitch range, giving the impression of a monotone (pitch range is narrower in Spanish than in English)

- Lower pitch at the beginning of many utterances (typical of Spanish) that would normally be started at higher pitch in English

Strategies for Assessing Hispanic Children

In assessing Spanish-English bilingual children, it is important to note that English may also influence their Spanish language (Goldstein, 2004). It has been noted, for example, that a child may aspirate the normally unaspirated Spanish stop sounds. Possibly, certain English consonants may be substituted for Spanish consonants. Also, the general speech community in which a bilingual child lives may influence either or both languages. It has been noted that Hispanic children who regularly interact with AA children may acquire some of the AAE characteristics. The opposite is also likely to happen. This may be true of all bilingual children regardless of their primary language.

A careful analysis of an extended speech-language sample will be one of the most important assessment tasks. As noted before, Spanish-English bilingual children may be more accurate in producing shared phonemes than unshared phonemes (Goldstein, 2004). Generally error patterns in English and Spanish are similar, with a higher frequency of errors on consonants than on vowels, and similarly higher frequency of errors on clusters than on singletons. The 5 Spanish vowels are mastered by age 18 months. Phonologic patterns that may still be evident at the end of preschool include cluster reduction, unstressed syllable deletion, stridency deletion, and tap or trill /r/ deviations. To the contrary, processes that disappear by the end of preschool include velar and palatal fronting, prevocalic singleton omission, stopping, and assimilation. A majority of English-Spanish bilingual children with phonological disorders tend to exhibit cluster reduction, unstressed syllable deletion, stopping, liquid simplification, and assimilation. The speech-language sample will help make an assessment of such phonologic patterns. In addition, clinician may administer selected standardized tests listed in Table 4–2.

Chapter 7 (Speech Production) and Chapter 9 (Language Skills) offer protocols to assess speech and language features of Spanish-influenced English. These protocols should be combined with those that are commonly used (e.g., case history, interview, orofacial examination).

Table 4–2. Spanish Language Assessment Instruments

Assessment Instrument	Age Range	Skills Assessed
Clinical Evaluation of Language Fundamentals-Second Edition, Spanish (CELF Preschool-2 Spanish) Wiig, Secord, & Semel (2009)	3 years to 6;11 years	Concepts, vocabulary, sentence structures, phonological awareness, and early literacy rating.
Clinical Evaluation of Language Fundamentals-Fourth Edition, Spanish (CELF-4 Spanish) Wiig, Secord, & Semel (2006)	5 years to 21 years	Vocabulary, word structure, sentence structure, semantic relationships, pragmatic skills, and other Spanish language skills.
Preschool Language Scale-5 Spanish Screening Test (PLS-5 Spanish Screening Test) (Zimmerman, Steiner, & Pond, 2012)	Birth to 7;11 years	Emerging interaction, comprehension, and expressive language skills; includes articulation, voice, and stuttering screening items.

(continues)

Table 4–2. *(continued)*

Assessment Instrument	Age Range	Skills Assessed
Preschool Language Scale, Fifth Edition Spanish (PLS-5 Spanish) (Zimmerman, Steiner, & Pond, 2012)	Birth to 7;11 years	Auditory comprehension of spoken language and expressive language skills in both Spanish and English to assess bilingual children.
Bilingual Spanish Proficiency Questionnaire (Mates & Santiago, 1985)	Varies	Not a standardized test, but parent interview questionnaire to gather information on Spanish and English articulation, language, voice, fluency skills.
Bilingual Vocabulary Assessment Measure (Mates, 1995a)	3 years and up	Expressive vocabulary screening in English, French, Italian, Spanish, and Vietnamese.
Dos Amigos Verbal Language Scale-Revised (Critchlow, 1996)	5 to 13 years	English and Spanish language skills; a screening test.
Expressive One-word Picture Vocabulary Test: Spanish-Bilingual Edition (EOWPVT-SBE) (Brownell, 2000)	4 years to 12 years	Spanish and English vocabulary; total acquired vocabulary in the two languages.
Receptive One-Word Picture Vocabulary Test: Spanish Bilingual Edition (ROWPVT-SBE) (Brownell, 2001)	4 years to 12 years	Spanish and English receptive vocabulary.
Spanish Test for Assessing Morphologic Production (STAMP) (Nugent, Shipley, & Provencio, 1991)	5 years to 11 years	Spanish morphological features.
Spanish Language Assessment Procedure, Third Edition (SLAP) (Mates, 1995b)	3 years to 9 years	Basic concepts and needs, following directions, story retelling, requesting, describing events, and so forth.
Test of Early Language Development-Third Edition: Spanish (Ramos & Ramos, 2007)	2 through 7;11 years	Receptive and expressive language, overall spoken language.
Spanish Articulation Measures, Revised Edition (SAM) (Mates, 1994)	3 years and up	Spanish speech sound production in word production, word repetition, and conversational speech.

Assessment of Native American Children

Children of Native Americans (American Indians) may be either bilingual or native English speakers depending on their family and living conditions. Children who speak a Native American language exclusively are rare and those who speak it as one of their languages are dwindling in number. Native American languages are being extinguished at a distressing rate as most of the youngsters do not speak their parents' language (Crystal, 1987; Highwater, 1975).

Native American languages are not a product of a single linguistic community; they were spoken by people who were dispersed in wide geographic areas: all the way from the northern tip of Canada and Alaska to the southern tip of South America. Languages spoken by people in widely spread and isolated geographic areas tend to belong to different language families with divergent language properties.

Many Native American children in the United States acquire English as their first, and only, language. Most Native American languages are now spoken by a few elderly; some languages are pronounced dead with the death of a few older people (Bayles & Harris, 1982; Crawford, 1996). To attend school, many Native American children live outside their reservation with non-Native American families that may not speak the child's native language (Robinson-Zanartu, 1996; Yates, 1987). Therefore, most Native American children are monolingual English speakers, or if they do speak their Native American language, they are essentially bilingual with their English being stronger than their native language. Such children and their families seek clinical speech-language services only in English.

It is essential to understand the Native American language and culture even if the Native American child being served is a monolingual English speaker. However, it is even more important to understand in depth the child's cultural and linguistic background if a Native American child is bilingual. The influence of the native language on English may be significant and the family may seek services in both the languages, especially when a disorder is diagnosed in both.

Strategies for Assessing Children Who Speak Native American Languages

Similar to Asian languages, Native American languages also belong to a variety of language families. In North, Central, and South America, Native Americans speak approximately 800 Native American languages; the North American continent has at least 200 Native American languages. The number of Native American language *families* varies from a high of 60 to a low of 3; and one classification of 8 language families include: Algonquian, Iroquoian, Caddoan, Muskogean, Siouan, Penutian, Athabascan, and Uto-Aztecan (Highwater, 1975). Therefore, it is not meaningful to list the phonological or morphosyntactic characteristics of "Native American languages" because both the languages and their characteristics vary widely.

Several useful Web sites on Native American culture and languages offer information on certain languages and their properties; clinicians may visit those Web sites and find information on the specific Native American language their clients speak (see, for example, http//www.indians.org/welker.americans.htm). Instead of trying to master the language characteristics of Native American Languages in general, clinicians should gain a deeper understanding of such languages spoken in their service area. This strategy is not only more practical, but also more meaningful than the general strategy of understanding the somewhat abstract "Native American languages." Local school districts or universities may have developed systematic information on the specific types of Native American languages spoken in their service area. Clinicians may access such databases or develop their own over a period of time.

The first and the major task in assessing a Native American child is to determine whether he or she is a bilingual speaker. If the child is not bilingual, assessment will then follow the more traditional guidelines. If bilingual, the child should be assessed in both English and the Native American language. The general guidelines offered in the first part of this chapter to assess bilingual children should then be followed. In addition, the general cultural pattern of Native Americans should be considered:

- Respect to each other is highly valued; children especially may show respect to older or authoritative persons by avoiding eye contact and looking down during conversation.

- Some Native American mothers may not talk much while caring for their infants; this has implications for assessment of infant-mother interactions.

- The main mode of learning from the parents and other adults is by listening and observing.

- Parents may report that their children have better auditory comprehension skills than expressive language skills.

- Some parents may discourage their children from speaking their native language until their articulation is judged acceptable; consequently, a long period of nonverbal communication (pointing and gesturing) may pass before children begin to use words.

- Silence or few spoken words may be viewed as more valuable than talking too much or talking in English, which are viewed as imitating the "White Man".

- Quick answers to questions may be considered undesirable; therefore, a pause before answering questions is normal and does not indicate a language problem.

- Responding to questions they do not understand fully is not encouraged.

- Children may have to earn their right, as judged by parents, to express their opinions.

- Public behavior is generally restrained; expression of strong feelings is discouraged; expression of public grief may be acceptable only during official mourning ceremonies.

Assessment of Native American children poses unique challenges. There are no standardized, norm-referenced tests to assess communication skills and disorders in varied American Indian languages. Traditional tests may be invalid for assessing American Indian children (Robinson-Zanartu, 1996). An extended language sample, analyzed in light of the child's first language and child-specific criterion-oriented tasks may be the best options. A sincere effort to understand the general Native American culture, its rich folklore and printed literature, and information on communication styles will usually produce good results. When this understanding is combined with a detailed description of the speech-language characteristics of the bilingual Native American child, the assessment may be fair and appropriate to the child.

Traditional and Alternative Assessment Approaches

We have so far described issues related to fair and appropriate assessment of children from ethnoculturally diverse backgrounds and specific communication characteristics of selected cultural minority groups that typically are served by speech-language pathologists in the United States. Certain aspects of the traditional assessment concepts and methods are inappropriate for assessing children of ethnocultural minority groups. We have taken note that the most inappropriate are the routine administration of normative tests that are not standardized on specific cultural minority groups to make clinical decisions. A mistake that may follow from this initial error is to misinterpret the results. Such misinterpretations typically stem from a lack of understanding of the ethnocultural minority child's unique communication patterns. The result may be either an overdiagnosis or an underdiagnosis of a communication disorder.

In recent years, there has been a search for alternative assessment approaches that may be especially suitable for children of ethnocultural minority. We describe and evaluate these approaches in Chapter 5. We also note in that chapter that assessment of children of ethnocultural minority is not entirely unique. Most traditional procedures, including the case history, orofacial examination, hearing screening, and speech and language sampling are needed in the assessment of all children. Therefore, what is needed is an integrated approach that includes the necessary components of the traditional assessment and the strengths of several alternative approaches that have been researched. We note in the next chapter that some of the strengths of alternative approaches that are forcefully advocated for children of ethnocultural diversity also are useful in assessing mainstream children.

CHAPTER 5

Alternative and Integrated Assessment Approaches

- Behavioral Assessment
- Criterion-Referenced and Client-Specific Assessment
- Authentic Assessment
- Dynamic Assessment
- Portfolio Assessment
- Efforts at Combining Different Approaches
- A Comprehensive and Integrated Assessment Approach

Traditional assessment procedures, described in Chapter 3, seek to identify and compare a child's level of performance to the average performance of his or her peers sampled during the test standardization to determine if there is a communication impairment. Historically, these procedures have relied heavily on the use of standardized, norm-referenced tests. Although such tests are convenient to use, they may not accurately reflect the skills and learning potential of most children. As discussed in the previous chapter, standardized tests have most often been criticized for their inappropriateness for assessing communication skills of children from low income or linguistically and culturally diverse backgrounds.

Standardized tests, however, are not free from limitations when administered to mainstream children. As noted in Chapter 3, standardized tests sample skills in an extremely limited manner; test items and the highly structured testing context may not reflect natural social communication. Furthermore, such variables as materials, setting, task, and conversational parameters may influence the results of assessment (Crais, 1995; McCauley & Swisher, 1984b; McFadden, 1996; Wetherby & Prizant, 1992). In addition, the procedures used in establishing a participant group from which to collect normative data may create different types of bias. For example, Peña, Spaulding, and Plante (2006) and Spaulding, Plante, and Farinella (2006) have demonstrated that standardized tests that have included children with language impairment in their normative sample are less accurate in identifying language disorders because of the resulting lower normative scores; consequently, language disorders may be underdiagnosed. These concerns, along with the influx of non-English dominant children over the past 10 years, have resulted in a search for alternative assessment procedures that will more accurately identify communication skills and their disorders, not only in minority children, but also in mainstream children. As we will see later, many features of alternative assessment approaches are relevant to a comprehensive assessment of all children.

An entirely different kind of problem exists with the traditional assessment procedures. The problem is an excessive reliance on the linguistic view of language and the assessment approach based entirely on *linguistic structures* with their attending problems discussed in the next section. Unfortunately, this problem is not generally understood, discussed, or researched in speech-language pathology. A different approach to assessment, different from the traditional and all the better known alternative approaches, is the *behavioral assessment* of communication disorders. To bring this entirely different perspective to speech-language pathologists' attention, we describe the basic elements of behavioral assessment and its relevance to speech-language pathology.

We begin with behavioral assessment, and then move on to criterion-referenced and client specific assessment, authentic assessment, dynamic assessment, and portfolio assessment. We finally propose a comprehensive and integrated approach that may be appropriate to assessing communication skills in all children, including mainstream and minority children. This approach includes the most desirable and essential features of the traditional approach and those of alternative approaches.

Behavioral Assessment

This chapter is about the well-known limitations of the traditional assessment and alternative procedures that may help overcome those limitations. The limitations of the traditional assessment, as summarized in the previous chapter (as well as the sections that follow), include the inappropriateness of standardized tests for ethnocultural minority children, their limited and contrived sampling of target communication skills, and their poor diagnostic value. The behavioral view of assessment of communication disorders would expand the list of disadvantages of traditional assessment.

Limitations of Linguistic Assessment

In a paper that might be the first of its kind, Esch, LaLonde, and Esch (2010) have demonstrated that assessment in speech language pathology is excessively concerned with the form of responses, not why speakers say what they say (the cause-effect relation). They point out that assessment should "provide both the *description* (topography) and the *explanation* (function) for any *given response*" (Esch et al., p. 167; italics in the original). Esch et al. also correctly point out that assessment in speech-language pathology is almost exclusively concerned with linguistic structures because of the way the language disorders are typically defined in the profession. For example, the American Speech-Language-Hearing Association (ASHA) (1993) defines language disorders as an impairment in "comprehension and/or use of spoken, written, and/or other symbol systems. The disorder may involve: (1) the form of language (the phonology, morphology, and syntax), (2) the content of language (semantics), and/or (3) the function of language in communication (pragmatics) in any combination" (p. 2). ASHA's definition is overwhelmingly structural; its reference to "symbol systems" removes speech and language from the realm of social communication. It refers to *function* in a different sense than what is meant in the behavioral analysis or natural science. *Function* in pragmatics is still a structural concept; pragmatic categories are structurally organized; a few potentially functional categories are described in unobservable mentalistic terms (e.g., "intentions" that lead to verbal responses). The definition, by its very nature, discourages a functional assessment of communicative behaviors and disorders.

As Esch et al. (2010) have pointed out, traditional tests of speech and language skills sample structures with no regard for their function; their analysis also revealed that most tests sample only naming (a *tact* in Skinner's analysis). Most of the tests fail to sample such basic yet important verbal skills as requests (*mand*, in Skinner's analysis).

An Overview of Verbal Behavior

Skinner (1957) analyzed verbal behaviors, not language, because the former is better analyzed with the methods of natural science than the latter, which is often thought of as a mental system beyond the scope of science. He was interested in an analysis of what people say, under what conditions they say it, what causes it, and what consequences maintains it. Skinner described three kinds of causes for verbal behaviors: environmental events, motivational variables, and verbal behaviors themselves (that cause other verbal behaviors). These three kinds of causes produce five kinds of primary verbal operants (classes of verbal behaviors): echoics, mands, tacts, intraverbals, and textuals. A special kind of effect exerted on verbal behavior is called the audience.

In addition to the primary verbal operants, Skinner also described a secondary verbal operant called *autoclitics*, which include what is traditionally called grammar (morphologic and syntactic features). Autoclitics also include any part of an utterance that makes a comment on some other part of the same utterance. For instance, the "regular plural inflection" of linguistics is an autoclitic, as well as the italicized portion of the utterance, "*I read in the newspaper that* it is going to rain today;" the nonitalicized portion is the primary operant, the italicized is the secondary autoclitic because it would not have been emitted had there been no reason to emit the primary response. Table 5–1 gives definitions and examples of Skinner's primary verbal operants and autoclitics. A *verbal operant* is a class of verbal behaviors; it is a cause-effect unit. For example a *tact* is a class of verbal behaviors with a physical event or object as their antecedent stimuli, certain topographic features that may vary from instance to instance, and a certain kind of consequence (usually social reinforcement) that follows the response. A variety of tacts may be collectively called a verbal operant, but a single instance (e.g., a child saying "ball" when asked, "what is this?") is an exemplar of that verbal operant.

Assessment of verbal behavior will include the linguistic structures, but those structures will be named and organized differently. Linguistic structures are topographic features of verbal behaviors; they need to be specified, but on a functional basis. Behavior assessment will inform the clinician the kinds of verbal behaviors the child can and cannot emit. It is similar to the traditional assessment except that the child's repertoire is specified in terms of functional units (such verbal operants as tacts, mands, etc.). To make this kind of assessment, speech-language pathologists will have to master a new "language" of describing the behavior of speakers and listeners. They may wish to begin with Skinner's (1957) *Verbal Behavior* and move on to many other sources available to understand and appreciate a natural science view of "language," or more precisely, verbal behavior (Barbera, 2007; Esch et al., 2010; Hegde, 2008c, 2010; McLaughlin, 2006, 2010; Palmer, 2006, 2008; Weitzman, 2010; Winokur, 1976).

Functional Behavioral Assessment

Functional behavioral assessment is designed to find out the cause-effect relations that control the topographic features of verbal behaviors. *Language* as a theoretical linguistic system may be structurally organized, but verbal behaviors (what speakers say) are not; they are functionally organized. The term *functional* implies a cause-effect relation, not the more typical pragmatic *use* or *intention*. It is the same cause-effect relations that the clinicians manipulate to teach missing verbal behaviors to children with communicative disorders, even if the treatment targets are labeled *language structures*. When it is understood that the same linguistic structure may have different multiple causes, and different linguistic structures may have the same single cause, the importance of functional analysis is appreciated. A word is always a word in the structural analysis, but in the functional analysis, it may be different kinds of responses under different conditions. For example, a girl with a language disorder who says "truck" in a traditional play-oriented assessment session is said to "posses the word" or "have it in her vocabulary." Not much more is done to understand this response. To fully understand the girl's response, the clinician should find out what *kind* of a response it was by determining what caused it. Her response could be any one of the cause-effect verbal operants Skinner described; the same single word may belong to different classes of verbal behaviors, with different causes:

> *Did the physical stimulus—a toy truck—evoke the response?* If so, it was a *tact,* and its cause was the physical feature of the immediate environment (the toy truck itself). In more general terms, the child "named" what she saw.

Table 5–1. Functional units of verbal behavior (verbal operants)

Skinner's Terms	Examples	Antecedents	Consequences
Tacts (Descriptions, comments, etc.) A primary verbal operant.	"Flower!" "It is a table." "He is John." "It is hopping."	Parts of the physical world (environmental events, persons, objects, etc.; external stimuli that cause sensory consequences); *plus a listener*	Listener's agreement or disagreement: "A beautiful flower!" "That's right, it is a table." "No, he is not John!" "Hopping fast!" Reinforcement is typically verbal.
Mands (commands, demands, requests, questions, etc.) A primary verbal operant.	"May I have some water please." "Shush!" ("Be quiet") "What do you mean?" "Your place or my place?"	A physiologic state of deprivation or aversive stimulation (hunger, thirst, discomfort, pain, sexual deprivation); different states of the body, as against the events outside the skin; *plus a listener*	Primary reinforcers that listeners offer to reduce deprivation or aversive stimulation. Presentation of food items; removal of aversive stimulation; opportunities for sexual behaviors; reinforced by nonverbal as well as verbal behaviors.
Echoics Imitative behaviors that reproduce their own stimuli. A primary verbal operant	Clinician: "Say, *book.*" Child: "Book." The child's response is an echoic.	Another person's verbal behavior (as against the physical aspects of the world around or internal states of the body); *plus a listener*	Presence or absence of reinforcement, depending strictly on whether the response reproduces the stimulus, approximates it, or moves in the right direction.
Intraverbals Verbal behaviors generated by the immediately prior verbal behaviors of the speaker. A primary verbal operant.	Almost all continuous and connected speech (and writing). Recitation of the alphabet; proverbs and common sayings; typical phrases (e.g., table—chair); history as recited; all sentence completion tasks; most academic talk; all narratives with sequence and temporal order.	Immediately preceding verbal responses of the speaker, that stimulate additional verbal responses. For example, in reciting the alphabet, naming the prior letters are the stimuli for the following letters; uttering the name of one president may stimulate the name of the next president; saying "table" may stimulate "chair;" *plus a listener*	Such simpler intraverbals as A-B-C-D or common sayings (table—chair) are explicitly socially reinforced; more complex intraverbals, such as a lecture that describes sequenced historical events, reinforcement is more subtle; both social reinforcement and subtle discriminative kinesthetic cues may play a role; delayed social reinforcement that comes after an extended period of speech also may strengthen intraverbals.

(continues)

Table 5–1. *(continued)*

Skinner's Terms	Examples	Antecedents	Consequences
Autoclitics Parts of verbal operants that tact the controlling variables of primary verbal operants. A secondary verbal operant, a special kind of tacts; called secondary because their emission depends on the primary verbal operants.	All grammatical morphemes plus any part of an utterance that tacts the controlling variables of primary verbal operants. "I see *two* cups." "The boy *is* walking." "*I heard it over the radio that* the democratic Presidential candidate is coming to town."	Primary verbal behaviors, without which there will be no need for the secondary autoclitics. For instance, the primary reason why the quantifier *two* and the plural *s* in the first example are emitted is that the speaker is currently tacting a stimulus complex (two cups). The primary tact is the antecedent of *two* and the morpheme *s; plus a listener*	Social reinforcement typically in the form of listener agreement or discriminated verbal and nonverbal behavior. For instance, the listener may react differently to the second example depending on whether the boy *is* or *was* walking. Autoclitics are for the benefit of the listener, not speaker.
Textuals (Reading and writing)	Naming the printed alphabets Naming the words and sentences (oral and silent reading). Writing: copying the letters, writing to dictation, writing under intraverbal control ("spontaneous writing" or composition)	Printed stimuli for reading. Printed stimuli for copying. Oral speech for dictated writing. Intraverbal control for "spontaneous writing;" listeners play variable role; typically present while teaching someone to read and write	Social reinforcement for a progressively better correspondence between reading and the printed stimuli ("correct reading."). Social, conditioned generalized, or primary reinforcers (monetary gain) for "spontaneous writing."

Did a state of motivation or deprivation evoke the response? In general terms, perhaps the girl "wanted" to play with the truck that she saw, but couldn't reach it; maybe it was a request. In behavioral terms, it was a *mand*; as such, its cause was a state of deprivation in the girl (not having access to something for a duration, thus causing the mand).

Did a modeled stimulus evoke the response? Perhaps the child said "truck," immediately after the clinician said the same word. If so, the girl's response was an *echoic*, evoked by the clinician's modeled verbal stimulus; its cause was clinician's verbal response, not the physical stimulus, nor a state of motivation.

Did a string of clinician's verbal responses evoke the response? If so, the girl's response is an *intraverbal* (a verbal response evoked by other verbal responses). The girl may have said "truck" in the manner of a better known "sentence completion" task (e.g., the clinician may have asked, "Ice cream is being brought to a store by a . . ." or something similar).

Did the clinician show the printed word TRUCK, *and ask, "what does this say?"* If so, the child read the word correctly, and therefore, the response was a *textual.*

Note that the response category changed every time the evoking condition (the cause) of the child's response changed; but topographically (and linguistically) the response remained the same. When clinicians consider what causes a verbal response, they will reclassify the same topographic response as either an echoic, a mand, a tact, an intraverbal, or a textual. This kind of assessment or analysis informs much more than the linguistic description that the child *"knows the word truck."* There is no parallel to the functional (cause-effect) analysis of verbal behaviors in the linguistic analysis.

It is important to know what kind of functional response the child's production was for several reasons. The most important, however, is that the child who produces a word, a phrase, or a sentence as an echoic may not produce it as a tact or a mand; a response produced as a tact may not be produced as a mand or vice versa; a response produced as an intraverbal may not be produced as a mand or a tact. Responses produced as all of theses may not be produced as a textual. In terms that are more familiar to speech-language pathologists, a child who can imitate a response may not produce it under other conditions; a child who names an object may fail to request the same object; a child who names or requests an object may not complete an incomplete sentence that requires the same response; and so forth. Therefore, the traditional conclusion that the girl in our example has the word *truck* in her vocabulary, and therefore, there is no need to teach it, is invalid. The word the child produced may just belong to one or two response classes, and the response in other classes may still have to be taught. To take another example, the clinician may find in a boy's language sample the word *book* was produced on one or more occasions. The clinician then may conclude that the word book need not be a treatment target. The problem with this conclusion is that the same word *book* may be produced when the child wants a book; names a physical stimulus book; repeats after the clinician who said "book;" responds "book" when asked, "you read a . . . ?" or reads "book" when shown the printed word. Although the linguistic analysis is insensitive to the differences in stimulus conditions that produce different kinds of verbal responses, there is evidence to show that the same response ("book" in our example) given under those different stimulus conditions are indeed functionally independent, needing separate teaching. This means that the boy who said "book" when the clinician said "book" (echoic) may not respond correctly or not respond at all when shown a book and asked "What is this?"(tact), may not request a book when wanted (mand), may not respond in a sentence completion format (intraverbal), and may not read the printed stimulus (textual). This should make it clear to the clinician that the traditional structural analysis does not clearly identify treatment targets whereas the functional analysis does.

In Skinner's (1957) analysis of verbal behavior, echoics, mands, tacts, and intraverbals have different causes, hence may be acquired independent of each other. This claim has generally been supported in the experimental analysis of children with communication disorders (Duker, 1999; Hall & Sundberg, 1987; Kelley, Shillingsburg, Castro, Addison, & LaRue, 2007; Kelley, Shillingsburg, Castro, Addison, LaRue, & Martins, 2007; Lamarre & Holand, 1985; Lerman et al., 2005; Oliver, Hall, & Nixon, 1999; Reichle, Barrett, Tertile, & McQuarter, 1987; Twyman, 1996). In these studies, teaching mands did not result in tacts and teaching tacts did not result in mands. This lack of generalized production may be more evident in very young children and children with language disorders who often fail to show generalized learning. In verbally competent children and adults, there may be more generalized learning than in the very young, as suggested by a few other studies (LaFrance, Wilder, Normand, & Squires, 2009; Petursdottir Carr, & Michael, 2005). Generally, research has shown that mands and tacts may be independent of each other during acquisition, but once acquired, verbal operants begin to be multiply controlled and that their independence may not be maintained (Hall & Sundberg, 1987; Petursdottir et al., 2005; Skinner, 1957).

Past treatment research on teaching language structures, especially grammatic features, have demonstrated additional limitations with the structural analysis that often leads to confused language treatment targets. McReynolds and Engmann (1974) found that subject noun and object noun phrases, though separate linguistically, are functionally the same: teaching either subject noun phrases or object noun phrases was sufficient to generate the production of the untrained noun phrase. A child language treatment efficacy study demonstrated that each English irregular plural is a treatment target, because a child who has been taught to produce a set of such words (e.g., *men, women, children*) will not produce other words in the same linguistic category (e.g., *sheep, teeth, feet*) without specific training (Hegde & McConn, 1981). Therefore, irregular plural is a collection of different and independent verbal responses; that they form a grammatic class is of little relevance to target behavior selection in treatment. Experimental treatment studies also have demonstrated that verbal auxiliary (*is* and *are* forms) and copula (*is* and *are* forms), though separate linguistically, are the same behaviorally (Hegde, 1980; Hegde & McConn, 1981). Teaching either one is sufficient to generate the other on the basis of generalization. The regular plural is a collection of different response classes, created by allomorphic variations (e.g., the *s* and *z* plural morphemes); the regular past tense similarly breaks down into different response classes based on the *t, d,* and *ed* endings (e.g., *buzzed, baked,* and *counted*) (see Guess & Bear, 1973 for studies).

Treatment is always functional in the sense that it manipulates the causal variables to teach some response classes, even under uncontrolled conditions. Structural-linguistic analysis is never functional, so the structures identified may or may not be empirically real. Note that the subject-noun phrase and object noun phrase distinction is not real; verbal copula and auxiliary distinction is not real; regular plural as a single grammatic category is not real; regular past tense as a single category is not real; irregular past as a single category is not real; irregular plural as a single category is not real. Regular possessive as a single category is not real (Hegde, 1998; Hegde & Maul, 2006). Unfortunately, many other linguistic distinctions remain untested; Skinner's (1957) functional analysis of verbal behavior predicts that most linguistic distinctions would prove empirically invalid. Therefore, the typical assessment conclusion that a child produces a word, a sentence, a passive, or a possessive means little if one is interested in describing true treatment targets that need to be taught and the targets that need not be taught because they are based on pseudo distinctions; teaching some other target (considered linguistically different) will have produced those targets based on false distinctions. These observations question the validity of linguistic structural categories as treatment targets.

A definitive functional assessment of verbal operants requires an experimental method, which may be impractical for routine assessment. A commonly used experimental method to distinguish mands from tacts includes manipulation of putative causal variables under controlled conditions (Kelley, Shillingsburg, Castro, Addison, & LaRue, 2007; Lerman et al., 2005). Conditions are controlled so that that the variable that causes a mand is absent during the tact testing, and the variable that causes a tact is absent during the mand testing. Note that a mand is produced when access to something is denied for a period of time, causing a state of deprivation or establish motivation for a mand; for example, a girl who has not had access to her favorite toy for a while is likely to mand for it. A tact production is not caused by such motivational states; it is evoked more directly by a physical stimulus (plus a listener who will reinforce it). Therefore, to asses a relatively "pure" mand, the clinician should limit access to an object (known to reinforce the child in the past) for a period of time to establish motivation for mand. This procedure is generally called the *establishing operation* (Michael, 2000). When the motivation is established, and the child, as in our previous example, says "truck," and the clinician hands the toy truck, and the child begins to play with it, it is concluded that the child manded the toy truck, not tacted (named) it. Similarly, to assess a relatively pure tact, the child should have free access to the object to remove the potential deprivation and the state of motivation, so when the child says "truck," it is not a mand, but a tact. The clinician's typical response to a tact would have been such social reinforcement as, "Yes! It is a truck isn't it!," and not handing the object to the child. This basic procedure has been used with appropriate controls in single-subject experimental designs to separate mands from tacts (Kelly et al., 2007; Lerman et al., 2005).

Mands and tacts are difficult to distinguish from each other partly because they often are a part of the same utterance, multiply controlled. For instance, the boy who says, "May I have that red, big, piece of puzzle?" is manding (requesting) a piece of puzzle, while also responding to its physical property (*red* and *big*); the portion of the response controlled by that physical property is a tact. This is what is meant by multiple controls of verbal responses. Another difficulty is that a girl with limited verbal repertoire may produce a mand which may be misinterpreted as a tact. For instance, the girl with language disorder may say, "red piece" or even telegraphic "red" to mand a piece of puzzle of that color, but a listener may think that the child just named it (a tact). Had she been verbally proficient, she may have said, "Please give me that red piece of puzzle."

It is generally not too difficult to distinguish simple echoics, intraverbals, and textuals from other verbal operants. Clinicians who ask a child to imitate their verbal model will have delivered the controlling stimulus (their own model) for the echoic; clinicians who offers a partial verbal string (e.g., "you write with a . . .) to evoke the intraverbal "pencil" from the child will have delivered a controlling stimulus; clinicians who show a printed word and ask the child to read it will have similarly delivered a controlling stimulus for a textual response. Controlling variables of complex forms of these verbal operants, especially those of the intraverbals in conversational speech, may be difficult to determine as well, but this may not pose a serious challenge in the initial assessment of children with language disorders because they lack complex verbal behaviors. The controlling stimuli may be obscure in cases of even simple mands and tacts, especially in children with limited verbal repertoire, and more so when they are combined in a single utterance.

Practical Assessment of Verbal Behaviors

A good language sample and verbal behavioral assessment tasks the clinician develops will help describe the child's verbal repertoire in nonlinguistic terms. The clinician's analysis of the recorded language sample from a child would result in a description of the frequency of such verbal operants as echoics, mands, tacts, textuals, intraverbals, and autoclitic. One might contrast these with the description of such linguistic structures as words, grammatic morphemes, syntactic features, and pragmatic structures that clinicians typically offer in their assessment report.

To be able to assess potential verbal operants instead of linguistic structures, the clinician needs to modify the manner in which language samples are traditionally recorded. The traditional language sample fails to give enough information on the potential antecedent stimuli and the consequences that followed a child's response, both of which are essential to understand the kind of verbal operant the child emitted.

The targets of routine behavioral assessment of child language are the frequency with which a child emits the verbal operants, their potential antecedents, and consequences. The questions for assessment include the following:

- What is the frequency with which the child produces echoics, mands, tacts, intraverbals, textuals, and autoclitics?
- What kinds of verbal operants are present and what kinds are absent in the child's verbal repertoire?
- Does the child produce the verbal operants under typical stimulus conditions or does the child need additional stimulus support to produce them?
- What kinds of additional stimulus support are successful? What kinds are unsuccessful?
- What kinds of consequences seem to maintain the verbal operants the child does emit?
- Does the child have a verbal operant (skill) deficit requiring a clinical diagnosis?
- What might be the initial and subsequent treatment targets?

To better assess the verbal operants a child emits during language sampling, the clinician may take the following steps:

1. Record an extended naturalistic language sample. Collect such stimulus materials as toys, picture books, puzzles, paper, crayons, simple words printed on sheets of paper, and so forth.
2. Engage the child in conversation. Manipulate the stimulus items to evoke specific kinds of verbal operants.
3. Deny access to toys, specific pieces of a puzzle, picture books, edibles (if found appropriate to use), and so forth to evoke mands from the child.

4. Let the child have free access to those and other objects to evoke tacts.

5. Prepare some modeling stimuli to evoke echoics.

6. Prepare some simple and brief sentence completion tasks to assess intraverbals as well as specific sentence forms (e.g., saying "the ball was . . ." may prompt the child to say "kicked by the boy" to evoke passive sentences).

7. Prepare pictures and verbal stimuli to assess autoclitics (especially the 14 basic grammatic morphemes Brown's 1973 study described).

8. Hold a conversation with the child to assess conversational skills.

Manipulate the response consequences to assess the potential verbal behavior categories. Note that verbal operants not only have their unique or typical antecedents (e.g., modeling, deprivation, physical stimulus, verbal stimulus), but also the consequences. Therefore, in addition to manipulating the putative antecedents, the clinician also should manipulate putative consequences to find out what kind of a verbal operant the child just exhibited. For example, if the clinician thought that a child's verbal response was a mand, she would hand an object to the child, even though the child may not have specified it because of limited verbal skills. On the other hand, if the clinician presumed that the response was a tact, she would verbally reinforce it (not hand anything to the child), by saying, for example, "Yes, that is a *ball.*"

The clinician's guesses as to what the response was might be wrong, however. Therefore, the clinician will have to check the match between the response and the consequence delivered to it:

1. *The response and the consequence the clinician delivered matched.* The clinician gave something to the child (for a mand) or verbally reinforced it (for an echoic, a tact, an intraverbal, a textual) by praise or agreement. This means that the response met its typical consequence. If so, the child may not emit any further response that suggests a mismatch, as described in #2.

    a. If the response was indeed a mand, and the clinician handed an object to the child, then the child might interact with the object (e.g., will play with the object handed, consume, or save for later consumption if the clinician gives a food item).

    b. If the response was indeed a tact, and the clinician said "That is right!," "You are correct," "I think so, too," or something to that effect, the child will move on to emit other responses.

    c. If the response was an echoic, an intraverbal, or a textual, the clinician will have manipulated the appropriate stimuli with minimum ambiguity, will have delivered verbal praise or agreement, and the child will move on to emit other responses.

2. *The response and the consequence the clinician delivered mismatched.* Thinking that the response was a mand, the clinician gave something to the child (e.g., a toy or a cup of water), but the child's response was indeed a tact, an echoic, an intraverbal, or a textual, though such mismatches are more likely to occur in the case of mands and tacts. Thinking that the response was a tact, the

clinician verbally praised or agreed with the child, but the response was a mand. This means that the response did *not* meet its typical consequence.

    a.   If the response was indeed a mand (e.g., "Juice" as a proxy for "I want juice"), and the clinician only offered verbal reinforcement (e.g., "Yes, that *is* juice"), the child is likely to emit other verbal or nonverbal responses to suggest the mismatch. The child might whine, point to the juice, say "No!," repeat the word "juice," or emit a similar response that informs the clinician of the mismatch.

    b.   If the response was indeed a tact (e.g., "Juice"), and the clinician handed a cup of juice to the child thinking it was a proxy for a mand, the child will emit one or more responses to suggest the mismatch. The child might push the cup toward the clinician, whine, say "No!" (as a proxy for "I don't want juice"), point to the juice, repeat the word "juice," or emit a similar response that informs the clinician of the mismatch.

    c.   If the response was an echoic, an intraverbal, or a textual, the chances of a mismatch are minimal, because the clinician herself will have controlled the stimuli, and will have reinforced verbally; the child will move on to respond to other stimuli.

Although these practical strategies help identify the functional categories of verbal behaviors less definitively than the experimental strategies (Kelley et al., 2007; Lerman et al., 2005), they are still an improvement over the typical strategies that describe only the linguistic structural properties of child's utterances. Potential functional verbal operants thus identified may be better suited as treatment targets than the structural categories that are often not independent response classes (treatment targets).

In addition to the primary verbal operants (mands, tacts, echoics, intraverbals, and textuals), the clinician may analyze the frequency of various autoclitics (especially those that are described as morphologic features in linguistics) evident in the language sample. Different patterns of word productions that result in "different kinds of sentences" also may be noted in the sample.

Functional Assessment of Problem Behaviors

Some children with communication disorders exhibit problem behaviors during assessment and treatment sessions. Both verbal and nonverbal problem behaviors children with communication disorders exhibit during treatment need to be reduced to effectively teach desirable communicative behaviors. Such undesirable verbal behaviors as asking frequent questions (e.g., "are we done yet?") and such nonverbal behaviors as leaving the chair, crawling under the table, playing with the stimulus materials, and so forth should be understood for their causes to effectively reduce them. Aggressive verbal and nonverbal behaviors and self-injurious behaviors of children with autism also are in this category. A behavioral analysis helps determine what kinds of antecedents trigger such behaviors and what kinds of consequences, typically unintended, maintain them. Although not generally practiced by SLPs, functional analysis of problem behaviors, including aggression and self-injurious behaviors, is quite advanced.

To make a functional assessment of problem behaviors, the clinician needs to manipulate their putative controlling variables. It is more likely that the speech-language pathologist will make this analysis in initial treatment sessions than during assessment (Hegde, 1998). We only briefly mention a few of the available strategies and refer the clinician to other sources to better understand them (Carr et al., 1994; Denno, Carr, & Bell, 2010; Hegde, 1998; Reichle & Wacker, 1993). In essence:

- *Some problem behaviors may be maintained by incidental (unintended) positive reinforcement, often the clinician's attention.* To find out if this is the case, the clinician may alternately present and withhold the presumed reinforcer to see if it increases and then decreases. Positive reinforcement maintains the undesirable behavior if its frequency changes as expected. The behavior may then be reduced by withholding the reinforcer (Iwata, Vollmer, & Zarcone, 1990). For instance, a child's frequent verbal interruptions (e.g., "Are we done yet") of assessment or treatment tasks may be reinforced when the clinician promptly responds by saying "Not yet," "In a little while," and so forth. Ignoring such interruptions may result in a decrease in their frequency.

- *Other problems behaviors may be maintained by negative reinforcement.* Some behaviors help the child escape from aversive events or situations; if so, the behaviors are negatively reinforced. Assessment or treatment tasks may be aversive to some children, especially when the task is too difficult for them. To escape from such aversive tasks (e.g., responding to a series of difficult test items or treatment trials), the child may exhibit an undesirable behavior (e.g., playing with the stimulus material, being fretful), causing the clinician to verbally reprimand the child ("No, don't play with that" or "Sit quietly"). Such verbal reprimands terminate the assessment or treatment task, even if briefly, and thus negatively reinforce the problem behavior. To assess this possibility, the clinician may terminate the task on hand at the earliest sign of an undesirable behavior to observe its increase in frequency during the subsequent segments of the session. Alternately, the clinician might continue to present the tasks with no interruptions to see if the behavior frequency decreases. If these expected changes do occur, then the behavior is negatively reinforced (Iwata et al., 1990; Repp & Singh, 1990). It may be reduced by preventing escape (i.e., continued and uninterrupted presentation of the task on hand). Another strategy, often used in treatment sessions, is to make the task easier or model more often (Hegde, 1998).

- *Some problem behaviors may be maintained by automatic reinforcement.* Some undesirable behaviors generate sensory consequences to the child, and thus maintain those behaviors. Some children with intellectual disabilities or autism may bang the desk, clang materials, or clap incessantly. With no environmental event reinforcing them, it is presumed that the sensory consequences are their maintaining causes. To assess this possibility, the clinician may alternately allow and remove the sensory consequence to see if the behavior increases and then decreases. For instance, the clinician may place soft, padded material on the desk to eliminate or greatly reduce the auditory as well as kinesthetic sensations the child receives from banging on the desk to see if the behavior decreases and then remove the padded material to see if the behavior increases. These changes in the behavior, if observed, suggests that the behavior was maintained by sensory consequences (automatic reinforcement). From then on, the clinician would design and apply strategies to eliminate sensory consequences to extinguish the problem behaviors.

The essence of functional assessment of verbal or nonverbal behaviors is to understand their causes. A successful functional assessment is more powerful than a mere structural analysis because the former will have identified potential treatment strategies. An ultimate goal of assessment is to suggest not only what skills are present or absent, but what strategies might work during treatment. This goal is effectively met only by a functional assessment.

Criterion-Referenced and Client-Specific Assessment

Criterion-based or *client-specific assessment procedures* are two similar procedures that are practical alternatives to standardized test-based assessment procedures. Both avoid an evaluation of a child's communication skills in light of norms derived from a standardization sample (Hegde, 1998; McCauley, 1996). Therefore, the two approaches, more similar than different, help avoid the pitfalls of standardized tests. The criterion-referenced approach may use existing nonstandardized assessment tools and interpret data in terms of whether the measured skills meet certain mastery criterion (e.g., morphologic or phonemic productions at 90% accuracy). When appropriate, a criterion-referenced approach may use items from a standardized test with the assurance that the children who share a particular client's ethnocultural and socioeconomic backgrounds were included in the standardization sample. But the results may still be analyzed in terms of mastery level, not the test's norms. Similarly, the results of a standardized test administered to mainstream children on whom the test was standardized also may be interpreted for mastery levels demonstrated, with no regard for norms established through the test.

The client-specific procedure, on the other hand, will simply avoid all standardized tests as well as individual items from tests, even when assessing the skills of a child for whom appropriately standardized tests are available. The client-specific procedures are strictly developed for a given client, in view of what needs to be assessed and how (Hegde, 1998). Care is taken to ensure that each skill is assessed with sufficient exemplars. For instance, instead of asking the child to produce given grammatic morphemes or phonemes in the context of just one or two (or only a few at the most) words, phrases, or sentences, the client-specific measurement requires a sufficient number of exemplars that will permit a meaningful and reliable calculation of percent correct response rate. Typically, 15 to 20 exemplars may be needed to calculate the correct response rate of most language structures and phoneme productions. This is not a typical and explicit concern in the criterion-referenced assessment.

The client-specific approach requires that the clinician develop stimulus materials that are especially relevant for the child. The criterion-referenced approach, too, may work better and will be more similar to the client-specific approach if standardized stimulus items are avoided and stimulus materials relevant to the child are chosen. The goal of making reliable and nonbiased assessment of communication skills is better served if the criterion-referenced approach also samples the skills adequately in multiple contexts, so the child's existing or projected mastery levels of skills may be objectively stated in terms of percent correct response rate. If this is accepted, then in both procedures the clinician specifically designs assessment procedures, including stimulus materials, for a given client. This approach is appropriate for any child, including mainstream children for whom standardized instruments are available.

In using the criterion-referenced or client-specific approach as described, the clinician uses the case history information to understand the cultural background, bilingual/multilingual status if any, education, occupation, and general level of sophistication of the client and the family. The clinician then makes an initial judgment about potential assessment tools that need to be developed for the client. During the interview, the clinician asks questions about the child's interests, hobbies, and social activities. The clinician obtains information about the child's favorite toys, books, activities, academic curricula, and academic and social demands made on the child. The clinician then selects target speech and language skills to be assessed and designs procedures that are unique to those skills and the child and the family's background.

In assessing language skills, the clinician determines the specific grammatic morphemes produced in words, phrases, or sentences (e.g., the regular and irregular plural morphemes, past tense inflections, the verbal auxiliary and the copula, the present progressive-*ing*); specific syntactic structures (e.g., active declarative sentences, questions, requests, complex sentences); narrative skills (telling a story or retelling a story the clinician narrates); conversational skills including topic initiation, turn-taking, topic maintenance; repair strategies during a conversational episode involving the clinician (e.g., request for clarification, response to request for clarification); and such other relevant skills. In assessing speech production, the clinician may select target sounds or sound patterns. In assessing fluency disorders, the clinician may measure the frequency of dysfluencies or stuttering in conversational exchanges. In assessing voice, the clinician may select specific voice parameters. In assessing literacy skills, the clinician may select writing skills (writing to dictation, spontaneous writing, copying a printed paragraph, copying geometric shapes) and reading skills (reading printed passages).

The clinician then prepares the stimulus materials that are relevant to the child's ethnocultural and educational background. The clinician may write words, phrases, or sentences that help assess the various targets. The client's interest, hobbies, literacy levels, cultural background, and linguistic variation will determine the nature of the stimulus material prepared. Ethnoculturally appropriate and familiar gestures or signs that will be useful in evaluating the target behaviors or skills also may be selected.

The stimulus items to be used in assessment will be selected, preferably from the child's home environment. Stimulus items (objects and pictures) that are used in the home, familiar in the culture, and accepted by the client or the family will be especially useful in making a client-specific assessment. Whenever practical, the clinician may select the stimulus items from everyday sources, familiar magazines, and colorful pictures. Many parents are willing to bring a collection of child's toys, storybooks, pictures of family members, and frequently used objects (e.g., the child's favorite cup or shirt) to the assessment session if requested in advance of the assessment session. During assessment, the clinician freely substitutes stimuli that are found to be inappropriate for the client (something not done when using standardized assessment tests). Additional exemplars and stimulus items may be added as found appropriate; again, this is typically not done in administering standardized tests.

Beginning clinicians may find the task of developing assessment targets and stimuli for each child anew a daunting task. It is certainly not the case that the clinician will have to develop new stimulus materials for each child. But if this is done consistently for a few children initially, the load of preparing new stimulus materials for subsequent children will be significantly less. Also, if the stimulus materials developed for treatment of children are classified and stored carefully, the same materials may be used in assessment. Multiple target skill exemplars (e.g., 15 words with plural /s/, present progressive -*ing*, etc.) and specialized stimuli may be cataloged and stored. For each child, only a few new and relevant stimuli may need to be developed; most of these child-specific stimuli may be supplied by the parents.

The results of client-specific or criterion-referenced assessment are interpreted to be informative of the child's current skill level. The clinician may make judgments whether the skill level that is present is adequate to meet the oral, gestural, written, or academic communication needs of the child. If the skill levels fall below what is required of such needs, a deficiency or disorder is diagnosed, and treatment is recommended.

Advantages of client-specific or criterion-referenced approach include the following:

- The two approaches avoid the pitfalls of standardized tests
- The behaviors to be assessed are sampled more adequately in all children
- The results of assessment are uniquely relevant to the child being assessed
- The assessment results directly lead to treatment planning
- The approach provides more reliable and valid data than standardized tests or several other alternative approaches.

Potential disadvantages of the approaches include the following:

- The two approaches will not allow a comparison of an individual child's performance with the performance of a normative sample; indeed, the approaches were designed to avoid this comparison
- The approaches do not allow for a diagnosis of a disorder made strictly on the basis of normative comparison of an individual child's performance; this may be a significant limitation if the education policy of schools require such a diagnosis to qualify children for services
- The approaches are, at least initially, more time consuming than the standardized test-based assessment because they require more time to prepare or select stimulus materials for assessment.

Authentic Assessment

Another alternative to traditional approach is called *authentic assessment*. Udvari and Thousand (1995) define *authentic assessment* as occurring "when students are expected to perform, produce, or otherwise demonstrate skills that represent realistic learning demands . . . the contexts of the assessment are real-life settings in and out of the classroom without contrived and standardized conditions" (p. 95).

Traditionally, children are removed from the classroom and relocated to a small office or "speech therapy room" for their assessment. The clinician is often unfamiliar to the children, and the testing environment likely contains materials and activities that are equally unfamiliar. One or more standardized tests might be administered. The child is then asked to respond to a number of questions or complete a series of tasks. The child's responses are recorded and scores are calculated for comparison to normative data. A speech-language sample might be collected as part of the assessment, but it is generally evoked by showing the child pictures and asking questions about them, or by asking the child to respond to a prepared set of questions. Once a language sample is transcribed, the traditional approach emphasizes a comparison of the results to normative data on speech and language development.

In making an authentic assessment, standardized tests are avoided. Instead, a sample of the child's speech and language is collected in such familiar environments as the classroom or home. Preferably, the sample is collected during an everyday activity resulting in naturally occurring communication. This sample is then analyzed to determine if there is a need for intervention. Speech-language pathologists have long recognized the value of language sample analysis; however, it was traditionally used as a complement to norm-referenced tests rather than as the sole assessment method. Authentic assessment depends mostly on language samples recorded in naturalistic contexts.

According to Stockman (1996b), language sample analysis (LSA) is a valuable assessment procedure for use with a linguistically diverse population because it "legitimizes the ordinary talk of every community as a clinical resource" (p. 356). "Ordinary" language is described as language that is familiar and a routine part of daily life and interactions. Stockman (1996b, 2008) added that using naturally displayed language behavior brings cultural sensitivity, validity, accessibility, and flexibility to the language assessment. Two major concerns regarding LSA are that it lends itself to subjective analysis and that the collection and analysis of the samples are time consuming. In an attempt to deal with these concerns, researchers have explored the idea of identifying and analyzing a *minimal competency core (MCC)* (Schraeder, Quinn, Stockman, & Miller, 1999; Stockman, 1996b, 2008).

Minimal Competency Core

A minimal competency core reflects "the least amount of linguistic skill or knowledge that a typical speaker would display for a given age and context" (Schraeder et al., 1999, p. 196). For example, Stockman (1996b, 2008) described a common (minimal) core of 15 word initial consonants included in the repertoire of normal 33- to 36-month-old African American children: /m/, /n/, /p/, /b/, /t/, /d/, /k/, /g/, /f/, /s/, /h/, /w/, /y/, /l/, and /r/. Stockman used this criterion in a retrospective analysis and found it to be successful in identifying those who were diagnosed with a speech disorder. In addition, Stockman demonstrated the application of an MCC to the analysis of children's pragmatic, semantic, and morphosyntactic features. Core competencies were identified for African American children in each of these language areas. Stockman replicated her 1996 study which involved only 7 children with a larger study with 120 Head Start students (2008), confirming the value of the minimum competency core in assessing speech sound competency in African American children.

Schraeder et al. (1999) developed an authentic assessment protocol for screening language in preschool children. They used an MCC to construct a criterion-referenced protocol that included semantic, pragmatic, and phonological core features for 3-year-old children. Children were observed during spontaneous conversations, play activities, and interactions at preschool. At least 50 intelligible and spontaneous utterances were recorded for each child, and the occurrences of behaviors on the minimal competency core protocol were noted. In addition, the children's mean length of utterance (MLU) was calculated. The authentic assessment procedures used in this study were successful in separating the children with language disorders from those with the least proficient age-appropriate communication skills. Figure 5–1 presents an example of an MCC.

Contrastive Analysis

Another alternative assessment method that has been used in analyzing language samples of children with diverse backgrounds is *contrastive analysis*. The goal of contrastive analysis is to separate dialectical speech and language differences from clinically significant speech and language errors. McGregor, Williams, Hearst, and Johnson (1997) describe four components of contrastive analysis:

1. The clinician needs to become familiar with the dialect spoken by the client.
2. A speech-language sample is collected.
3. The sample is evaluated to identify any differences from Mainstream American English, (MAE).
4. Based on knowledge of the client's dialect, the clinician determines if the identified differences are dialectical variations or "true errors."

Seymour, Bland-Stewart, and Green (1998) used the contrastive analysis to compare children who spoke MAE to those who spoke African American English (AAE). They defined contrastive features as those that differed between AAE and MAE, and noncontrastive features as those that were shared between AAE and MAE. Noted noncontrastive errors were more indicative of a language disorder than the contrastive features because the former features should not vary significantly as a function of the child's dialect. Seymour et al. (1998) found that the features that were most problematic for children with language disorders in their study were prepositions, present progressive-*ing*, conjunctions, articles, modals, and complex sentences.

Schrader et al. (1999) highlighted several advantages of authentic assessment:

- It may help the speech-language pathologist arrive at a valid diagnosis with fewer false positives
- Speech-language samples collected in a familiar, natural context may be more representative of the child's skill level than those evoked during contrived circumstances
- There is no need for expensive standardized tests
- It can be used to assess children of different cultural backgrounds.

Language Form Categories

- **Morphologic and syntactic skills**
  - MLU (2.7-3.6) ☐
  - Elaborated Simple Sentence (subject+verb+compliment) ☐
  - Noun Modifiers (*the, a, an, that, this, other*) ☐
  - Inflections (*ed, ing,* other) ☐
- **Semantic skills (Major)**
  - Existence ☐
  - State ☐
  - Action ☐
  - Locative Action ☐
  - Locative State ☐
  - Dative ☐
- **Semantic categories (Coordinated)**
  - Specifier ☐
  - Possession ☐
  - Negation ☐
  - Time ☐
  - Attribution ☐
  - Quantity ☐
  - Recurrence ☐
- **Superordinate**
  - Coordination ☐
  - Causality ☐
- **Pragmatic categories**
  - Initiates Interactions ☐
  - Elicits Language ☐
    - comments on objectives / events ☐
    - asks questions ☐
    - requests objects, actions ☐
  - Responds to Language ☐
    - relates comments to prior speaker turn ☐
    - answers questions ☐
    - imitates spontaneously ☐
  - Clears Communication Channel ☐
    - requests repetitions ("huh?") ☐
    - repeats words on request ☐
    - closes interactions ("bye-bye") ☐
- **Phonological Skills**
  - Nasals: /m/, /n/ ☐
  - Stops: /p/, /t/, /k/, /b/, /d/, /g/ ☐
  - Fricatives: /f/, /s/, /h/ ☐
  - Glides: /w/, /j/ ☐
  - Final Consonants ☐
  - Initial Blends ☐

Figure 5–1. Example of a Minimal Competency Core (MCC) for 3-year-old children. Adapted from Stockman (1996) and Schraeder, Quinn, and Stockman (1999).

Possible disadvantages of authentic assessment include:

- It usually takes more time than the traditional, standardized test-based assessment

- The results may be more subjective

- Results obtained from authentic assessment procedures may not always fit neatly into the criteria utilized by some institutions for qualifying a child for clinical services

Dynamic Assessment

Dynamic assessment has been advocated as an alternative or supplement to traditional standardized testing. The main objective of dynamic assessment is to understand how the child would perform on treatment tasks, sometime described as a test of *modifiability* (Gutierrez-Clellen & Peña, 2001; Kapantzoglou, Restrepo, & Thompson, 2012; Larsen & Nippold, 2007; Olswang, Bain, & Johnson, 1992; Peña, 1996; Peña et al., 2006; Ukrainetz, Harpell, Walsh, & Coyle, 2000; Wade & Haynes, 1989). In dynamic assessment, clinicians go beyond the traditional task of assessing the client's existing skills; they provide brief periods of intervention to assess whether the child's performance can be modified or improved on a given task. Because of the brief treatment included in assessment, dynamic assessment better leads to treatment targets and strategies than the traditional assessment (Haynes & Pindzola, 2004).

The dynamic assessment model has been used by school psychologists for some time (Lidz, 1987, 1991) and is now being adapted by other members of the multidisciplinary assessment team in school settings. The diagnostic session can be used to determine a client's readiness for treatment and to evaluate different treatment variables for their feasibility. Dynamic assessment procedures have the potential to be a meaningful and unbiased way to assess children from different cultures or linguistic backgrounds because the procedure seeks to evaluate *how* a child learns and what works or does not work for an individual child rather than comparing a child's performance to the norms derived from standardized tests.

Dynamic assessment has also been advocated as a valid way to differentiate between cultural or dialectical language differences and language disorders (Gutierrez-Clellen & Peña, 2001; Kapantzoglou et al., 2012; Lidz & Peña, 1996) by assessing modifiability of children's speech or language differences. For example, Lidz and Peña (1996) described an adaptation that showed promise for accurately discriminating between Latino children who were language different versus language deficient. The authors were concerned with picture naming or labeling tasks that are frequently a large part of standardized language tests. Studies have shown that low income or minority students typically obtain low scores on these tasks (Dunn & Dunn, 1981; Washington & Craig, 1992). This may be because their language experience has been different. For example, Heath (1983) found that African American parents in the rural South were more likely to seek comparisons, explanations, and nonverbal responses from their children than non-African American parents. Mainstream Americans, however, often use single words and labeling when communicating with their young children. Likewise, Lidz and Peña (1996) discussed similar differences in communication styles between Puerto Rican mothers and their children, and Mexican American parents and their children. These different experiences may explain why children from diverse cultural backgrounds may not do as well on tasks that require labeling or other communication strategies they are not familiar with. This could lead to an overidentification of language deficiencies because these children are at risk for being inappropriately labeled as having a language disorder.

To explore a solution to this problem, Lidz and Peña (1996) presented two case studies in which they offered brief treatment as a part of their assessment. The children in these studies were (3;11 and 4;1 years, months), and were bilingual Puerto Rican and English speaking. For pretest and posttests, the authors used the *Expressive One Word Picture Vocabulary Test (EOWPVT)*. On the pretest, both received a standard score of 55. Following the pretest, the authors provided two 20-minute interventions with the goal of increasing the children's awareness of labels as "special names" to use when identifying pictures or objects rather than just providing a function or category. Tasks consisted of stories, classification, and puzzles. The clinician noted strategies used by the child, the responsiveness of the child to the feedback, and instructions of the clinician, the effort required from the clinician, level of attention, and evidence that the child could transfer new learning. Posttests, administered after this intervention, showed significant improvement in one child (+ 2 SDs), indicating good modifiability, where as the other child showed very little improvement, suggesting negligible modifiability. Lidz and Peña concluded that children who were less responsive, less modifiable, and showed little or no transfer of new learning, may be at a high risk for having a language disorder.

Presumably, dynamic assessment may assist in differentiating those children who will require therapeutic intervention from those who do not. Children who show little to no change during modifiability assessment are more likely to need intervention to facilitate improved language; therefore, they would be good candidates for language treatment. On the other hand, children who improve significantly during the assessment (high modifiability), and maintain those improvements, may not require intervention (Gutierrez-Clellen & Peña, 2001). There are several dynamic assessment protocols that differ somewhat in how the selected skills are stimulated or taught. They generally fall into one of three categories: graduated prompting, testing the limits, and test-teach-retest.

Graduated Prompting

In graduated prompting, the clinician uses a hierarchy of prompts designed to facilitate the child's responses during the assessment. The clinician analyzes the number and level of prompts needed to evoke a target response and to facilitate generalization of learning to a new task. For example, in their dynamic assessment of children with specific language impairment, Bain and Olswang (1995) used a progressive hierarchy of "supportive cues," which consisted of: (1) general statement (least supportive); (2) questions designed to elicit a specific response; (3) sentence completion tasks; (4), indirect models; and (5) direct models (most supportive).

Larsen and Nippold (2007) used a hierarchy of increasingly explicit prompts to teach word meanings to typically developing children and found that the children differed in their rate of learning. The simplest prompt might be asking the child to say what a given word means; the more explicit prompt might be to give an example of a sentence in which the target word is used; and the most explicit prompt might be to give the correct meaning as one of three choices and asking the child to chose the correct answer (Larsen & Nippold, 2007). Similar prompting hierarchies have been successfully used to teach naming skills in adults with aphasia (Hegde, 2006).

Such cues might be used to evoke specific vocabulary and language structures or to increase mean length of utterance (MLU). The cues need to be designed specifically for the behavior being targeted. The clinician would start with the least supportive cue, and then progress as needed until the desired response is evoked. A scoring system takes into consideration the level of prompting needed. This analysis allows the clinician to determine the level at which a child's skills may be modified (Campione & Brown, 1987). Graduated prompting has been used in child language assessment (Bain & Olswang, 1995; Olswang & Bain, 1996; Olswang, Bain, & Johnson, 1992) and in phonemic awareness assessment (Spector, 1992).

Testing the Limits or Task Variability

Traditionally administered, a standardized test procedure is not modified to suit the needs of an individual child. However, in the *testing the limits* approach of dynamic assessment, the clinician modifies traditional test procedures by providing elaborated feedback to the child on his or her performance on test items (Carlson & Wiedl, 1978, 1992). Elaborated feedback may include commenting on the correctness of a response, providing the reasons why the answer was correct or incorrect, and explaining the principles involved in a task. Task variability may involve other modifications in the way a test is administered, such as using a more naturalistic environment or letting the child demonstrate a skill. An example of a more naturalistic environment would be incorporating it as part of "snack time" or "craft time" in the classroom. An example of allowing a child to demonstrate a skill might be to ask the child to group objects into categories.

A few studies report that these procedures may reduce a child's test anxiety and be more effective than standardized tests in estimating cognitive and academic ability of children from diverse ethnic groups (Carlson & Wiedl, 1978, 1992; Fagundes, Haynes, Haak, & Moran, 1998; Ginsburg, 1986). In contrast, those children who do not perform better with these modifications may be at a higher risk for academic or linguistic problems (Paul, 2001). This may indicate a greater need for intervention. Although results obtained through testing the limits procedures have high face validity, their effectiveness for differentiating language disorders from language differences has not been empirically evaluated.

Test-Teach-Retest

Another variation of dynamic assessment, the test-teach-retest procedure requires the clinician to first assess, then teach, and then reassess a skill. In this approach, the clinician: (1) administers a pretest to identify deficient or emerging skills, (2) provides an intervention designed to modify the client's level of functioning in a given skill, and (3) administers a posttest to assess the modifiability of the client's skill level as a function of intervention. The method has been found to be useful in differentiating language disorders from culturally based language differences in children from diverse ethnic groups (Budoff, 1987; Feuerstein, 1979; Gutierrez-Clellen, Peña & Quinn, 1995; Kapantzoglou et al., 2012; Lidz & Thomas, 1987; Peña, 1996; Peña et al., 2006).

Peña, Quinn, and Iglesias (1992) reported that with a group of Latino American and African American preschool children, the test-teach-retest procedure was successful in differentiating children with possible language disorders from those with normal language skills. The authors concluded that children with high verses low language ability were differentiated by their posttest scores and the modifiability scores. Ukrainetz, Harpell, Walsh, and Coyle (2000) found similar results when they used test-teach-retest dynamic assessment procedures to separate language differences from language disorders in Native American kindergartners. In their study, Kapantzoglou et al. (2012) offered brief treatment sessions to teach nonwords to Spanish-English speaking bilingual children. Treatment involved imitation-oriented cues that were somewhat hierarchical (e.g., immediate imitation of the nonword after a model, imitation after a gesture, and delayed imitation). The authors reported that typically developing children learned the nonwords faster than those with primary language impairment, thus supporting the use of the method to identify bilingual children with language disorders. In an experimental study involving a no-treatment control group, a group of school-age children with language impairment (14 children), and a group of typically developing children, Peña et al. (2006) demonstrated that two brief treatment sessions could help identify language impairment. The target skills taught were narrative skills (storytelling). The experimental part of the study included a total of 71 children of whom 38% were African American, 34% were European American, and 28% were Latino American. The children were drawn from three school districts in Texas and one in California. These and other studies generally show that language impairment may be diagnosed on the basis of a slower improvement rate under brief treatment sessions, contrasted with a relatively faster rate typically found in children with normal language skills.

Advantages of the dynamic assessment include:

- Low modifiability scores on the posttest may indicate the presence of a language disorder
- The brief treatment offered in the procedure may assist the clinician in assessing the child's rate or the extent of improvement; this might help predict the type and intensity of treatment that might be needed
- Because the brief treatment requires target behavior specification, the assessment procedure directly leads to some initial treatment targets
- High modifiability scores may help identify children who do not need treatment because of their ready response to treatment, even though they show some skill deficiencies at the time of assessment
- The testing-the-limits variation of dynamic assessment allows the clinician to use standardized tests in a flexible manner.
- The method is especially useful in assessing children with varied ethnic, linguistic, and socioeconomic backgrounds

Disadvantages of the dynamic assessment approach include:

- Many of these procedures have high face validity but their reliability is difficult to establish. Experimental approaches of the kind used by Peña et al. (2006), however, are likely to overcome this limitation, and produce more reliable (as well as valid) data on this promising method.

- The procedures demand extraordinary time and effort because assessment is not completed unless some treatment is executed.

- Modification of procedures prescribed for standardized test administration may make it difficult to interpret the results.

- Clinicians in many public schools may face a dilemma: treatment, even if experimental, may not be authorized unless a valid diagnosis justifies it; a valid diagnosis within the approach cannot be made unless some treatment is offered.

- In many studies, language disorders in participating children were diagnosed with other traditional methods (including standardized tests) before they were assessed with the dynamic procedures (e.g., see Peña et al., 2006); it is not clear if the method may be routinely used with no assistance from any other assessment procedures.

- There is insufficient evidence to fully accept the claim that children whose speech-language errors or deficiencies are readily modifiable within dynamic assessment do not need further intervention. To support the claim, we need predictive studies that take time to complete. The claim may eventually prove to be unsupported, but in the meanwhile, many children may be denied needed services.

Portfolio Assessment

The Individuals with Disabilities Education Act (P.L. 94-142) does not mandate specific assessment tools or require that standardized measures be used when assessing children. The act does require that tools of assessment have characteristics of equity, validity, and nondiscrimination. The law requires the use of a team assessment approach that incorporates multiple measures. The assessment procedures should be based on specific educational needs and look at "the whole child." A *portfolio assessment* can be designed to meet these requirements.

DeFina (1992) defined portfolio assessment as a "systematic, purposeful, and meaningful collection of students' work in one or more subject areas" (p. 13). Obviously, such a portfolio goes much beyond the results a standardized test can generate; the portfolio collection is larger than the typical clinical folder maintained for most children. The approach requires a multidisciplinary team that might include the classroom teacher, classroom aide, parents, school psychologist, and any other person having frequent contact with the child. In addition to the standard items, Kratcoski (1998) recommends the following to be included in a child's portfolio:

- Story retell samples
- Observation notes of class participation, work observation, and social interaction
- Work samples of tests, papers, assignments, and speeches

- Teacher, parent, and peer interviews; interviews of the child
- Audiotapes/videotapes
- Writing samples or journal entries
- Peer evaluations
- Case conference notes

The speech-language pathologist may use several of the items just listed to collect multiple sources of data that would enable the multidisciplinary team to construct a valid profile of the communication skills and deficiencies of the child. Over time, treatment progress notes and qualitative observational reports can be added to the portfolio. The portfolio can be reviewed to determine whether current treatment is successful and to plan the next step. For example, a child's communication problem may be a difficulty in responding to questions; the child may often provide a nonspecific or inappropriate answer. For this kind of difficulty, such strategies as providing a multiple choice format to choose from, repeating the question in a different way, having the child repeat the question prior to formulating a response, and providing part of the answer may be potential solutions. The teacher and aide would then be asked to use these strategies in the classroom and make notes as to how the child responds. The speech-language pathologist would also be working on these skills. Notes from the teacher, the aide, and the clinician could then be placed in the portfolio. The notes may support the success or failure of these strategies, indicating a need for changes in them.

Research on portfolio assessment is limited, and better researched evidence is available for authentic and dynamic approaches. Adding additional items to a child's clinical file (portfolio) seems to be a good idea, but how effectively can the clinician use portfolios is something for the researchers to investigate.

Advantages of portfolio assessment include (Haynes & Pindzola, 2004; Kratcoski, 1998):

- Documentation of improvement in the child's communication skills over time because the portfolio includes items entered at regular intervals over a period of time
- Facilitation of interdisciplinary collaboration by involving teachers, special educators, psychologists, and parents in the process
- Assessment of the child's production of targeted communication skills in various contexts
- Evaluation of the child's communication in a holistic and educationally relevant manner
- Assistance in developing treatment goals and strategies, something not achieved through standardized testing.

Despite its advantages, portfolio assessment has not been widely used, possibly due to some of the drawbacks:

- Lack of quantitative information; the qualitative nature of information portfolios provide may not be in line with the criteria established for determining eligibility to receive services

- Time-consuming process; collection and analysis of portfolio items require much more time than is required by the traditional assessment; merely placing different items in a portfolio is of little consequence
- Difficulty in managing and coordinating the contents of each portfolio, especially when the clinician has an unusually high caseload
- Problems related to analysis of the contents and communicating the results of analysis to interdisciplinary team members
- Limited storage facilities available to the clinicians in public schools; storing and retrieving portfolio information for large number of students can be especially challenging.

Compared to the traditional approach, the several alternative approaches described so far have different strengths and limitations, as summarized in Table 5–2. Some of the approaches, although trying to solve certain problems, create new problems. Clinicians, however, combine the strengths of certain alternative approaches with the useful and nondiscriminatory features of traditional approaches to develop a comprehensive and fair assessment approach. We explore this possibility in a later section.

Table 5–2. Comparison of Traditional and Alternative Assessment Procedures

	Description	Advantages	Disadvantages
Traditional Assessment	May incorporate language sample analysis (LSA) and other naturalistic observations; rely heavily on standardized and norm-referenced procedures; seek to compare a child's performance to the performance of his or her peers (norms) to diagnose a communication disorder; highly structured; seek statistical data based on normal distribution of skills in the population.	• Less time consuming • Normative evaluation of individual performance may help qualify children for services • Cleary defined administration and objective scoring procedures • Reliability and validity assessed during test construction • Possible comparison of results across various test administrations, clients, and examiners • Limits variations in assessment procedures	• Administered in an unfamiliar environment, by an unfamiliar person (SLP), using unfamiliar tasks and materials; the results may not represent typical social communication • Stimulus items or procedures may be discriminatory or inappropriate for children of diverse cultural or socioeconomic backgrounds • The normative sample may not be representative of the child being tested

Table 5–2. *(continued)*

	Description	Advantages	Disadvantages
Traditional Assessment *(continued)*			• Limited sampling of behaviors to be assessed • Results may not translate into treatment goals • Tests can be expensive
Behavioral Assessment	Makes an analysis of functional verbal response categories and seeks to specify a cause-effect relation; requires more or less precise experimental manipulations to determine such functional verbal operants as echoics, mands, tacts, intraverbals, textuals, and autoclitics.	• Helps identify causes and effects in communication • Functional verbal operants may be better treatment targets than the linguistic structures • Samples a wider variety of verbal behaviors than the traditional assessment • Capable of identifying the controlling variables of problem behaviors as well	• My be time consuming because of a need for experimental manipulations • Somewhat limited research on autoclitics and different "forms of sentences" SLPs wish to assess • Unfamiliarity of the conceptual and methodological basis of the approach
Authentic Assessment	Based on LSA, not standardized test. The sample is collected in familiar and naturalistic contexts or environments. Analysis may suggest a need for intervention. • Minimal competency may be established for speech and language skills • Contrastive analysis offers a nonbiased diagnosis of communication disorders in culturally diverse children.	• May help arrive at a valid diagnosis with fewer false positives • Samples collected in a familiar, natural context may better represent the child's skill level • May be less biased in assessing culturally diverse children • Eliminates the need for expensive tests • Minimal competency core may further help avoid a normative comparison	• The collection and analysis of language samples can be time consuming • Analysis may be more subjective • Information obtained may not help qualify a child for services • Minimal competency cores are not well established for all communication skills • Adequacy of minimal competency for academic success not yet established

(continues)

Table 5–2. *(continued)*

	Description	Advantages	Disadvantages
Dynamic Assessment	Includes a test-teach-retest format to assess improvement in deficient skills. The child is encouraged to participate by asking questions, thinking aloud, etc. Emphasizes qualitative data. Graduated prompts and providing feedback on the child's responses to test items are additional features.	• Provides information on *how* the child learns, in addition to *what* the child learns • Engages the child in a learning experience and tries to promote positive changes in the child's performance • Offers an opportunity to evaluate different treatment variables • Provides the child with greater opportunity for success • May help reduce cultural bias by giving systematic feedback on responses	• Qualitative results may not help qualify a child to receive services • Results may be more subjective • Reliability problems because of the variability in procedures • Difficulty interpreting test results because of procedural alterations • Test-teach-retest format is time consuming • No diagnosis without some teaching
Portfolio Assessment	A collection of the student's work and related information that helps to understand the child's background and skill level. Involves a multidisciplinary team approach. Helps identify the communication problem and tries to determine the potential causes of the problem. Contents are reviewed periodically to determine whether the treatment is successful and what the next step might be.	• Promotes collaboration of team members • Provides a picture of the child's strengths and limitations • Contributes to the development of treatment goals and strategies • Involvement of teacher, SLP, aide, and parents might improve progress and promote generalization and maintenance • Helps demonstrate improvement over time because of periodic entries	• The collection and organization of information is extremely time consuming • Practical problems of storage of portfolios of large numbers of children • Requires a great deal of coordination and communication between the team members—may be impractical

Efforts at Combining Different Approaches

Because of the limitations of the traditional assessment approach with an emphasis on standardized tests, alternative approaches have been researched. Many elements of the traditional approach are essential, however. Therefore, speech-language pathologists have begun to use a combination of standardized, norm-referenced tests and newer, alternative procedures. Some have proposed a strategy of combining norm-referenced tests and descriptive procedures. For instance, Kelly and Rice (1986) described a protocol that included the following items: parent-clinician interview, parent-child observations, clinician-directed formal assessment procedures (e.g., norm-referenced tests), nonformal assessment procedures (e.g., speech-language samples), and parent-clinician interpretations.

Several other clinical researchers have also described a combination of standardized, norm-referenced tests and "informal" procedures (Bleile, 2002; Hodson, Scherz, & Strattman, 2002; Hoffman & Norris, 2002; Miccio, 2002; Tyler & Tolbert, 2002; Williams, 2002). The estimated total time required to complete these types of assessments may range from 60 to 172 minutes. Khan (2002) described a "Quick and Dirty" (p. 253) assessment approach for use in a school setting where assessment time is often limited to one or two 45-minute sessions. Khan recommended that the clinicians concentrate on the primary area of concern and on obtaining the information required to determine eligibility for services through standardized tests. She suggested that the speech-language sample and other information could be obtained later, during the first few therapy sessions.

The combined approaches described above still may not meet the needs of culturally diverse children, and the inclusion of norm-referenced tests may render them culturally biased. In response to this concern, Kayser (1989) proposed a framework for the assessment of Spanish-English speaking students that uses such qualitative and quantitative measures as interviews, questionnaires, standardized test instruments, and naturally evoked language samples. In addition, she suggested that the clinicians modify testing procedures and adapt test instruments to reduce cultural bias. Other authors have also suggested the use of modified standardized tests with culturally diverse clients (Fagundes, Haynes, Haak, & Moran, 1998; Laing & Kamhi, 2003; Rhyner, Kelly, Brantley, & Krueger, 1999).

As discussed earlier, modifications may affect the reliability and validity of standardized tests. Therefore, instead of modifying standardized test items, one might as well use child-specific assessment exemplars the clinician might write; just reporting the modifications made to a test will not help other clinicians interpret the results in a valid manner. Anything that is "dirty and quick" may be practical, but might sacrifice reliability and validity and might result in misdiagnosis or missed diagnosis. Clinicians may take note that all alternative approaches, considered better suited to make a valid diagnosis, actually take more time than the traditional. Balancing the need to make a valid diagnosis and the time constraints within which to do that has always been a difficult goal to achieve. It is likely that a valid assessment takes more time than what most clinicians have. Regardless of practical restraints, there still is a need to develop a comprehensive and integrated approach to assessment that includes the major desirable aspects of most alternative approaches and the mandatory features of the traditional approach. A description of such an approach follows.

A Comprehensive and Integrated Assessment Approach

The previous discussion makes it clear that in recent years, much thinking and research have gone into finding alternatives to a standardized test-based traditional approach to assessing communication disorders in children. The advocated alternative approaches, though diverse in certain respects, are united in their effort to eliminate, limit, or modify the negative consequences of standardized tests and the predominantly linguistic structural assessment. Each approach has its own attractive features and offers unique information on the child's communication skills. Unfortunately, no alternative approach is free from significant limitations. More importantly, a majority of speech-language pathologists do not seem to routinely use any of the alternative approaches. The reasons for this lack of acceptance are several.

First, alternative approaches are used less frequently, possibly because of the belief that such approaches are necessary only in the case of minority children or children with intellectual disabilities and autism, and that they are not useful for mainstream children. Most alternative approaches researched in speech-language pathology are often advocated for minority children, which reinforces that mistaken belief. In fact, aspects of alternative approaches are good for all children, regardless of their ethnocultural or linguistic status. For instance, an assessment of what causes or maintains the deficient communicative behaviors of children—a hallmark of the behavioral assessment—is more scientific and useful than the traditional structural assessment. Selection of assessment stimuli from the child's natural environment and multiple exemplars to assess a skill: both aspects of the client-specific strategy, will enhance the reliability and relevance (validity) of measures in case of all children. Similarly, as suggested in the criterion-referenced approach, assessment of skill mastery instead of an evaluation against norms will help determine treatment goals more efficiently and quickly. Using everyday activities to collect "ordinary language" samples in real-life situations, a strength of the authentic assessment, will provide more valid measures of social communication skills than the standardized tests or contrived language sampling techniques. Brief and informal experimental assessment of response to treatment, the main thrust of the dynamic assessment, will provide more definitive suggestions for treatment. Finally, the portfolio assessment expands the database on which to make diagnostic as well as treatment decisions, and as such, is useful for all children.

Second, clinicians receive a relatively uniform training in the use of standardized test-based linguistic structural assessment than they do with any of the alternative approaches that only researchers seem to use. Most training programs especially ignore the behavioral assessment strategies that offer a better bridge to treatment decisions. Most clinicians see alternative approaches as truly alternative, not mandatory, preferable, or distinctly advantageous to all children they serve. The clinicians continue to use the standard and well-established procedure based on standardized tests and linguistic analysis in which they are better trained than the alternative approaches.

Third, each approach is offered not only as an alternative to the traditional approach, but as an alternative to all other alternative approaches as well. As the alternative approaches multiply, the clinicians become increasingly unsure of a single practical as well as valid approach to take. Clinicians may find it difficult to choose from competing alternative approaches that may imply, incorrectly, that traditional approaches should be completely abandoned.

Fourth, and perhaps the most important, is lack of an integrated approach that includes the strengths of the traditional as well as alternative approaches in which the alternative approaches are not competing with each other or with the traditional approach. No alternative approach has been designed to completely replace the traditional approach because the latter consists of elements that are essential to all assessment approaches. For instance, the case history, interview, orofacial examination, hearing screening, language sampling (though there are variations on how this is done), diagnosis, prognostic statements, and postassessment counseling are common to all assessment approaches. No alternative approach can dispense with these traditional components.

It is possible to incorporate the major strengths of several suggested alternative approaches into a single comprehensive approach that retains the strengths of the traditional approach as well. In such a comprehensive approach, the clinician would, regardless of the child's ethnocultural or linguistic background:

- Retain the case history format, orofacial examination, and hearing screening more or less in the traditional manner

- Conduct the interview in the traditional format for the most part, except that the clinician would make some modifications. The clinician would spend more time asking questions about the child's interests and hobbies, the child's favorite books and games; daily activities, including peer play; family communication styles and any bilingual or bidialectal status; times the parents spend with the child on a daily basis; emergent literacy skills of the child and literacy activities the parents and the child engage in at home; sibling communication interactions; and academic strengths, limitations, and demands. Such in-depth interviews will help construct a more personal (the child- and family-specific) profile of individuals seeking services.

- Select standardized tests prudently, use them sparingly, and interpret the results cautiously. The clinician would select standardized tests that are highly reliable, valid, and have included in the normative sample children of the ethnocultural background the child is being served. Preferably, the clinician will select a test that samples the dialectal variation the child speaks. Positive findings on the test will always be interpreted in relation to the child's dialectal variation. The clinician will use only a minimal number of tests, and consider standardized tests as supplemental to measures described in various alternative assessment approaches. This would be a trend that is opposite to the traditional approach in which nonstandardized assessments are considered supplemental to standardized measures.

- Sample speech and language through client-specific and criterion referenced measures. The clinician would take naturalistic language samples, record language samples in classrooms or the child's home, sample ordinary and everyday language usage, have the child narrate stories from his or her own books or experiences, repeat samples, and offer multiple opportunities to produce each target skill (as against just one or two opportunities that typify standardized tests) to enhance reliability and validity of measures.

- Design client-specific stimulus materials to evoke speech and language samples. The clinician may ask parents to supply stimulus materials from home;

have parents bring the child's favorite toys, books, and play materials to the assessment session; and write multiple exemplars of phoneme and language structures to be evoked with the help of the child's own stimulus materials.

- Conduct a functional (behavioral) assessment during language sampling as suggested under the *Behavioral Assessment* section. This analysis will help identify such functional verbal response classes as echoics, mands, tacts, intraverbals, and autoclitics as well as their evoking stimuli and reinforcing consequences.

- Conduct informal teaching experiments to see if the lacking skills are modifiable; this is similar to the traditional stimulability test; however, this test-teach-retest feature of dynamic assessment (Gutierrez-Clellen & Peña, 2001) goes beyond the traditional stimulability assessment and there is a need to develop brief treatment protocols for dynamically assessing speech and language skills.

- Expand the traditional child's clinical folder to include materials typically not included in it. The clinician may place in the child's folder the entire transcribed interview, or an interview protocol that may have been used with the parents with additional notes taken during the interview. The clinician may include such other items as the transcribed language sample or periodically audio-recorded brief conversational speech samples that document the current speech-language skills (including intelligibility) to contrast with the skills recorded at the time of assessment. Items such as the child's handwriting sample, a brief oral reading sample, samples of the child's art work or math work, and any notes taken during the clinician's observation of the child's communication skills in naturalistic settings (the classroom, cafeteria, or the playground) also may be included. Additional entries may consist of any comments or requests from the teachers and academic vocabulary the child needs to master.

- Make emergent literacy and more traditional literacy skill assessment a part of speech-language assessment. A comprehensive assessment of communication disorders in children should include literacy skills with a view to later integrating literacy and academic skill training with speech and language training. Make literacy assessment a part of the behavioral assessment in which textual responses, their controlling variables, and reinforcing consequences are identified.

- Offer postassessment counseling in which the results of assessment are described to the parents and the child (to the extent appropriate). The clinician would offer a tentative diagnosis, state a reasonable prognosis, and describe recommended evidence-based treatment options.

- Write an integrated clinical report. The clinician would take into consideration the child and his or her family background, the child and the family's strength and limitations, and resources needed to remediate the diagnosed problem.

In the case of children who belong to ethnoculturally diverse backgrounds and are bilingual and bidialectal, the clinician would take additional steps to make the assessment meaningful, fair, and appropriate. The clinician once again would borrow from various alternative approaches because such approaches have as their main concern a nonbiased and culturally appropriate assessment of diverse children. The clinician would:

- Further limit the use of standardized tests or altogether eliminate their use; any test selected for administration will be standardized on the minority group to which the child belongs, and the test items are written specifically to evoke the dialectal variations; use stimulus materials that are child-specific.

- Alternatively, refrain from giving feedback to the child on his or her performance and provide such feedback to contrast the performance under these two conditions; contrast feedback with no feedback only when client-specific stimulus materials are used, not when items from standardized tests are used.

- Analyze the assessment results not in terms of statistical norms, but only in terms of the individual child's performance levels and the academic and social demands made on the child. The clinician may:

  - analyze the child's speech and language skills and functional verbal units in the context of the child's primary (home) language or primary social dialect

  - use the skill mastery criterion; for example, consistent with the client-specific and criterion-referenced approaches, the clinician may calculate the percent correct for each of the target skills assessed

  - use the minimal competency core concept for assessing speech production in African American children (Schrader et al., 1999; Stockman, 1996b, 2008); although more research is needed to establish the general validity of the minimal competence core, the method seems to help avoid a normative comparison of minority children's performance; this would be consistent with authentic assessment

  - Make a contrastive analysis; the clinician would first identify the differences found in the speech and language skills of a minority child and determine whether those differences are a part of the child's own linguistic background; if the differences are not part of the child's linguistic background, a disorder would be diagnosed; this would be consistent with authentic assessment (McGregor et al., 1997)

Table 5–3 summarizes the main features of an integrated and comprehensive assessment procedure. While retaining the necessary components of the traditional approach, the integrated approach includes the most desirable features of alternative assessment approaches.

There is a need for more research on clinical validity, reliability, and applicability of alternative assessment models and the recommended comprehensive and integrated approach. Clinicians need to continue to look at ways in which validity, reliability, relevancy, and efficiency of assessment procedures can be increased by incorporating useful features of newer approaches into a comprehensive and yet practical assessment procedure.

Table 5–3. An Overview of Comprehensive and Integrated Assessment Approach

Elements	Traditional	Special Features	Source
Case History	Yes	Greater attention paid to family communication, ethnocultural background, and preliteracy and literacy environment	All alternative assessment approaches including literacy concerns
Hearing Screening	Yes	None	All assessment approaches
Orofacial Examination	Yes	None	All assessment approaches
Interview	Yes	Concentrate on the child's favorite activities, hobbies, interests, family communication, home literacy environment; academic demands and curricula	All alternative assessment approaches including literacy concerns
Standardized Testing	Yes; may be limited, modified, or eliminated	Select tests carefully; limit the use of standardized tests in all cases; consider eliminating them in the case of minority children	All approaches; traditional when used in the standard format
Speech/Language Sample	Yes; significantly modified	Construct child-specific stimuli; select stimuli from the child's home; record naturalistic, everyday conversations; record samples in everyday situations; assess each skill with multiple exemplars; experiment informally to identify functional verbal operants	Traditional when used without modifications; client-specific, criterion-referenced, behavioral, and authentic assessment approaches
Expanding the Database	No	Include such additional materials as the child's academic or artistic work samples, transcribed speech or interview samples	Portfolio assessment
Analysis of Speech/Language Samples	Yes, with additional features for minority children	Analyze in terms of the minority child's unique language features; distinguish mastered and yet-to-be-mastered skills; make the minimal competency core analysis and contrastive analysis; possibly, consider the test-teach-retest method; identify verbal operants, not just linguistic structures	Traditional without modifications; client-specific, criterion-referenced, behavioral, authentic, and dynamic approaches

Table 5–3. *(continued)*

Elements	Traditional	Special Features	Source
Preliteracy and Literacy Skill Assessment	No	Document the home literacy environment and take oral reading and writing samples consistent with the child's academic level; include a functional analysis of textuals	Literacy concerns
Postassessment Counseling	Yes	Counsel the child, family, or both about the results of analysis, suggest a diagnosis and prognosis, and discuss treatment options	All assessment approaches

PART II

Assessment of Speech Sound Production

CHAPTER 6

Assessment of Speech Sound Production: Resources

- Overview of Speech Sound Production
- Speech Sounds and Their Acquisition
- Phonologic Analysis of Speech Sounds
- Speech Sound Disorders
- Dysarthria Associated with Cerebral Palsy
- Childhood Apraxia of Speech
- Overview of Assessment of Speech Sound Production
- Screening for Speech Sound Disorders
- Standardized Tests of Articulation and Phonologic Skills
- Spontaneous Speech Sample
- Stimulability of Speech Sounds
- Assessment of Speech Sound Production in Ethnoculturally Diverse Children
- Analysis and Integration of Assessment Results
- Diagnostic Criteria and Differential Diagnosis
- Postassessment Counseling

Speech sound disorders, a general term that includes articulation and phonologic disorders, are among the most common communication disorders found in children, and often make up a large percentage of the speech-language pathologist's caseload, particularly in an educational setting. The prevalence rate of speech sound disorders in 6-year-old children is about 3.8%; a higher, 4.5% is observed in boys, and a lower 3.1% is observed in girls (Shriberg, 2010 ; Shriberg et al., 2005). A severe difficulty in producing the sounds of speech can significantly reduce a child's intelligibility and may have negative effects on the child's social and academic life. The purpose of completing a speech evaluation is to describe the speech sound production skills of the child and to determine whether there is an articulatory or phonologic disorder that requires treatment. As noted later in this chapter, this assessment is always done in the context of the child's cultural and linguistic background.

Speech sound production, also known as articulation, is a complex act that requires precise placement, sequencing, and timing of the articulators. This has to occur in coordination with airstream management, phonatory control, and velopharyngeal functioning. Therefore, assessment of speech sound production requires an understanding of the dynamics of speech production. To diagnose a speech sound disorder, the clinician should have knowledge of how children learn to produce their speech sounds.

Overview of Speech Sound Production

For a more thorough understanding of factors that contribute to speech sound production and learning, clinicians should consult other sources (Bernthal & Bankson, 2009; Peña-Brooks & Hegde, 2007). In this section we briefly summarize the basic information on speech sound production, the classification of speech sounds, and normative information on speech sound learning in children.

Speech sound production is made possible by a better-understood neuroanatomic system and somewhat inadequately studied environmental variables that influence how children learn their speech sounds and language. After all, speech sounds gain their importance because they help build a more complex verbal repertoire. Normal neuroanatomic structures and hearing and intellect within the normal range are among the factors that influence the acquisition of language and its speech sounds.

Although the neurophysiological factors provide the foundation for learning, it is the cultural milieu of the child and the family that offers a learning environment for the child. Variations in the child's learning environment affect the rate at which children learn their speech sounds and the topographic features with which they produce them.

Peripheral Anatomic Systems

Speech production requires intact vocal and articulatory structures, and normal neural regulation of those structures. Speech sounds themselves are a physical phenomenon as well. Therefore, to gain an understanding of the anatomy, physiology, physics, and neurology of speech production, clinicians should consult other sources (Bhatnagar, 2008; Raphael, Borden, & Harris, 2011; Seikel, King, & Drumright, 2010).

Significant structures directly involved in speech production include the soft and hard palates, the tongue, the teeth, and the lips. The lungs provide the air supply needed to set the vocal folds into action. Healthy vocal folds that vibrate normally generate the sounds that are articulated into speech sounds. The oral and nasal cavities add resonance characteristics to speech produced by these structures. Significant structural deviations that negatively affect speech production include cleft palate, a short or malformed velum, ankyloglossia (tongue tie), poor nasal patency, severe dental abnormalities, and a severe malocclusion. Depending on their severity, these deviations may cause mild sound distortions to extremely unintelligible speech. For example, an unrepaired cleft palate or short velum may not allow the child to direct airflow orally, and will significantly affect his or her production of all oral sounds. Poor nasal patency, for whatever reason, may prevent or reduce nasal resonance during speech production, thus affecting the quality of nasal sounds.

Ankyloglossia refers to a lingual frenulum that is too short, thus anchoring the tongue to the floor of the mouth. A heart-shaped tongue upon attempted tongue protrusion is a typical sign of ankyloglossia. In severe cases, the child may not be able to elevate portions of the tongue to make contact with the palate, as needed for producing many speech sounds.

A severe dental malocclusion may affect the shape of the oral cavity. An extreme degree of malocclusion may reduce the degree of contact between articulators. For example, a severe underbite or Class III occlusion may make it difficult or impossible to achieve the labiodental contact needed to produce /f/. These types of peripheral anatomic problems often require medical or orthodontic management. The speech-language pathologist may teach compensatory speech production before or during medical or orthodontic management to facilitate the best possible articulation given the structural limitations. Following the completion of medical or orthodontic treatment, the clinician may teach more normal or refined manners of speech production.

Neurophysiologic Systems

The peripheral speech production mechanism is under a complex neurophysiological control system. Therefore, an intact neurophysiologic system is essential to acquire normal speech production.

A complex set of nerves control the structures directly or indirectly involved in speech production, including the muscles of breathing, vocal folds, soft palate, tongue, and the lips (Seikel et al., 2010). For speech as well as language functions, several cerebral centers are important, but the most significant are the frontal and temporal lobes. The primary motor cortex, the premotor area, and Broca's area are especially important for speech production. The primary auditory cortex is critical for normal hearing functions and Wernicke's area is important for language planning and comprehension.

Among the peripheral nerves, several cranial nerves control the speech production mechanism. The most important of them include the trigeminal (V), facial (VII), hypoglossal (XII), vagus (X), glossopharyngeal (IX), and the accessory (XII). In addition, the auditory branch of the vestibuloacoustic (VIII) serves the hearing function and is thus important for learning and producing the speech sounds. For details on innervations and functions of these nerves, see other sources (Peña-Brooks & Hegde, 2007; Seikel et al., 2010).

Neurophysiologic problems that cause speech difficulties arise from faulty musculature or a damaged nervous system which causes neuromotor problems (Bhatnagar, 2008). A speech sound disorder that is due to muscle weakness and incoordination associated with one or more central or peripheral nervous system pathology is called *Dysarthria,* one of the motor speech disorders (Duffy, 2005; Hegde, 2008a, 2008b). In children, dysarthria is frequently associated with *cerebral palsy*, described in a later section in this chapter.

In contrast to dysarthria, *apraxia of speech* (AOS) results when a central nervous system pathology affects speech motor programming or speech motor sequencing in the absence of peripheral muscle weakness or paralysis. Also known as *verbal apraxia,* AOS is less common and more controversial in children than in adults, and pure apraxia is rare even in adults. Severe articulation disorders in children are currently diagnosed, although not without controversy, as *childhood apraxia of speech*, described in a later section.

Auditory System

Normal hearing of speech and language produced in the child's environment is essential to acquire the verbal repertoire, including specific speech sounds. Normal hearing serves a dual role in speech sound acquisition: it enables the child to hear speech, and when the child begins to produce speech sounds, it enables self-monitoring of productions. With a significant hearing loss, which eliminates these two kinds of assistance, the child will not have the optimum conditions for learning speech and language of the verbal community.

Severe-to-profound hearing loss is an obvious causal factor of poor speech (and language) learning. In addition, mild-to-moderate hearing loss and a history of recurrent otitis media may also contribute to delayed or impaired speech learning if they occur prior to, or during, the period of speech sound acquisition. The degree to which a hearing loss might affect speech development is dependent on multiple factors. Whether the loss was congenital or acquired, or whether it was chronic or intermittent are obvious factors. Congenital and chronic hearing loss affects speech acquisition more negatively than loss acquired later or loss that was intermittent.

The type of hearing loss is another important factor. The loss may be *congenital,* producing the greatest effect on oral communication skills, especially if severe. It may be *acquired* during or after speech and language learning. The hearing loss may be *conductive,* caused by middle ear or outer ear pathologies. It may be *sensorineural,* caused by impaired inner ear structures or reduced neural transmission of the sound. Sensorineural loss, which tends to be more severe than conductive loss, produces greater negative effects on speech than conductive loss. The timing at which intervention was initiated and the quality and intensity of services offered also are critical. Generally, the earlier the initiation of effective and intensive speech-language training services, the greater the chances of improved oral communication skills.

The range of normal hearing varies from 0 dB HL to 15 or 25 dB HL. Hearing loss, also known as *hearing impairment,* varies in severity. Auditory thresholds that exceed 25 dB in the case of adults and 15 dB in the case of children may be classified as a hearing loss. A person with a hearing loss that is low enough to permit oral language acquisition, although with the help of a hearing aid, is considered *hard of hearing.* A person whose hearing loss offers no help in acquiring oral speech and language skills is known as *deaf.* Severity is often classified as follows:

- Slight impairment: 16 to 25 dB HL
- Mild impairment: 26 to 40 dB HL

- Moderate impairment: 41 to 70 dB HL
- Severe impairment: 71 to 90 dB HL
- Profound impairment: 91+ dB HL

Severe to profound hearing loss produces significant effects on all aspects of oral communication. Oral speech and language acquisition may be delayed and the acquisition of morphologic and syntactic aspects may be severely affected. In addition, an individual with significant hearing loss may exhibit poor pitch control and a hoarse or breathy vocal quality. Hypo- or hypernasality also may be common, along with disturbed speech prosody or rhythm. The main speech characteristics that are typically associated with the presence of a significant hearing loss include the following:

- Reduced speech rate, pauses, and slower articulatory transitions
- Voiced-voiceless speech sound confusion
- Oral-nasal speech sound confusion
- Distorted vowels
- Omission of final consonants, especially the omission of /s/
- Weak production of final consonants
- Truncated diphthongs
- Insertion of a schwa (e.g., "səlow" for *slow*)
- Aspirated release of an unaspirated final consonant (e.g., "mopʰ" for *mop*)
- Inappropriate stress patterns.

In assessing a child with a hearing loss, a careful history that documents the onset of hearing loss is essential. In addition, the results of otologic and audiologic examination, and a detailed assessment of speech, language, voice, prosody, and fluency are needed.

Linguistic, Cultural, and Familial Factors

Speech and language skills are typically a product of a verbal and cultural environment in which children are raised. As we have seen in Chapter 4, speech and language skills of children (or of adults) should be understood in the context of their immediate home environment and the larger cultural context in which the skills are acquired.

In assessing the speech production skills of a child to diagnose a potential speech disorder, clinicians should investigate the immediate environmental variables that affect the child's speech production patterns. For instance, the child's speech sound production may be a function of a dialect other than the clinician's. Another variable is the effect a primary language has on English spoken as a second language. As discussed in a later section, assessment of children who belong to diverse ethnocultural backgrounds should take such variables into consideration.

An additional factor related to the child's family is the *familial prevalence* of communication disorders in general, and speech sound disorders in particular. Some evidence suggests that familial prevalence of speech sound disorders is higher than that in the general population. Up to 39% of children with an articulation disorder may have another member of the family with the same or similar speech disorder (Shriberg & Kwiatkowski, 1994). Although the full diagnostic and prognostic significance of this finding is not clear, clinicians should investigate the familial prevalence in all cases.

Intellectual Disability

Whether children's intelligence exerts a significant effect on the acquisition of speech sounds has been a matter of much research in the past (Bernthal & Bankson, 2009; Peña-Brooks & Hegde, 2007). The results of studies generally have shown that within the normal range of variations, intelligence does not make a difference in the speech skills of children. Nonetheless, it cannot be concluded that intelligence is unrelated to articulatory proficiency in children (Peña-Brooks & Hegde, 2007).

Intellectual level that significantly falls below the normal limit can have a significant effect on speech and language learning in children. Articulation disorders are more prevalent in children whose IQ scores fall below 70 than in children whose scores are above 70 (Peña-Brooks & Hegde, 2007). The lower the level of intelligence, the greater the chances of observing speech and language disorders in children. With a significant intellectual disability, clinicians can expect a substantial speech and language disorder. Therefore, it is essential to ascertain the intellectual level of the child to complete a speech and language assessment.

Most school-age children with an articulation disorder have normal intellectual skills. However, if the child has been diagnosed with an intellectual disability, it is essential to get the report from the child's psychologist. Speech-language assessment results are interpreted in light of the child's measured intellectual level. One of the questionable clinical views of the past, which may still linger in some schools, is that if the child's communication skills match what are expected of his or her mental age (as against the chronologic age), then the child is doing as well as possible, and therefore, no intervention is necessary. This view would prevent children with intellectual disabilities from receiving much needed intervention for their speech and language problems, unless there is a discrepancy between their observed skills (lower) and their mental age (higher, though still lower than their chronologic age).

The discrepancy model of qualifying (mostly disqualifying) children with intellectual disabilities for speech-language and other special services has had a negative effect on many children who could have benefited from systematic intervention. A more beneficial and productive approach is to assess speech and language skills from the standpoint of social and educational demands the child faces and design and qualify the child for services to improve the skill levels. Such a nontraditional approach, often described as *client-specific* or *criterion-referenced,* is fairer to children with intellectual disabilities than the discrepancy model. Chapter 5 offers additional information on several nontraditional assessment approaches.

Speech Sounds and Their Acquisition

Phonetics, the study of speech sounds, provides a traditional way of classifying speech sounds. Phonetic principles describe how people produce the sounds (especially the consonants) of their language. Phonetically, consonants are classified according to their place of articulation, manner of articulation, and voicing feature (Edward, 2003; Shriberg &

Kent, 2003; Small, 2005). The place of articulation refers to the *dynamic location* in the vocal tract where a consonant is formed. Manner of articulation describes *how* a consonant is produced. The final voicing feature refers to whether the *vocal fold vibrations* are involved in the production of a consonant. The same consonants are classified and reclassified according to these three phonetic principles. Table 6–1 shows the manner, place, and voicing features of English consonants.

Table 6–1. Manner, Place, and Voicing Features of English Consonants

Sound	Voicing	Manner	Place
NASALS			
m	+	Nasal	bilabial
n	+	Nasal	alveolar
ŋ	+	Nasal	velar
STOPS			
b	+	Stop	bilabial
p	–	Stop	bilabial
d	+	Stop	alveolar
t	–	Stop	alveolar
g	+	Stop	velar
k	–	Stop	velar
FRICATIVES			
z	+	Fricative	alveolar
s	–	Fricative	alveolar
v	+	Fricative	labiodental
f	–	Fricative	labiodental
ð	+	Fricative	linguadental
θ	–	Fricative	linguadental
ʒ	+	Fricative	palatal
ʃ	–	Fricative	palatal
h	–	Fricative	glottal
hw	–	Fricative	glottal/bilabial
AFFRICATES			
dʒ	+	Affricate	palatal
tʃ	–	Affricate	palatal
GLIDES			
w	+	Glide	velar/bilabial
j	+	Glide	palatal
LIQUIDS			
r	+	Liquid, rhotic*	palatal
L	+	Liquid, lateral*	alveolar

*Distinctive feature term.

The classification based on *place of articulation* yields the following categories of consonants:

- Bilabial: Mutual contact of the upper and lower lips
- Labiodental: Placement of the upper front teeth over the lower lip
- Linguadental or interdental: Placement of the tongue tip between the upper and lower front teeth
- Lingua-alveolar or alveolar: Contact of the tongue tip against the alveolar ridge
- Linguapalatal or palatal: Contact of the tongue blade against the hard palate
- Linguavelar or velar: Contact of the tongue dorsum against the velum
- Glottal: Vibration of air at the level of the vocal folds

The classification of consonants based on the *manner of articulation* provides the following categories of consonants:

- Stops: Produced by stopping the airflow in the oral cavity and suddenly releasing it
- Fricatives: Produced by forming a constricted channel through which air is forced
- Affricates: Produced by an obstructed airstream which is quickly released
- Nasals: Produced by lowering the velum to keep the velopharyngeal port open
- Glides: Produced by a relatively unrestricted and transitory point of constriction in comparison to other consonants (/w/ and /j/)
- Liquids: Produced with a vocal tract that is obstructed only slightly more than for vowels (/l/ and /r/ are the two English glides).

The classification of consonants based on the *voicing feature* results in the following categories:

- Voiced: Produced while the vocal folds are vibrating
- Voiceless: Produced without the vocal fold vibrations

Normative Data on Speech Sound Learning

Normative data on speech sound learning have been generated by two types of research studies: Cross-sectional and longitudinal. Cross-sectional studies simultaneously sample a fairly large number of children in different age groups whereas longitudinal studies follow a relatively smaller number of children as they grow older. Cross-sectional studies will have different children at different age levels whereas the longitudinal studies will see the same children as they pass their chronological milestones. Most studies on speech sound acquisition in children have used the cross-sectional method (Peña-Brooks & Hegde, 2007).

Since the early 1930s, at least 8 often cited cross-sectional studies have reported normative data on speech sound learning in children (Arlt & Goodban, 1976; Fudala & Reynolds, 1986; Poole, 1934; Prather, Hedrick, & Kern, 1975; Sander, 1972; Smit, Hand, Freilinger, Bernthal, & Bird, 1990; Templin, 1957; Wellman, Case, Mengert, & Bradbury,

1931). Normative data from those 8 studies are shown in Table 6–2. Because of methodologic differences in the studies, the norms generated from the studies do not entirely agree. In addition to potential influence of variations in evoking sounds and unequal sampling of children from different socioeconomic strata, the use of different sound mastery criterion may have played a significant role in generating divergent data. In some studies,

Table 6–2. Developmental Norms for Phonemes

Phonemes	Wellman et al. (1931)	Poole (1934)	Templin (1957)	Sander (1972)	Prather et al. (1975)	Arlt et al. (1976)	Fudala & Reynolds (1986)	Smit et al. (1990)
m	3	3½	3	≤ 2	2	3	2 ½	≤ 3½
n	3	4½	3	≤ 2	2	3	2	≤ 3½
h	3	3½	3	≤ 2	2	3	1½	≤ 3
p	4	3½	3	≤ 2	2	3	2	3 to 3½
f	3	5½	3	3	2 to 4	3	2 ½	3½ to 4
w	3	3½	3	≤ 2	2 to 8	3	1½	≤ 3
b	3	3½	4	≤ 2	2 to 8	3	2	≤ 3
ŋ	—	4½	3	2	2	3	—	≥ 9
j	4	4½	3½	3½	3	3	3	3½ to 4
k	4	4½	4	2	2 to 4	3	2½	≤ 4
g	4	4½	4	2	2 to 4	3	2½	3 to 4
l	4	6½	6	3	2 to 4	4	5	5 to 6
d	5	4½	4	2	2 to 4	3	2½	≤ 3½
t	5	4½	6	2	2 to 8	3	3	≤ 3½
s	5	7½	4½	3	3	4	11	9
r	5	7½	4	3	3 to 4	5	5½	8
tʃ	5	—	4½	4	3 to 8	4	5½	5½ to 7
v	5	6½	6	4	4+	3½	5½	4½ to 5½
z	5	7½	7	4	4+	4	11	≥ 9
ʒ	6	6½	7	6	4	4	—	—
θ	—	7½	6	5	4+	5	5½	6 to 7
dʒ	—	—	7	4	4+	4	5	6 to 7
ʃ	—	6½	4	4	3 to 8	4½	5½	6 to 7
ð	—	6½	7	5	4	5	5½	4½ to 7

90% children were required to produce a sound correctly before it was deemed mastered, whereas in other studies, the similar percentage used was 75. The higher percentage would result in later mastery age levels.

It should be noted that generally speaking, earlier studies (e.g., Poole, 1934; Wellman et al., 1931) show older ages of mastery than the more recent studies (e.g., Fudala & Reynolds, 1986, Smit et al., 1990). It may be appropriate now to use the younger age levels shown in more recent studies (e.g., Arlt & Goodban, 1976; Fudala & Reynolds, 1986; Prather et al., 1975; Smit et al., 1990). Data from Fudala and Reynolds shown in Table 6–2 are from their study on standardizing the second edition of the *Arizona Articulation Proficiency Scale*. Both the Smit et al. study and the Fudala and Reynolds study used the mastery criterion of correct production in 90% of children tested. One interesting observation made by Fudala and Reynolds (1986) is that /s/ and /z/ may initially reach the mastery criterion at around 6 years of age, but as the children lose their central incisors, this mastery may be lost as well, only to be regained around age 11. Clinicians may need to consider this in assessing /s/ and /z/ productions in children, especially in the age range of 6 to 11 when any distortions noted in their production may or may not suggest an articulation problem.

Clinicians who wish to compare male and female children's sound mastery separately may consult Smit et al. (1990) who provide normative data separated for the two groups. The authors also provide normative data on intervocalic /r/ and /l/, syllabic /l/, postvocalic /ɚ/, and selected word initial consonant clusters. Fudala and Reynolds (1986) also provide data on some consonant clusters.

All norms must be cautiously interpreted. As can be seen in Table 6–2, some phonemes may be mastered within a range of 2 or more years; individual differences, therefore, will be significant. Norms rarely predict the precise age at which an individual child will attain mastery on given phonemes.

Phonologic Analysis of Speech Sounds

Phonology, the linguistic study of the sound systems of languages, proposes that children simplify the adult sounds and sound combinations during the time they are still learning to produce their speech sounds. It is not clear that children knowingly simplify the adult productions as claimed, but that children omit, substitute, transpose sounds and make other kinds of sound changes while learning to master their speech sounds is well documented. The various ways in which such simplifications of adult speech occur are known as *phonologic patterns (processes)*. In other words, patterns of speech sound productions that are different from those found in normal adult speech are phonologic patterns. As children gain mastery in producing the sounds of their language, phonologic patterns decline, and their productions begin to better approximate the adult model until the two match.

Phonologic patterns, therefore, are a part of learning to speak one's language. Normative studies have generally documented a general timeline for the disappearance of phonologic patterns in children. Children are said to have a *phonologic disorder* if phonologic patterns persist beyond the observed time lines when they normally decline or disappear.

Common Phonologic Patterns

There are varied classifications and descriptions of phonologic patterns. However, most commonly observed phonologic patterns are classified into three main categories: (a) the syllable structure patterns, (2) substitution patterns, and (3) assimilation patterns. As the following description of common phonologic patterns shows, there are several specific patterns within each category that help organize a child's multiple misarticulations.

Syllable Structure Patterns

These are patterns of sound productions that alter the syllabic structure of words:

- *Unstressed Syllable Reduction:* The deletion of a syllable, typically unstressed in words:
  - [nænə]   for *banana*
  - [pa]   for *pocket*
  - [medo]   for tomato
- *Final Consonant Deletion/Postvocalic Singleton Consonant Deletion:* The omission of a single consonant that terminates a word or syllable:
  - [hæ]   for *hat*
  - [da]   for *dog*
  - [bu]   for *book*
- *Initial Consonant Deletion/Prevocalic Singleton Consonant Deletion:* The omission of a single consonant that initiates a word:
  - [æt]   for *cat*
  - [ʌn]   for *sun*
  - [u]   for *shoe*
- *Intervocalic Singleton Consonant Deletion:* The omission of word-medial consonants:
  - [wæ ən]   for *wagon*
  - [bə ɚ]   for *butter*
  - [ke ən] for *Karen*
- *Cluster Reduction/Consonant Sequence Reduction or Deletion:* The omission of one or more segments in a cluster so that the cluster is omitted or reduced to a singleton:
  - [neɪk]   for *snake*
  - [peɪn]   for *plane*
  - [tɪŋ]   for *string*
- *Epenthesis:* The insertion of an unstressed vowel or a new phoneme into a word:
  - [pəleɪ]   for *play*
  - [fweɪs]   for *face*
  - [sθup]   for *soup*

- *Metathesis:* The transposition of two sounds:
  - [æks]   for *ask*
  - [bəskɛdɪ]   for *spaghetti*
  - [æmɪnəl]   for *animal*
- *Reduplication:* Repetition of a sound or syllable in place of all the others:
  - [wɑwɑ]   for *water*
  - [bæbæ]   for *basket*
  - [tɑtɑ]   for *television*

Substitution Patterns

In these patterns, one class of sounds replaces another class of sounds:

- *Fronting:* The substitution of a more anteriorly produced phoneme, such as alveolar for a velar:
  - [tændɪ]   for *candy*
  - [do]   for *go*
  - [bɪd]   for *big*
  - [wɑs]   for *wash*
- *Backing:* The substitution of a more posteriorly produced phoneme for an anteriorly produced phoneme:
  - [ku]   for *shoe*
  - [bok]   for *boat*
  - [gɑg]   for *dog*
- *Alveolarization:* The substitution of an alveolar sound for a labial or linguadental phoneme:
  - [taɪ]   for *pie*
  - [deɪ]   for *they*
  - [bæs]   for *bath*
- *Palatalization:* Adding a palatal component to a nonpalatal phoneme:
  - [kop]   for *soap*
  - [wɪŋ]   for *win*
- *Depalatalization:* The palatal component is deleted from a palatal phoneme:
  - [wats]   for *wash*
  - [su]   for *shoe*
  - [dʒu]   for *cue*
- *Affrication:* The substitution of an affricate for a nonaffricate sound:
  - [tʃu]   for *shoe*
  - [tʃup]   for *soup*
- *Deaffrication:* The substitution of a fricative or a stop for an affricate:
  - [ʃɛr]   for *chair*

- ○ [tɛr]   for *chair*
- ○ [keɪʒ]   for *cage*
- ○ [keɪd]   for *cage*
- *Denasalization:* Substitution of a stop for a nasal phoneme:
  - ○ [do]   for *no*
  - ○ [baɪ]   for *my*
  - ○ [rig]   for *ring*
- *Gliding:* The substitution of a glide for a liquid:
  - ○ [wɛd]   for *red*
  - ○ [pweɪ]   for *play*
  - ○ [dʒɛwo]   for *yellow*
- *Stopping:* The substitution of a stop for a nonstop phoneme, usually a fricative or affricate:
  - ○ [tʌm]   for *thumb*
  - ○ [wat]   for *watch*
  - ○ [top]   for *soap*
- *Vowelization:* The substitution of a vowel for a liquid phoneme.
  - ○ [ka]   for *car*
  - ○ [bato]   for *bottle*
  - ○ [hɛ ə]   for *hair*
  - ○ [bɛ ot]   for *belt*
- *Stridency Deletion:* The omission of a strident or the substitution of a nonstrident sound for a strident sound:
  - ○ [ta]   for *saw*
  - ○ [wʌd]   for *was*
  - ○ [kɪ]   for *kiss*
  - ○ [up]   for *soup*

Assimilation Patterns

Assimilation is the alternation of a phoneme that is influenced by, and thus becoming more like, the surrounding phonemes:

- *Labial Assimilation:* Production of a nonlabial sound instead of a labial because of another labial in the word:
  - ○ [wæp]   for *wax*
  - ○ [mab]   for *moss*
  - ○ [bom]   for *bone*
- *Velar Assimilation:* Production of a velar sound instead of a nonvelar:
  - ○ [kek]   for *take*
  - ○ [gog]   for *goat*
  - ○ [kik]   for *keep*

- *Nasal Assimilation:* Production of a nasal sound instead of a nonnasal because of another nasal in a word:
  - [non]   for *nose*
  - [mam]   for *mop*
  - [maim]   for *Mike*
- *Prevocalic Voicing:* A voiceless sound preceding a vowel is changed into voiced:
  - [deɪk]   for *take*
  - [bɛn]   for *pen*
  - [baɪ]   for *pie*
- *Postvocalic Devoicing:* A voiced sound following a vowel is devoiced:
  - [bis]   for *bees*
  - [pɪk]   for *pig*
  - [sæt]   for *sad*

Most children who are normally learning their speech sounds may exhibit some or most of these patterns, although some patterns occur less frequently than others. As pointed out in a later section, these phonologic patterns constitute a phonologic disorder if observed beyond certain age levels.

Speech Sound Disorders

Speech sound disorders are various kinds of errors in producing speech. These errors may occur only on one or two sounds with essentially normal intelligibility, or they may occur on multiple sounds with significantly reduced speech intelligibility. Difficulty in producing individual speech sounds with no specific error patterns are known as *articulation disorders* and multiple sound errors that form patterns based on phonologic patterns are described as *phonologic disorders*.

As noted earlier, articulation disorders may have an *organic* etiology (e.g., neurologic or motoric deficiencies, structural abnormalities, or hearing loss). In the absence of a clear organic etiology, the disorder may still exist, and does in many children. In fact, articulation disorders in a majority of children may be described as *functional* in the sense that no specific peripheral-organic or neurophysiologic pathology explains them. It is sometimes assumed that functional disorders are due to faulty learning, but there is often no positive evidence of that.

There are different ways of describing or classifying speech sound disorders (Paul & Flipsen, 2010). Some are traditional, and others are newer. Some classifications are etiologic, although mutually exclusive etiologic factors have been difficult to identify (Shriberg, 2010; Tyler, 2010). Genetic influence on speech sound disorders seems evident, although no single gene or specific genes that cause speech sound disorders have been identified (Lewis, 2010; Shriberg, 2010). At a concrete level, each individual phonetic error may be evaluated as *correct* or *incorrect*. At a more abstract level, errors thus evaluated may be classified on the basis of some principle. Either phonetic production principles or phonologic process principles may help organize individual errors into larger patterns.

Distinctive features provide yet another method of classifying speech sound errors, but the use of this method has declined since the advent of phonologic patterns.

Classification of Individual Sound Errors

In the oldest and the most traditional approach, the clinician evaluates the production accuracy of each phoneme the child produces, although no new approach can skip this evaluation. The clinician prepares individual words, phrases, or sentences in which the phonemes are either in the word-initial, word-medial, or word-final positions. The child is asked to produce the target words, phrases, or sentences. The clinician also may use a traditional fixed-position standardized test of articulation in which the child is typically asked to name pictures. A carefully designed and evoked speech sample may serve the purpose of assessing the correct production of individual sounds in running speech.

Regardless of how the sounds are evoked, the clinician scores the accuracy of each sound production to judge whether it is correct or incorrect. Incorrect productions are then classified as *distortions, substitutions,* or *omissions.* A distorted sound is recognized for what it is; it is just not accurately produced. A substituted sound is also easily recognized, but it is judged to be in the wrong phonetic context. A substituted sound, though correct if produced in other contexts, wrongly replaces a different sound that is expected in the phonetic context. Omissions are sounds that are simply absent where they are expected to be present.

It may be sometimes useful to know whether the sounds misarticulated are the ones that occur more or less frequently in the language. The effect of even a few misarticulations on speech intelligibility may be noticeable if the sounds misarticulated are the ones that occur more frequently than the ones correctly produced. If the same numbers of misarticulations occur on sounds least frequently used in the language, the effect on intelligibility may be less. Table 6–3 lists the rank order of frequency of occurrence of English consonants.

The method of classifying individual sound errors into distortions, substitutions, and omissions is simple and accurate; it serves the clinical purpose well when the errors are few and there is no concern about potential patterns that may be extracted from the errors. Such newer methods as phonologic process analysis that seek to identify patterns of errors seem to have overshadowed this basic approach, but it still has merits. Even to identify patterns, the clinician should first judge the accuracy of each phoneme production. Therefore, the pattern analysis does not avoid the traditional evaluation of the accuracy of each phoneme production; it just goes beyond it, and that too, only when necessary (Peña-Brooks & Hegde, 2007).

Classification of Speech Sound Errors Based on Phonetic Principles

Using another traditional approach, errors may be classified on the basis of well-established phonetic principles that describe how speech sounds (especially the consonants) are normally produced. Recall from the previous discussion that phonetic principles classify sounds according to place and manner of production, and voicing features of each sound.

Table 6–3. Rank Order of Frequency of Occurrence for English Consonants

Consonant	Rank Order of Frequency of Occurrence
n	1st
t	2nd
s	3rd
r	4th
d	5th
m	6th
z	7th
ð	8th
l	9th
k	10th
w	11th
h	12th
b	13th
p	14th
g	15th
f	16th
ŋ	17th
j	18th
v	19th
ʃ	20th
ɵ	21st
dʒ	22nd
tʃ	23rd
ʒ	24th

Source. Adapted from Computer-Assisted Natural Process Analysis (NPA): Recent Issues and Data, by L. D. Shriberg and J. Kwiatkowski, 1983, *Seminars in Speech and Language*, 4, pp. 397–406.]

Examples of speech sound errors classified on the basis of those features follow:

- *Place*
  - /tæt/ for "cat"   /t/ for /k/ = substituting a front sound for a back sound
  - /bæg/ for "bad"   /g/ for /d/ = substituting a back sound for a front sound
  - /θi/ for "see"   /θ/ for /s/ = substituting an interdental sound for a linguadental sound

- *Manner*
  - ○ /top/for "soap" /t/ for /s/ = stopping of a continuant sound
  - ○ /du/ for "zoo" /d/ for /z/ = stopping of a continuant sound
  - ○ /no/ for "toe" /n/ for /t/ = nasalizing a plosive sound
- *Voicing*
  - ○ /sɪpɚ/ for "zipper" /s/ for /z/ = substituting an unvoiced sound for a voiced sound
  - ○ /gar/ for "car" /g/ for /k/ = substituting a voiced sound for an unvoiced sound

Analysis of errors based on place-manner-voice features is a traditional pattern-based approach to grouping misarticulations. A more elaborate method of finding patterns in articulatory errors involves an analysis of phonologic patterns in which misarticulations are considered phonologic disorders.

Classification of Speech Sound Errors Based on Phonologic Patterns

A child with a severe speech sound disorder with multiple sounds in error and significantly reduced speech intelligibility is a candidate for diagnosing a phonologic disorder. The speech of such a child will allow a classification of errors in terms of phonologic patterns described earlier.

As noted previously, the age of the child and the normative data regarding the disappearance of specific phonologic patterns are the two important considerations in diagnosing a phonologic disorder. Various research studies have shown that different patterns normally disappear at different age levels, thus offering a diagnostic guideline for evaluating clinically significant phonologic patterns in children. Based on the results of various studies and often cited sources (e.g., Grunwell, 1987; Khan & Lewis, 2002; Lowe, 1995; Smit, 1993a, 1993b, 2004), disappearance of individual patterns that apply to at least 75% of sampled children may be suggested as follows (Peña-Brooks & Hegde, 2007):

Phonologic Patterns	Likely Age of Disappearance
Denasalization	2;6
Assimilations	3
Affrication	3
Context-sensitive voicing change	3
Final consonant deletion	3
Fronting of initial velar singles	4
Deaffrication	4
Derhotacization	4
Cluster reduction (without /s/)	4
Depalatalization of final singles	4;6

Phonologic Patterns	Likely Age of Disappearance
Depalatalization of initial singles	5
Alveorization	5
Final devoicing	5
Cluster reduction (with /s/)	5
Labialization	6
Initial voicing	6
Gliding of initial liquids	7
Vocalization of prevocalic liquids	7
Epenthesis	8
Consonant cluster substitution	9

The clinician should be cautious in using the guidelines on ages at which phonologic patterns normally disappear. There are significant individual differences; patterns persist longer in some children than in others. The ages will be different if different phoneme mastery criteria are used. For instance, if the criterion is expected to apply to 90% or more of the sampled children, the ages at which the patterns disappear will be higher than what is just summarized.

Additional Problems in Children with Speech Sound Disorders

Many children with speech sound production problems also may experience other difficulties. For instance, such problems in some children may be associated with expressive language disorders. The actual percentage of children in whom the two kinds of disorders may coexist varies between 40 and 80% (Rescorla & Lee, 2001; Tyler, Lewis, Haskill, & Tolbert, 2002). About 10 to 40% of children may have language comprehension problems (Shriberg & Kwiatkowski, 1994).

Children with severe speech sound disorders, especially when combined with a language disorder, may be expected to have academic difficulties (Felsenfeld, Broen, & McGue, 1994; Lewis & Freebairn, 1992). Overall, children with speech sound disorders have poor reading and spelling skills as compared to their peers. These academic difficulties are generally attributed to the children's limited language skills.

A thorough assessment of children with speech sound disorders should include an assessment of language skills as well as literacy skills. The extent to which these additional skills are assessed will depend on the case history information, information gathered during the parent interview, and the impressions the clinician gains from talking with the child.

Dysarthria Associated with Cerebral Palsy

Children with cerebral palsy exhibit a complex set of motor speech disorders due to an injury to the still developing brain. *Cerebral palsy* is a congenital nonprogressive neuromotor disorder caused by prenatal, perinatal, and postnatal factors (Mecham, 1996). *Prenatal factors* that cause brain injuries are many and range from maternal radiation, a variety of maternal infections (including HIV infection), drug toxicity, fetal anoxia, and premature detachment of the fetus. *Perinatal factors* include trauma to the brain during delivery, fetal cerebral hemorrhage, and anoxia. Varied *postnatal factors* include asphyxia, sepsis (blood toxicity), head trauma, and such diseases as encephalitis and meningitis.

Neuromotor disorders are prominent in children with cerebral palsy. The child may be quadriplegic (paralysis of the trunk and all four limbs), diplegic (paralysis of the corresponding extremities on both sides of the body), paraplegic (paralysis of the lower trunk and both the lower extremities), hemiplegic (paralysis of one side of the body), or monoplegic (paralysis of a single extremity). The severity of communication disorders a child with cerebral palsy exhibits will depend on the extent and severity of these neuromuscular deficits. The total clinical picture will vary across children (Love, 2000).

On the basis of neuromotor symptoms, cerebral palsy has been routinely classified into the following 5 groups: (1) *spastic,* with increased muscle tone and slow, effortful, jerky movements caused by pyramidal system lesions; (2) *athetoid,* with slow, writhing involuntary movements when initiating voluntary movements, caused by extrapyramidal lesions; (3) *ataxic,* with disturbed equilibrium and balance, caused by cerebellar lesions; (4), *rigid,* with simultaneous contraction of all muscles and slow and effortful movement, caused by damage to the higher motor control centers; and (5) *mixed,* with symptoms of other varieties (especially the spastic and athetoid), caused by pyramidal and extrapyramidal lesions.

Dysarthria associated with cerebral palsy in children may affect all aspects of speech production. Depending on the severity of the neuromotor deficits, a child may exhibit articulatory, phonatory, respiratory, and resonance problems.

Generally, more severe *articulation problems* are associated with athetosis than with spasticity. Inefficient or imprecise articulation, slurred speech quality, difficulty with tongue-tip sounds, and difficulty phonating or prolonging sounds may be observed in many children. There is a predominance of omissions over substitutions or distortions. Most children have greater difficulty with sounds in word-final positions than in other positions. Such phonologic patterns as cluster reduction, stopping, depalatalization, fronting, and gliding also may be observed. Errors may be more noticeable in connected speech than in single-word productions.

Resonance problems associated with cerebral palsy include hypernasality and nasal emission due to velopharyngeal dysfunctions and poor oral resonance due to difficulties with controlling intraoral breath pressure. *Phonatory problems* include a weak voice, low vocal intensity or poor control of intensity (resulting in irregular bursts of loudness); loss of voice toward the end of sentences and phrases, high pitch and strained vocal quality due to hyperadduction of the vocal folds; and breathiness due to hypoadduction of the vocal folds.

Respiratory problems generally include persistence of a rapid breathing rate beyond the first year of infancy. Additional problems include excessive diaphragmatic activity and reduced activity of the chest and neck muscles, flattening or flaring of the rib cage, indented (sucked-in) sternum, and air wastage during speech production resulting in short phrases or weak productions of final segments of sentences.

Prosodic problems may be significant in some children. Monotone, monoloudness, lack of smooth flow of speech, and general dysprosody may be evident. Most of these prosodic problems are a result of respiratory, phonatory, and resonatory problems associated with the neuromotor deficits.

Although an assessment of dysarthric speech is the main concern in evaluating children with cerebral palsy, the clinician needs to consider the language skills as well. Cerebral palsy may affect language development and some children's morphosyntactic skills may be limited (Hegde, 2008b).

Childhood Apraxia of Speech

Also known as *developmental apraxia of speech* (DAS), childhood apraxia of speech (CAS), though now generally accepted as a diagnostic category, is still controversial. The term *apraxia* refers to a presumed motor programming deficit. The neuropathology of apraxia of speech in adults (AOS) is well documented (Duffy, 2005); however, it is mostly presumed in children. In adults, the features and diagnostic criteria of apraxia of speech are generally agreed on; but in children, they are highly variable across clinicians (Forrest, 2003; Hall, 2000; Hall, Jordan, & Robin, 1993; Hegde, 2008a, 2008b; Lewis, Freebairn, Hansen, Iyengar, & Taylor, 2004a, 2004b; Love, 2000; Marquardt, Sussman, & Davis, 2001; Peña-Brooks & Hegde, 2007; Shriberg, Aram, & Kwiatkowski, 1997).

CAS is an articulation disorder of unknown etiology, although it is generally defined as an articulatory motor programming disorder. Neuropathology parallel to those found in AOS has not been demonstrated in CAS. No consistent or significant brain lesion has been identified. Theoretically suggested etiologies include faulty speech programming, a faulty sensory feedback mechanism, faulty sequencing of movements, a faulty schema of speech production, and problems in developing timing control (Hall et al., 1993; Hegde, 2008a, 2008b).

CAS may be a more heterogeneous disorder with multiple etiologies than the traditional articulation or phonologic disorder. CAS tends to be associated with several genetic and nongenetic conditions. It may be associated with Down syndrome or Fragile X syndrome, inborn metabolic disorders, sensorineural hearing loss, intellectual disabilities, ataxic cerebral palsy and generalized hypotonia, and attention deficit disorders (Hegde, 2008a, 2008b). In addition, a higher familial incidence of speech and language disorders associated with CAS suggests the influence of genetic factors. More prevalent in boys than in girls, the affected children may be described as generally clumsy or uncoordinated. CAS is not the most severe form of an articulation disorder, though often described as such. As it does with any disorder, severity can range from mild to severe.

Speech development is usually delayed in children with CAS. Speech production skills lag behind language comprehension and cognitive skills. In general, speech sound errors in CAS and in typical articulation and phonologic disorders are similar, although there are some unique features associated with the former. As in the typical form of articulation disorders, speech sound omissions and substitutions are common; distortions may be prominent in some older children, however. Children with CAS have greater difficulty producing more complex sound combinations (e.g., blends, or multisyllabic words that are greatly simplified). Vowels may be distorted and diphthongs may be reduced to single sounds. The most frequent speech errors occur on consonant clusters followed by fricatives, affricates, stops, and nasals. In general, speech deteriorates as the length and complexity of the utterance increases.

A noteworthy feature of CAS is that the errors may be highly inconsistent. Children with CAS may correctly produce a sound in one context but not in another. Inconsistency and variability of errors may occur on repeated attempts of the same word or utterance. Children with CAS have difficulty with purposeful movements of the articulators. Therefore, they may demonstrate silent posturing, groping, or searching behaviors during the orofacial examination or when trying to produce specific sounds or words. It is these features that suggest an *apraxic* speech problem.

Additional features of CAS that may help distinguish it from the usual speech sound disorder include some atypical errors. For instance, transposition or reversal of phoneme sequences (e.g., "maks" for *mask* or "soun" for *snow*) and addition of phonemes (e.g., "applesacks" for *applesauce*) are noted in CAS. Other unique features of CAS may include prolongation of speech sounds, and repetition of sounds, even the final sounds or syllables in words. Consequently, a higher rate of dysfluency than normal may be observed in children with CAS. Some children may produce nonphonemic speech that cannot be transcribed.

Variable and inconsistent resonance problems also characterize CAS. Hypernasality, hyponasality, and nasal emission may all be observed to some extent in most children with CAS. Prosodic deviations not typically found in children with other kinds of speech sound disorders also may characterize CAS and may assist in differential diagnosis. Abnormal linguistic stress, variable rate of speech, lack of intonation, and unusual patterns of pauses in speech are among the main prosodic deficits. Orofacial examination, diadochokinetic tasks, standardized tests, and speech samples may all reveal these characteristics of CAS. An assessment protocol that helps document the main features of CAS is presented in Chapter 7.

Overview of Assessment of Speech Sound Production

As the previous discussion suggests, a child's speech sound production may be impaired to various degrees, and for different reasons. Furthermore, what is initially thought of as an impairment may simply be due to a linguistic and cultural difference, not a disorder. Therefore, assessment of speech sound production in children suspected to have a speech sound disorder has multiple goals, the most important of which include the following:

- Determine whether a speech sound disorder exists in the cultural and linguistic context of the child and the family
- Suggest possible contributing or etiologic factors
- Assess articulatory performance in single word contexts and in conversational speech
- Catalog the child's phonemic inventory
- Describe error patterns that may reveal inappropriately persisting phonologic patterns
- Evaluate the effect of the child's speech sound disorder on social and academic communication

- Analyze the child's performance in light of developmental norms, expected and criterion-referenced skill levels, and the child and the family's ethnocultural background including bilingual and bidialectal status
- Suggest prognosis for improved speech under specified conditions
- Describe potential treatment targets
- Make recommendations.

To meet these multiple goals of speech assessment, the clinician takes several steps to understand the child's communication skills and the family background. The clinician conducts a variety of examinations and uses several assessment procedures. In general, a thorough assessment includes:

- A written case history
- Parent or caregiver interview
- Hearing screening
- Orofacial examination and diadochokinetic tasks
- Standardized assessment instruments that are appropriate to the child
- Spontaneous speech sample
- Alternative assessment procedures
- Stimulability
- Differential diagnosis
- Recommendations
- Postassessment counseling

Several of these components are common to assessment of all types of communication disorders. Common procedures such as a case history, parent interview, hearing screening, diadochokinetic tasks, and orofacial examination that apply across disorders were described in Chapter 1. The clinician needs to implement these procedures in assessing speech production skills as well. To complete these common assessment tasks, the clinician may use the specific protocols given in Chapter 2.

The case history and the parent interview in the case of a child with suspected speech sound disorder will concentrate on the child's speech development and production, while not ignoring other aspects of communication. A critical aspect of this part of assessment is to obtain information on the child and the family's ethnocultural background to rule out a difference in speech production as opposed to a disorder. An interview protocol specific to the assessment of speech production in children is presented in Chapter 7. If found appropriate, the clinician may administer standardized tests of articulation and obtain a speech sample to evaluate the production of speech sounds in fixed word positions and continuous speech. In the case of children of ethnocultural diversity, the clinician may replace standardized tests with alternative assessment strategies as described in Chapters 4 and 5 as well as in a later section in this chapter. Finally, the clinician will assess stimulability for speech sounds that are in error.

Several detailed protocols for assessing speech production in children are provided in Chapter 7 and on the accompanying compact disk (CD). Specific protocols to assess speech production in African America, Asian American, and Hispanic American children also are provided. The clinician may use these protocols to make a thorough assessment of speech production in a systematic manner. The protocols can be printed out individually or compiled for a complete, ready-to-use evaluation.

Screening for Speech Sound Disorders

A speech screening is a relatively quick, pass or fail procedure that can be administered to a large number of children in a short time. It generally takes 10 to 20 minutes, and can be conducted using a standardized protocol or a number of informal activities. Speech screenings are generally conducted in preschool or public school settings to identify children who are at risk for an articulation or phonologic disorder and require further assessment. Elementary schools typically conduct speech-language screenings in kindergarten or first grade. If a child fails the screening, he or she is generally referred for an in-depth speech assessment. If a child passes the screening, no further assessment is warranted.

A number of standardized speech screening instruments are available. Some of them are standalone screening protocols, whereas others are part of a larger speech-language assessment instrument. Table 6–4 contains a list of several standardized screening protocols.

Some clinicians might prefer to design a nonstandardized screening protocol that can be tailored to a specific age group, setting, dialect, or ethnocultural background. A nonstandardized speech sound screening can be made up of the following components:

1. Engage the child in a brief conversation, or ask specific questions to evoke several spontaneous verbalizations. Document any speech sound production errors.

2. If the child is old enough, have him or her read an appropriate passage such as the *Rainbow Passage* or *Grandfather Passage* that contains a representative sample of speech sounds. Document the errors.

3. Have the child produce a number of words, phrases, or sentences containing a representative sample of age-appropriate speech sounds. Use pictures, written stimuli, or imitation, if needed.

The criterion for passing or failing an informal speech screening is specified by the examiner, and is typically based on established developmental norms and the phonologic system of the child's linguistic community (Peña-Brooks & Hegde, 2007). Results of the screening may result in a determination that no further assessment is warranted, or that an in-depth speech assessment is recommended. If the results of the screening are not clear cut, it is prudent to recommend further assessment to make sure that a potential speech sound disorder is not overlooked. Early identification and intervention can greatly facilitate speech sound and phonologic development in young children. Speech screenings can be an efficient tool that is used to facilitate this process.

Table 6–4. Standardized Speech Screening Protocols

Screening Instrument	Age Range	Description
Denver Articulation Screening Test (DAST) (Drumwright et al., 1973)	2½ years to 7 years	Uses imitation to screen 30 speech sounds in initial and final word positions; contains a 4-point intelligibility rating; tailored for use with Anglo, African American, and Mexican American children
Fluharty Preschool Speech and Language Screening Test-Second Edition (Fluharty, 2000)	2 years to 6 years	Uses real objects to screen 19 speech sounds
Joliet 3-Minute Speech and Language Screening (Revised) (Kinzler & Johnson, 1993)	2½ years to 4½ years	A quick screening for speech and language skills
Phonological Screening Assessment (PSA) (Stevens & Isles, 2001)	Children and adults	Screens phonological processes with 100 most commonly used words
Preschool Language Scale (PLS) (Zimmerman, Steiner, & Evatt-Pond, 2002)	1 year to 7 years	The PLS contains an articulation screening for 18 speech sounds and one consonant cluster
Templin-Darley Screening Test (Templin & Darley, 1969)	3 years to 8 years	50 items are used to screen 22 consonants, 26 consonant clusters, 1 vowel, and 1 consonant-vowel combination
Test of Minimum Articulation Competence (T-MAC) (Secord, 1981)	School-age children	The T-MAC contains a 3- to 5-minute screening test which uses pictures to screen all English consonants; also contains a *Rapid Screening Test* for preschool children

Standardized Tests of Articulation and Phonologic Skills

A large number of standardized tests are available to assess speech production in children. Within their well-recognized limitations, standardized tests can be helpful in getting an initial impression of the child's phonemic inventory, assessing the number and type of speech sound errors, and identifying error patterns based on place, manner, and voicing features or phonologic patterns. Results of standardized tests may supplement more naturalistic and more valid measures, including conversational speech samples and systematic and detailed baserates that may be obtained sometime later. To suggest or rule out the existence of an articulation disorder, the speech performance data obtained through standardized tests can be compared to normative data on speech sound acquisition, described previously, and presented in Table 6–5.

Table 6–5. Traditional Speech Sound (Articulation) Tests

Assessment Instrument	Age Range	Skills Assessed
Arizona Articulation Proficiency Scale, Third Revision (Arizona-3) (Fudala, 2000)	1;5 years to 18 years	Uses word-level stimulus cards to assess all consonant, blends, vowels and diphthongs
Bankson-Bernthal Test of Phonology (Bankson & Bernthal, 1990)	3 years to 9 years	A test of both traditional articulation and phonological processes
Clinical Assessment of Articulation and Phonology (CAAP) (Secord & Donohue, 2002)	2;6 years to 8;11 years	Uses word-level stimulus cards and sentences to assess consonants, blends and vocalic /ɚ/; contains a *phonologic process checklist* for 10 common phonologic processes
Fisher-Logemann Test of Articulation Competence (Fisher & Logemann, 1971)	3 years to adult	Uses color picture, word-level stimuli to assess 25 consonants, 23 blends, 12 vowels, and 4 diphthongs; errors are classified according to manner, place, and voicing; contains a sentence test for consonant productions
Goldman-Fristoe Test of Articulation-Second Edition (GFTA-2) (Goldman & Fristoe, 2000)	2 years to 21 years	Uses large, color picture, word-level stimuli to assess 39 consonants and blends; contains a *stimulability assessment*; contains 2 picture stories that the child is asked to paraphrase in order to elicit connected speech
Photo Articulation Test-Third Edition (PAT-3) (Lippke, Dickey, Selmar, & Soder, 1997)	3 years to 8;11 years	Uses colored photographs of word-level stimuli to assess 27 consonants and blends, 18 vowels, and diphthongs; 3 pictures are designed to assess connected speech; individual picture cards for *contextual testing* or for use with the visually impaired
Smit-Hand Articulation and Phonology Evaluation (SHAPE) (Smit & Hand, 1997)	3 years to 9 years	Uses colored photographs of word-level stimuli to assess 108 target phonemes and blends; contains an inventory to analyze phonologic processes
Structured Photographic Articulation Test-II (SPAT-D II) (Dawson & Tattersall, 2001)	3 years to 9 years	Uses colored pictures of word-level stimuli to assess consonants and blends; materials for sentence level productions; stimulability assessment; vowel screening; evaluation of 9 common phonologic processes
Templin-Darley Test of Articulation (Templin & Darley, 1969)	3 years to 8 years	Uses drawings of word-level stimuli and a carrier phrase to assess 141 speech sounds, including consonants, blends, vowels and diphthongs; contains *Sentences for Testing in Older Subjects*; a 50-item *Screening Test;* and the *Iowa Pressure Test* for assessing velopharyngeal adequacy

(continues)

Table 6–5. *(continued)*

Assessment Instrument	Age Range	Skills Assessed
Test of Minimal Articulation Competence (T-MAC) (Secord, 1981)	3 years to adult	Uses color illustrations of word-level stimuli to assess 24 consonants, blends, 12 vowels, and 8 diphthongs; a reading version of the test for older children; a sentence test to assess connected speech; and a rapid screening test
Weiss Comprehensive Articulation Test (WCAT) (Weiss, 1980)	All ages	Uses pictures of word-level stimuli to assess consonants and consonant blends; materials for sentence level productions

Some of the commonly used standardized tests of articulation, phonologic skills, and childhood apraxia of speech are respectively presented in Tables 6–5, 6–6, and 6–7. Several of the devices address more than one area, as noted in the table. In selecting a suitable test or tests to assess a child, the clinician should consult the respective manuals. Some manuals give more detailed information than others. The clinician should avoid tests for which the manuals do not specify such basic information as the standardization sample, reliability, and validity.

An important factor in selecting a standardized test is the child's ethnocultural background. Most speech tests are standardized on mainstream children and mainstream speech and language skills. Even if they included a certain number of children from minority groups, most standardized tests will not have been normed to *speech diversity due to ethnocultural variables*. A later section offers more details on assessing ethnoculturally diverse children.

Spontaneous Speech Sample

Spontaneous speech samples offer several advantages over standardized articulation tests. They help sample speech sound production in continuous speech more validly than the structured tests with standard stimuli. Speech samples also provide an insight into speech production under naturalistic conditions. Speech samples provide multiple opportunities to produce the same sounds, thus making it possible to calculate percent correct production of phonemes. In addition, a speech sample provides an opportunity to assess coexisting language, fluency, and voice disorders. Finally, natural speech intelligibility and the prosodic characteristics of speech may be assessed more fully through speech samples than standardized tests.

The speech sample should be collected using the procedures described in Chapter 1. The context of the speech sample should be as naturalistic as possible. A minimum of 50 utterances should be collected. Later on, the clinician should write out the utterances, and phonetically transcribe any words that contain speech errors, using the *International Phonetic Alphabet*. A dash may be used (—) to denote any unintelligible words. Once this transcription is done, the clinician should list any articulation errors that occurred in the sample,

Table 6–6. Phonologic Assessment Instruments

Assessment Instrument	Age Range	Skills Assessed
Assessment Link Between Phonology and Articulation-Revised (ALPHA-R) (Lowe, 2000)	3 years to 8 years	Uses line drawings and delayed imitation to evoke 50 target words; uses whole-word phonetic transcription; phonologic analysis or traditional (omission, distortion, substitution) format
Bankson-Bernthal Test of Phonology (BBTOP) (Bankson & Bernthal, 1990)	3 years to 9;11 years	Pictures are used to evoke 80 target words; analysis of phonologic processes, consonant productions, blends, and vocalic /ɚ/ and /ɝ/
Clinical Assessment of Articulation and Phonology (CAAP) (Secord & Donohue, 2002)	2;6 years to 8;11 years	Uses word-level stimulus cards and sentences to assess consonants, blends and vocalic /ɚ/; contains a *phonologic process checklist* for 10 common phonologic processes
Computerized Articulation and Phonology Evaluation System (CAPES) (Masterson & Bernhardt, 2001)	2 years to adult	Uses color photographs presented on a computer screen to assess target phonemes and phonologic processes; contains a screening tool and a dialect filter for African American English and Spanish-influenced English
Hodson Assessment of Phonological Patterns-Third Edition (HAPP-3) (Hodson, 2004)	2 years to adult	Uses objects, pictures and body parts to evoke 50 target words; assesses 25 phonologic processes, consonants and blends; analysis of the severity of unintelligible speech; 2 screening tools for preschoolers or older children
Interactive System for Phonological Analysis (Masterson & Pagan, 1994)	All ages	A computer analysis program used to generate quantitative data including percentage of phonologic process occurrence, frequency of phonemes in the phonetic inventory, analysis of consonant substitutions, and percentage of consonants correct
The Khan-Lewis Phonological Assessment-Second Edition (KLPA-2) (Khan & Lewis, 2002)	2 years to 21 years	A companion tool for use with the *GFTA-2* described in Table 6–5; uses target words evoked by the *GFTA-2* to assess 10 phonologic processes; a computer software program is also available for the analysis of results
Smit-Hand Articulation and Phonology Evaluation (SHAPE) (Smit & Hand, 1997)	3 years to 9 years	Uses colored photographs of word-level stimuli to assess 108 target phonemes and blends; contains an inventory to analyze phonologic processes
Structured Photographic Articulation Test-II (SPAT-D II) (Dawson & Tattersall, 2001)	3 years to 9 years	Uses colored pictures of word-level stimuli to assess consonants and blends; materials for sentence level productions; stimulability assessment; vowel screening; evaluation of 9 common phonologic processes

Table 6–7. Tests of Childhood Apraxia of Speech

Assessment Instrument	Age Range	Skills Assessed
The Apraxia Profile (Hickman, 1997)	2 years to 12 years	Describes and identifies the apraxic characteristics present in a child's speech
Kaufman Speech Praxis Test for Children (KSPT) (Kaufman, 1995)	Preschool	Measures a child's imitative responses, locates where the speech system is "breaking down," and identifies a systematic course of treatment
The Screening Test for Developmental Apraxia of Speech-Second Edition (Blakely, 2001)	4 years to 12 years	A screening instrument designed to assist in the differential diagnosis of childhood apraxia of speech and to identify children in further need of speech and/or neurologic assessment
Test of Oral and Limb Apraxia (Helm-Estabrooks, 1992)	All ages	Designed to identify, measure, and evaluate the presence of oral and limb apraxia in individuals with developmental or acquired neurologic disorders

note the contexts in which otherwise misarticulated sounds were produced correctly, calculate the percent intelligibility, and comment on any significant observations regarding fluency, prosody, and voice.

It is important to make a comparative analysis of errors noted in the spontaneous speech sample versus those at the word level sampled by standardized tests. Inconsistencies across these tasks may have differential diagnostic significance. For instance, incorrect production of sounds in spontaneous speech, although they are correctly produced in words included in a standardized test, would reduce speech intelligibility. Such a finding may be an indication of apraxia of speech. A formula for the calculation of percent intelligibility is presented below, as well as in the *Speech Sample Analysis Protocol* described in Chapter 7.

Children become more intelligible as they get older. In general, by the age of 3 years, a child should be intelligible, even to strangers. Difficulty understanding a child over the age of 3 would support the diagnosis of a speech sound disorder and subsequent recommendation for treatment (Bernthal & Bankson, 2009). A measure of intelligibility may be calculated for words and for utterances. Table 6–8 shows the methods of calculating these two types of intelligibility.

In addition, it may be necessary to calculate the rate of speech. A child's speech rate may affect articulation, overall intelligibility, fluency, and voice. When they measured the speaking rates of children in first through fifth grades, Purcell and Runyan (1980) found that average speaking rates increased from each lower to the next higher grade level, and that overall rates ranged from 125 words per minute to 142 words per minute. It is important to note, however, that speech rates vary tremendously across speakers and speaking situations; some can speak at a relatively fast rate and yet be intelligible; others may be relatively unintelligible at a slower rate. Therefore, the purpose for measuring

Table 6–8. Methods for Calculating Speech Intelligibility

Information Needed:

Total # of Utterances = _____

Number of Intelligible Utterances = _____ (*Note:* For this measure, if any part of an utterance is unintelligible, then the whole utterance is unintelligible.)

Total Number of Words = _____

Number of Intelligible Words = _____

Calculations:

% Intelligibility on a Word-by-Word Basis:

$$\frac{\text{\# of intelligible words}}{\text{total \# of words}} = \underline{\hspace{2cm}} \times 100 = \underline{\hspace{2cm}}\%$$

% Intelligibility on an Utterance-by-Utterance Basis:

$$\frac{\text{\# of intelligible utterances}}{\text{total \# of words}} = \underline{\hspace{2cm}} \times 100 = \underline{\hspace{2cm}}\%$$

Examples:

$$\frac{\text{\# of intelligible words}}{\text{total \# of words}} = \frac{150}{250} = \frac{.60}{} \times 100 = \text{60\% intelligible on a word-by-word basis}$$

$$\frac{\text{\# of intelligible utterances}}{\text{total \# of words}} = \frac{40}{50} = \frac{.80}{} \times 100 = \text{80\% intelligible on an utterance-by-utterance basis}$$

---

speech rate is not to compare it to norms, but to evaluate its effect on the child's communication. Does the child's rate of speech affect his or her production of speech sounds, intelligibility, fluency, or vocal quality? Would a change in the speech rate improve the child's intelligibility? Can a different rate be established and maintained? The answers to these questions will determine whether speech rate is an important variable and possible target for treatment. The procedure for calculating the rate of speech is given in Table 6–9.

The *Speech Sample Analysis Protocol*, presented in Chapter 7 may be used to record and analyze the results of the speech sample collected. Results of standardized tests and spontaneous speech sample analysis can be compared to each other and to normative data (see Table 6–2) to determine if the child's speech production is within normal limits for his or her age or whether the errors are clinically significant, requiring intervention.

Stimulability of Speech Sounds

The term stimulability refers to the client's correct or improved imitative production of an erred speech sound following the clinician's model or instruction. Typically, the clinician will model the sound production in isolation or in a C-V syllable and ask the child to

Table 6–9. Method for Calculating Rate of Speech

Procedure:

1. Tape-record a connected speech sample that does not contain interruptions or unusual pauses. This may consist of conversational speech, oral reading, or both. The sample should be at least 1 minute long. A longer sample is better; however, it may be difficult to get a lengthy sample of continuous speech with a child. If needed, the sample length can be adjusted by subtracting any time that passes during an interruption or lengthy pause, or by combining the results of several shorter samples. The sample should represent the amount of time speech was being produced.

2. Count the number of words produced in the sample and divide it by the length of the sample (number of minutes). This will give you the child's rate of speech as measured in words per minute (WPM).

Calculation:

# of words in the sample(s) ÷ total amount of time (minutes) = speech rate (wpm)

Example:

280 words (length of sample) ÷ 2 minutes (time of sample) = 140 words per minute (wpm)

repeat what was modeled. A mirror might be used so the child can monitor tongue and lip movements. If the child did not produce the sound with simple modeling, then the clinician may provide some basic instruction regarding the place, manner, or voicing of the phoneme. Instruction may include verbal, tactile, or visual cues. For example, if the target sound is /s/, the clinician might instruct the child to keep the tongue back behind his or her teeth or the clinician might use an applicator to touch the alveolar ridge telling the child to place the tongue tip on that spot. If the child's production following modeling, instruction, or both is correct or improved, the child is considered stimulable for that sound (Rvachew & Brosseau-Lapre, 2012). In this manner, stimulability may be tested for each error sound in all word positions. A detailed *Speech Sound Stimulability Assessment Protocol* is provided in Chapter 7.

Stimulability is assessed routinely, mostly as a basis to provide prognostic information to parents or caregivers. Children who are highly stimulable are presumed to respond better or faster during treatment; some clinicians believe that highly stimulable sound errors should be treated before nonstimulable sounds, or that the stimulable sounds may be corrected without treatment. These prognostic implications of a stimulability test have never been experimentally tested. Poor stimulability for a particular sound may not mean the child will respond poorly in therapy. Sounds with good stimulability may not mean that the child will improve without treatment or that they are the best initial treatment targets. In any case, only treatment can tell. Some evidence suggests that it may be more beneficial to teach the most difficult, least stimulable, and most consistently misarticulated sounds first to produce a much improved speech intelligibility (see Peña-Brooks & Hegde, 2007 for a review of studies). A less controversial advantage of stimulability testing, if done properly, is that it allows the clinician to experiment with several therapy techniques to determine which ones are more or less effective with a particular child. This information can be helpful in developing the treatment plan. Unfortunately, such a thorough stimulability test may take more time than is available in routine assessment sessions.

Assessment of Speech Sound Production in Ethnoculturally Diverse Children

As explored in Chapter 4, speech, language, and culture are inexorably intertwined. Most of the standardized articulation tests have been developed in the context of the mainstream culture and language. Therefore, many such tests are inappropriate in assessing speech production in ethnoculturally diverse children.

The assessment of speech and language skills of ethnoculturally diverse children is addressed in Chapters 4 and 5. Here we summarize a few main points that are specific to speech assessment:

- Tailor the interview questions designed to find out specific information about the child's and the family's cultural and linguistic background; use the *Interview Protocol* given in Chapter 7 and modify it to suit the individual child and the family.

- Find out if the child and the family members speak African American English (AAE), and if so, to what extent; ask whether the child speaks both mainstream English and AAE and whether the parents are concerned about the child's academic performance in school and whether they want their child to gain proficiency in mainstream English as well.

- Find out if the child speaks English as a second language, and if so, what is the primary language; ask questions about the child's and the family members' proficiency in either or both languages; question parents about the child's academic performance and the need to gain proficiency in English. It is essential to ask parents whether they can read and write English because if they do not, the child may not be receiving the needed support for English academic and literacy learning at home.

- Design the rest of the assessment procedures in light of the child's and the family members' ethnocultural and linguistic background; follow the guidelines offered in Chapters 4 and 5.

- Complete the standard procedures, including the case history, hearing screening, and orofacial examination; as mentioned before, tailor the interview questions to suit the child and the family.

- Use only those tests that have been standardized on a sample drawn from the child's ethnocultural group; because such tests are few or nonexistent, use alternative procedures.

- Select the best features from the alternative methods; for instance:
  - Create a child-specific speech assessment procedure by selecting words commonly used in the child's home to assess the production of individual sounds
  - Make your assessment as naturalistic as possible. For instance, structure the speech sampling minimally and invite family members to join-in. Obtain the speech sample with stimuli and storybooks that are relevant to the child's background; arrange for parents to bring the child's favorite books to the assessment session; and obtain a taped speech sample from home and include its transcription in the clinical file

- Expand the assessment data base by creating a portfolio; include comments on the child's speech by teachers, siblings, and playmates; results of teacher's assessment of language and literacy skills; the child's drawing and writing samples; observational notes on the child's speech intelligibility in the classroom, and so forth
- Informally teach the correct production of at least a few misarticulated sounds; systematically model and prompt the correct production of speech sounds the child misarticulates to see if the child's productions improve.

- Analyze the assessment data in the context of the child's speech and language features; see Chapter 4 for the speech characteristics of AAE, Spanish-influenced English, Asian language-influenced English, and English influenced by a Native American English; use one of the multicultural speech assessment protocols given in Chapter 7.

- Integrate the results of common assessment procedures (e.g., case history, hearing screening, diadochokinetic test) with those of alternative procedures to obtain a comprehensive profile of the child and the family

- Diagnose a speech sound disorder in an ethnoculturally diverse child (or in a child that speaks a different dialect of American English) only when:
  - The child's speech sound pattern (a) deviates from the child's own dialect (for example, the speech sound pattern of a Southern U.S. child deviates from Southern dialect)
  - The child's speech sound pattern deviates from the pattern of AAE when the child speaks AAE or when the child's speech pattern deviates from the expected patterns of mainstream English the child does speak, but the deviations are not due to the influence of AAE
  - The speech sound pattern of a second language deviates from the normal pattern of the child's primary language (e.g., Spanish or an Asian language)
  - The child's speech sound pattern deviates from the mainstream English, but the deviations are not due to the influence of the child's primary language.

In addition to a speech sound disorder, an ethnoculturally diverse child may also have a language disorder, a fluency disorder, or a voice disorder. Guidelines given in respective chapters on those disorders may be followed to make a comprehensive assessment of the child's communication skills.

Analysis and Integration of Assessment Results

Analysis and integration of assessment results obtained from various sources, including the case history, interview, speech samples, standardized tests, alternative procedures used, hearing screening, orofacial examination, and reports from other professionals is essential to make a diagnosis and differential diagnosis. Although this analysis will not be completed before conducting the postassessment interview, most experienced clinicians will have sufficient information to suggest a tentative diagnosis and prognosis, and make treatment recommendations. Thus, to achieve the goals of assessment as outlined in the initial portion of this chapter, the clinician may take the following steps:

1. Draw a profile of the child and the family. Consider information provided in the case history and interview when formulating a profile of the child's and the family's communication patterns; explore the family's ethnocultural background and any bilingual or bidialectal status; describe the onset and development of the disorder, associated clinical conditions, family's reaction to the child's speech problem, ethnocultural values and factors that affect the child's speech and the speech disorder, previous assessment or treatment results, and reports from other professionals; describe the family's preliteracy and literacy environment; describe the academic demands the child faces in school; describe the child's interests, hobbies, any special talents, and favorite activities.

2. Analyze the effects of the child's speech sound disorder on overall communication, academic achievement, and socialization. Use the information from the case history, interview, academic records, and information supplied from the teachers and other professionals to make this analysis.

3. Transcribe and analyze the speech sample. Use the *Speech Sample Analysis Protocol* provided in Chapter 7. Establish the phonetic inventory for the single consonants. List the speech sounds the child spontaneously and correctly produces, those the child produces correctly but only with the help of modeling and instruction, those the child produces incorrectly, and those the child omits; compare the speech sound errors noted on the spontaneous speech sample to those noted on the standardized tests; take note of any discrepancies between the two measures.

4. Establish the child's phonetic inventory for singleton consonants. This inventory will include the sounds the child produces reliably and the sounds the child does not produce reliably. Use the *Phonetic Inventory Analysis Protocol* in Chapter 7 for this purpose.

5. Establish the phonetic inventory for consonantal clusters. List the clusters the child produces correctly and spontaneously, those the child produces correctly with only modeling and instruction, and those the child produces incorrectly. Use the *Consonant Clusters Inventory Protocol* in Chapter 7 to complete this task.

6. Describe the speech sound error patterns and inappropriate phonologic patterns that might support the diagnosis of a phonologic disorder. Use the *Phonologic Pattern Protocol* in Chapter 7 to complete this task. If a less elaborate manner-place-voicing feature analysis seems sufficient to capture the child's pattern of errors, make such an analysis; use the *Manner-Place-Voicing Analysis Protocol* in Chapter 7.

7. Make an analysis of speech sound patterns that may be due to bilingualism or a dialect other than Mainstream American English, if warranted; select the appropriate protocol among the several *Multicultural Assessment Protocols* given in Chapter 7; develop similar child-specific protocols if necessary.

8. Determine the overall intelligibility of the child's speech. Use the *Speech Sample Analysis Protocol* given in Chapter 7 to describe the child's percent speech intelligibility.

9. Evaluate the child's performance in light of developmental norms, if found appropriate for the child. Make a normative evaluation flexibly, or not at all, if the child is from an ethnocultural minority group for whom valid and reliable norms are not available; use the *Speech Sample Analysis Protocol* in Chapter 7 to summarize the child's phonetic inventory. Table 6–2 specifies the typical ages of acquisition or mastery for listed English consonants.

10. Summarize the results of stimulability test; use the *Speech Sound Stimulability Assessment Protocol* provided in Chapter 7.

11. Make an analysis of apraxic speech, if warranted; use the *Childhood Apraxia of Speech Assessment Protocol* in Chapter 7.

12. Make an analysis of dysarthria, if warranted; use the *Dysarthric Speech Assessment Protocol* in Chapter 7.

Diagnostic Criteria and Differential Diagnosis

The steps listed so far will help determine the consonant singletons and clusters the child produces and those the child does not produce correctly. This summative information may support a diagnosis of a *speech sound production difficulty*. This difficulty may be associated with few or many errors, other clinical conditions, or may be relatively isolated. Therefore, the clinician needs to consider several criteria to make a definitive diagnosis and differentiate the child's disorder from other potential disorders that share common characteristics.

1. Diagnose an **articulation disorder** if:
    *   The child's difficulty is limited to a few sounds that may be summarized as omissions, substitutions, and distortions
    *   The difficulty seems to be purely phonetic
    *   There is no obvious pattern in the few errors noted in the child's speech
    *   There seems to be no neuromotor control problems
    *   There are no orofacial, laryngeal, and pharyngeal structural problems (e.g., cleft palate) that need special attention
    *   The difficulty negatively affects speech intelligibility
    *   The child's pattern of speech sound production is not due to ethnocultural factors.

2. Diagnose a **phonologic disorder** if:
    *   The child exhibits multiple speech sound errors that fall into patterns that can be described in terms of one or more phonologic patterns
    *   The phonologic patterns that are evident in the child's speech are typically absent in the speech of his or her peers
    *   There is significantly reduced speech intelligibility or the speech is nearly unintelligible

- The child's pattern of speech sound production is not due to ethnocultural factors.

3. Diagnose **dysarthria** if:
   - The child has been diagnosed with cerebral palsy or such a diagnosis seems appropriate
   - Neuromotor control problems found in children with cerebral palsy or other kinds of central nervous system damage do exist
   - The child's speech sound errors are consistent with central and peripheral nervous system injury
   - The orofacial examination reveals disturbed strength, speed, range of motion, tone, and accuracy of movements
   - The child's pattern of speech sound production is not due to ethnocultural factors.

4. Diagnose an **articulation disorder associated with hearing impairment** if:
   - An audiologic diagnosis of hearing loss has been made or is likely to be made
   - There is evidence of a history of chronic otitis media during the critical time for speech development
   - The pattern of speech sound disorder, including distorted vowels, suggests hearing loss
   - Significant resonance disorders are a part of the clinical picture (e.g., hyponasality or hypernasality)
   - Abnormal speech prosody is associated with the speech sound disorders (e.g., reduced speech rate, unusual pauses during speech, slow articulatory transitions, disturbed stress patterns, poor pitch control, and poor loudness control)
   - Deviant voice quality is also a part of the clinical picture (e.g., a hoarse or breathy vocal quality)
   - The child's pattern of speech sound production is not due to ethnocultural factors.

5. Diagnose **childhood apraxia of speech** if:
   - There is evidence of motor incoordination during the orofacial examination, including articulatory groping and searching behaviors
   - The child has poor imitative skills for oral movements and articulation
   - There are multiple speech sound errors with significantly reduced intelligibility
   - Errors of speech production are inconsistent and variable
   - The child's speech sound production skills deteriorate as the length and complexity of the utterance increases
   - The types of speech sound errors are not typical of a functional articulation disorder, but include speech sound sequencing problems, the transposition or reversal of speech sounds (metathetic errors), additions of phonemes, prolongation of speech sounds, and repetition of sounds or syllables

- The most frequent errors occur on consonant clusters followed by fricatives, affricates, stops, and nasals
- Automatic speech production is more successful than purposeful speech production
- Resonance problems are present, but variable and inconsistent
- The child's pattern of speech sound production is not due to ethnocultural factors.

6. Diagnose **articulation disorders associated with structural anomalies including cleft palate** if:
   - There is evidence of clefts, especially the palatal clefts (surgically closed or not)
   - The pattern of speech productions shows evidence of compensatory articulation as described in the chapter
   - There is evidence of resonance disorders associated with velopharyngeal incompetence associated with cleft palate
   - The child's pattern of articulation is not due to ethnocultural factors.

Postassessment Counseling

Conclude your assessment session with postassessment counseling. This is an opportunity to share information with the child's parents or other caregiver(s) who have accompanied the child. Although you will not have fully analyzed the results of the assessment, you will have gained clinical impressions that are valid enough to summarize the results, make a tentative diagnosis, offer recommendations, describe treatment options, suggest a prognosis, and answer the most frequently asked questions.

Make a Tentative Diagnosis

Summarize the results of your observations and your clinical impressions based on those observations. Make as clear a diagnosis as possible based on your preliminary analysis of the assessment results. In most cases you will be diagnosing an articulation disorder. For example, you might say that according to the assessment data, the child has a speech sound disorder that is often referred to as an *articulation disorder*. Describe the main features of the child's speech sound disorder that justifies your diagnosis. You might point out the child's speech sound errors and explain that they are not age-appropriate. If intelligibility is reduced, explain how the child's speech sound errors are contributing to this. If you diagnose a *phonologic disorder*, you might point out the child's multiple speech sound errors, error patterns, and significantly reduced intelligibility. If you suspect *childhood apraxia of speech,* you might point out the inconsistent nature of the child's multiple sound errors, significantly reduced intelligibility, and the occurrence of sequencing or transposition errors. Other types of speech sound disorders can be handled in a similar way.

   If the child's speech sound disorder is associated with other clinical conditions, point out their typical association. For example, you might say that children with cerebral palsy often have speech sound disorders associated with their muscle dystonia, or that children with hearing loss often have difficulty learning certain sounds. Avoid any implication that one clinical condition is the cause of another coexisting condition.

Make Recommendations

Although treatment is recommended in most cases, there may be times when it is not recommended or may be considered later, following a reassessment. The clinician should be prepared to discuss all options and counsel the parents or caregivers about a variety of issues that may be raised. The clinician should offer scientifically accurate information, answer all questions honestly and completely, and talk in terms of probabilities and not certainties. Depending on the assessment results, the clinician might say:

- That the child's speech appears to be within normal limits for his or her chronologic age; therefore, therapy is not recommended at this time.

- That the child's speech is "borderline," the errors are few, they are made on late-developing sounds, and the child may soon master them. The parents can be asked to watch for systematic improvement in the few misarticulated sounds over a period of several months. The parents may be asked to contact for a reassessment if no improvement is noticed in 6 months.

- That the child may need a brief period of *diagnostic therapy,* a feature of *dynamic assessment,* which includes test-teach-retest format (see Chapter 3 for details). This format helps evaluate how the child responds to treatment trials. If the child makes rapid progress, perhaps extended treatment may not be needed; on the other hand, a slow progress may mean that the treatment will be continued.

- That the child has an articulation or a phonologic disorder and treatment is recommended. The clinician then may discuss the intensity and length of treatment that the child is expected to need. The clinician may give a brief overview of treatment. For instance, the clinician might specify what sounds will be taught in which order and briefly describe such procedures as modeling, instructions on how to produce speech sounds, various kinds of prompts to get the correct production, verbal praise to strengthen the productions, and so forth. The caregivers may be offered additional information on the frequency and duration of treatment sessions, the cost, and so forth.

- That the child does *not* have a speech sound disorder, but speaks in a dialect that is different from his or her peers in the social and educational environment; intervention may be offered to teach speech pattern of mainstream English if the child and the family request it, but not to correct the dialectal variation.

- That the child needs to see an audiologist, otorhinolaryngologist, neurologist, psychologist, counselor, or another professional. The clinician would explain why such referrals are necessary and what the referred to professional will do.

- That the family may seek services at his or her facility or, if they prefer, seek help from another professional in the community. If they prefer to seek help from another facility, the clinician would give them a list of clinics in the area and offer to send reports to the clinician who would be serving the child.

Suggest Prognosis

Making a prognostic statement for improved speech production with or without treatment is a matter of judgment, not scientific accuracy. There is little or no research on such generally believed prognostic indicators as the subjectively judged severity of the disorder, vaguely understood family support, often presumed and rarely measured motivation of the client, generally undetermined effects of associated clinical conditions, and the effects of the never evaluated quality of previous treatment. There is, however, experimental evidence that treatment of articulation and phonologic disorders is effective (see Peña-Brooks & Hegde, 2007 for a review of studies). Nonetheless, clinicians consider both experimental evidence about treatment efficacy and subjectively judged variables that affect the course of the disorder in counseling the family about the prognosis for improved speech production under specified conditions (e.g., treatment versus no treatment). Based mostly on clinical experience and research evidence as noted, it is thought that:

- Most children's speech sound production skills improve with systematic treatment. This statement is supported by treatment efficacy research whereas the rest are a matter of clinical judgment. Therefore, generally, prognosis is better with treatment than without.

- Although no systematic experimental evidence supports it, it is likely that a child with an articulation disorder (fewer phonetic errors with no pattern) may require fewer treatment sessions than a child with a severe phonologic disorder with extremely limited speech intelligibility; however, the clinician needs to emphasize individual differences in response to treatment.

- With early and appropriate intervention, most children with childhood apraxia of speech will eventually learn to speak clearly. Some children may have minor differences in their speech patterns such as slightly distorted consonants or vowel sounds, and their intonation patterns may not be entirely normal. However, most children will speak in a way that is understood by others. Some children with severe apraxia of speech may not develop into primarily verbal communicators.

- The prognosis may be more guarded if the diagnosis is severe childhood apraxia of speech or dysarthria associated with severe neuromotor disorders, including cerebral palsy. *Guarded prognosis* may only mean that more intensive, prolonged, and regular treatment is needed to produce significant changes. It is probably not ethically justified to say that systematic and evidence-based treatment will have no effect, even on the most severe disorder. To the contrary, it is not ethical to promise any specific kind of outcome. Possibly, some errors may persist over time and the expectation of normal speech may not be reasonable in severe cases; this should be communicated to the caregivers. These children will make progress but may need augmentative or alternative methods (see Chapters 14 and 15) to help them communicate.

- Improvement under treatment may be faster if the family can observe treatment sessions and conduct home treatment sessions.

- Maintenance of treatment gains may be better if the family or caregivers implement generalization and maintenance procedures at home; long-term maintenance may require some booster treatment.

Answer Frequently Asked Questions

Most parents of children with speech sound disorders ask questions about the disorder and its treatment. The clinician should answer honestly using information that is scientifically justifiable. Research can be cited, as appropriate, to support the validity of the clinician's responses. Some commonly encountered questions and their answers follow; the clinician may need to modify the terms to suit the age, education, and general judged sophistication of clients and families in formulating the answers.

What Causes Speech Sound Disorders in Children?

Speech sound disorders may be associated with known physical conditions such as cerebral palsy, hearing loss, or cleft palate. At times, speech sound errors may be related to other structural problems of the mouth, jaw, or dentition. [*Give more details if the child has a known physical condition that is affecting his or her speech production.*] Speech sound disorders may also be associated with developmental disorders or certain genetic syndromes, such as Down syndrome. It is thought that in some children, an articulation problem called childhood apraxia of speech, may be due to neurologic impairments. [*Give more details on childhood apraxia of speech if the child has it.*]

Many speech sound disorders occur without a known cause, and are sometimes referred to as *functional articulation disorders.* A child may not learn how to produce sounds correctly—thought to be due to faulty learning—or may not learn the rules of speech sounds on his or her own. Some of these children may develop speech sounds over time, but most will need the services of a speech-language pathologist to learn correct speech production.

How Long Does It Take to Treat Speech Sound Disorders Effectively?

It depends on several factors such as the type and severity of the disorder, the existence or co-occurrence of other disorders, the age at which the child begins appropriate intervention, the child's willingness to participate in therapy activities, and the level of support available for practice outside of therapy time. The sooner the treatment is started, the more sustained and systematic the treatment, and the more involved the parents and family members are in working with the child at home, the faster is the progress. Generally, the more severe the disorder is, the greater is the length of treatment. [*Address the child's specific severity of the disorder and make comments on potential duration of treatment.*]

A child with one or only a few speech sound errors who consistently receives appropriate speech therapy at least twice a week may learn to produce those sounds correctly in a matter of months. Children with a severe articulation disorder, phonologic disorder, or childhood apraxia of speech may require intervention for one or more years. In addition, a child with apraxia of speech may need more frequent therapy (3 to 5 times a week).

Learning to speak clearly may be long and challenging for children with a diagnosis of apraxia of speech, but most can and do make great strides with speech therapy tailored to their individual needs.

Can Ear Infections Have Any Effect on Speech Development?

Ear infections can cause fluctuating hearing loss that may or may not be documented. Children learn their speech sounds by listening to the speech sounds around them. This learning begins very early in life. If a child has frequent ear infections during this important listening period then he or she may fail to learn some speech sounds correctly. Some children may develop these speech sounds over time but others will need the services of a speech-language pathologist to teach them.

What Are Some of the Treatment Options?

There are many well-researched treatment options available. Both individual and group teaching techniques are available, but individual one-to-one intervention is most effective in the initial stages. Articulation therapy may involve direct teaching of one or more error sounds at a time. This involves demonstrating how to produce the sound(s) correctly, learning to recognize whether a sound is correct or incorrect, and practicing the sound(s) in different words, phrases, sentences, and conversation.

Therapy for a phonologic disorder involves eliminating error patterns. For example, when a child does not produce several sounds in the word-initial position, we call it a pattern. To eliminate this pattern, we might teach the child to produce several sounds at the beginning position of words in the expectation that the child will then begin to produce other missing sounds in the same position with little or no therapy. If this didn't happen, we will teach all sounds that need to be taught, of course. Other patterns, such as missing several final sounds in words may be handled the same way. [*Describe other treatment options depending on the child's diagnosis, including cleft palate speech or childhood apraxia of speech.*]

When Do We Start Treatment?

We recommend that we start treatment sooner rather than later for better and lasting outcome. We can set up a date now or you can call me or the clinic office later to begin treatment. [*Depending on the service setting, the clinician offers additional information on when and how to begin a treatment program for the child.*]

CHAPTER 7

Assessment of Speech Sound Production: Protocols

- Note on Common Protocols
- Note on Specific Protocols
- Assessment of Speech Sound Production: Interview Protocol
- Speech Sample Analysis Protocol
- Phonetic Inventory Analysis Protocol
- Manner-Place-Voicing Analysis Protocol
- Consonant Clusters Inventory Protocol
- Phonologic Pattern Assessment Protocol
- Speech Sound Stimulability Assessment Protocol
- Childhood Apraxia of Speech Assessment Protocol
- Dysarthric Speech Assessment Protocol
- Selected Multicultural Assessment Protocols
- African American English: Speech Sound Assessment Protocol
- Asian American English: Speech Sound Assessment Protocol
- Spanish-Influenced English: Speech Sound Assessment Protocol

Note on Common Protocols

In completing a speech sound assessment, the clinician may use the common protocols given in Chapter 2, also available on the CD. To make a comprehensive assessment of speech sound disorders in children, the clinician may modify as needed and print for use the following common protocols from the CD:

The Child Case History Form

Orofacial Examination and Hearing Screening Protocol

Use this protocol along with the *Instructions for Conducting the Orofacial Examination: Observations and Implications.* If the preliminary findings of the orofacial examination suggests the possibility of velopharyngeal inadequacy or incompetence, use the *Resonance and Velopharyngeal Function Assessment* protocol in Chapter 13.

Assessment Report Outline

Expand the speech section in the outline to include all relevant information gathered through the case history, interview, assessment, and reports from other professionals.

Note on Specific Protocols

This chapter contains a collection of protocols that can be used individually or combined in a variety of ways to facilitate the evaluation of a child's speech sound production skills. Each of these protocols is also available on the CD.

The protocols on the CD may be individualized and printed out as a group and used for a complete speech sound assessment. Also, one or more protocols may be selectively printed out and used as needed. In assessing children with multiple disorders of communication, the clinician may combine these speech sound assessment protocols with protocols from other chapters. For example, the clinician may combine these with language assessment protocols (Chapter 7), fluency assessment protocols (Chapter 11), or voice assessment protocols (Chapter 13).

Speech Sound Assessment Protocol 1
Interview Protocol

Child's Name _____ DOB _____ Date _____ Clinician _____

Individualize this protocol on the CD and print it for your use.

Preparation

☐ Review the "interview guidelines" presented in Chapter 1.

☐ Make sure the setting is comfortable with adequate seating and lighting.

☐ Record the interview whenever possible.

☐ Find out if the parent is comfortable having the child in the same room during the interview. If so, have something for the child to do (toys, books, etc.). If not, make arrangements for someone else to supervise the child in a different room during the interview.

☐ Review the case history ahead of time, noting areas you want to review or obtain more information about.

Introduction

☐ Introduce yourself. Briefly review your plan for the day and how long you expect it to take.

Example: "Hello Mr. /Mrs. [parent's name]. My name is [clinician's name] and I am the speech-language pathologist who will be assessing [child's name] today. I would like to start by reviewing the case history and asking you a few questions. Once we are finished talking, I will work with [child's name]. Today's assessment should take about . . ." [estimate the amount of time you plan to spend].

Interview Questions

☐ What is your primary concern regarding your child's speech?

☐ Can you describe the problem?

☐ When was the problem first noticed? Has it gotten better or worse?

☐ Are there specific sounds or words that your child has difficulty with?

☐ Is it hard for you to understand your child? Approximately what percent of his [her] speech do you understand? How do you respond when you can't understand?

☐ Is it hard for other family members or close friends to understand your child?

☐ Approximately what percent of his/her speech do they understand?

☐ Is it hard for strangers to understand your child? Approximately what percent of his [her] speech do they understand?

(continues)

Interview Protocol (continued)

☐ How does your child react when others don't understand him/her?

☐ Are there times when your child's speech is better or worse?

☐ Do you feel that your child's speech problem is affecting his/her social interactions?

☐ Do you feel that your child's speech problem is affecting his/her school performance?

☐ Is English your child's first language? If not, what other language(s) does he [she] speak?

☐ Is the child easier to understand in one language or the other?

☐ If English is not the primary language, do you feel there is also a speech problem in the primary language?

☐ What language is spoken most often in the home?

☐ Has your child had a history of ear infections?

☐ Has your child ever had a hearing test? If yes, when and where? What were the results?

☐ Has your child seen any other specialists for this problem? If so, who and when? What were their recommendations? How have you followed up on this?

☐ Has your child received speech therapy before? If yes, when and where? What did they work on in therapy? Can you describe the types of activities that were used? How did your child respond? Do you feel the therapy was helpful? Why or why not?

Review the case history and follow up with any additional questions you need clarification on. Try to fill in any "blanks" in the medical, developmental, social and educational histories.

Closing the Interview

☐ Summarize the major points that you gathered from the interview, allowing the parent/caregiver to interrupt or correct information, as needed.

☐ Do you have any questions for me at this point?

☐ Thank you very much for you input. The information has been very helpful.

☐ Now, I will work with [child's name]. Once we are finished, I will sit down to share my findings with you.

Speech Sound Assessment Protocol 2
Speech Sample Analysis Protocol

Child's Name _____ DOB _____ Date _____ Clinician _____

Individualize this protocol on the CD and print it for your use.

Instructions
1. Collect a **minimum** of 50 utterances.
2. Write out each utterance, transcribing any words that contain articulation errors.
3. Use a dash (—) to represent unintelligible words.
4. Tasks to be completed:
   a. generate a *list of phonemic errors*
   b. calculate *% intelligibility on a word-by-word basis*
   c. calculate *% intelligibility on an utterance-by-utterance basis*

Record the Utterances and Speech Sound Errors on this Form

	List Phoneme Errors		
1. _____	**initial**	**medial**	**final**
2. _____			
3. _____			
4. _____			
5. _____			
6. _____			
7. _____			
8. _____			
9. _____			
10. _____			
11. _____			
12. _____			
13. _____			
14. _____			
15. _____			
16. _____			
17. _____			

(continues)

Speech Sample Analysis Protocol (continued)

18. _____

19. _____

20. _____

21. _____

22. _____

23. _____

24. _____

25. _____

26. _____

27. _____

28. _____

29. _____

30. _____

31. _____

32. _____

33. _____

34. _____

35. _____

36. _____

37. _____

38. _____

39. _____

40. _____

41. _____

42. _____

43. _____

44. _____

45. _____

46. _____

47. _____

48. _____

49. _____

50. _____

(add additional lines for any sample over 50 utterances)

Information Needed to Calculate Speech Intelligibility:

Total Number of Utterances = _____

Number of Intelligible Utterances = _____ (Note: For this figure, if any part of an utterance is unintelligible, then the whole utterance is unintelligible.)

Total Number of Words = _____

Number of Intelligible Words = _____

Calculations:

% Intelligibility on a Word-by-Word Basis:

$$\frac{\text{\# of intelligible words}}{\text{total \# of words}} = \text{_____} \times 100 = \text{_____}\%$$

% Intelligibility on an Utterance-by-Utterance Basis:

$$\frac{\text{\# of intelligible utterances}}{\text{total \# of words}} = \text{_____} \times 100 = \text{_____}\%$$

Other Observations Regarding Factors That Decrease Intelligibility

Speech Sound Assessment Protocol 3
Phonetic Inventory Analysis Protocol

Child's Name _____ DOB _____ Date _____ Clinician _____

Individualize this protocol on the CD and print it for your use.

- Sounds circled occurred at least three times in each position; they are part of the child's *productive* sound inventory.

- Sounds underlined occurred only one or two times in each position; they are *marginal*.

- Sounds that are neither circled nor underlined were not produced *in spite of the opportunity to produce them*. These sounds are *absent* from the child's phonetic inventory.

Initial Position

m	n	p	b	t	d	k	g	f	v	s	z
θ	ð	ʃ	tʃ	dʒ	w	L	r	j	h		

Medial Position

m	n	ŋ	p	b	t	d	k	g	f	v	s
z	θ	ð	ʃ	ʒ	tʃ	dʒ	w	l	r	j	h

Final Position

m	n	ŋ	p	b	t	d	k	g	f	v	s
z	θ	ð	ʃ	ʒ	tʃ	dʒ	l	r	ʃ		

Vowels and Diphthongs

ɑ	æ	e	e	o	ɔ	u	ʊ	i	ɪ	ə	ʌ
ɚ	ɝ	ai	au	ɔi	ju	eɪ	ou				

List of Absent phonemes:

Initial Position	Medial Position	Final Position

Speech Sound Assessment Protocol 4
Manner-Place-Voicing Analysis Protocol

Child's Name _____ DOB _____ Date _____ Clinician _____

Individualize this protocol on the CD and print it for your use.

Connected speech: _____ Single words: _____ Formal test: _____

Instruction: Circle the misarticulated sound and take note of the actual error response.

Analysis by Manner of Production

Stops	/p/	/b/	/t/	/d/	/k/	/g/
Fricatives	/f/	/v/	/s/	/z/	/θ/	/ð/
	ʃ	ʒ	/h/			
Affricates	/tʃ/	/dʒ/	Nasals	/m/	/n/	/ŋ/
Glides	/j/	/w/	Liquids	/l/	/r/	

Analysis by Place of Articulation

Bilabials	/m/		/b/		/p/		/w/
Alveolars	/t/	/d/	/s/	/z/	/n/	/l/	
Palatals	/ʃ/	/ʒ/	/tʃ/	/dʒ/	/j/	/r/	
Linguadentals	/θ/	/ð/	Labiodentals	/f/	/v/		
Velars	/k/	/g/	/ŋ/	Glottal	/h/		

Analysis by Voicing Feature

Voiced	/m/	/n/	/ŋ/	/b/	/d/	/g/
	/v/	/ð/	/z/	/ʒ/	/dʒ/	r
	/l/	/w/	/j/			
Voiceless	/p/	/t/	/k/	/f/	/θ/	/s/
	/ʃ/	/h/				

Summary of error patterns and comments:

_____

_____

_____

Speech Sound Assessment Protocol 5
Consonant Clusters Inventory Protocol

Child's Name _____ DOB _____ Date _____ Clinician _____

Individualize this protocol on the CD and print it for your use.

Key: ✓ = correct production ; X = incorrect production. The final column shows the age of mastery.

Instructions: *Ask the child to repeat after you; model the word productions and record the child's actual productions.*

Initial Clusters

/kw/	quick	_____	queen	_____	quack	_____	4;0
/tw/	twist	_____	twin	_____	twenty	_____	4;0
/sw/	swim	_____	swap	_____	sweat	_____	7;0
/pl/	play	_____	plan	_____	plate	_____	4;0
/kl/	clock	_____	clap	_____	clean	_____	4;0
/fl/	flat	_____	fly	_____	fleet	_____	5;0
/bl/	blip	_____	blame	_____	blow	_____	4;0
/gl/	glass	_____	glad	_____	glow	_____	4;0
/sl/	sleep	_____	slide	_____	sly	_____	7;0
/pr/	press	_____	prize	_____	prime	_____	4;0
/br/	brag	_____	brain	_____	brown	_____	4;0
/tr/	tree	_____	trap	_____	trick	_____	4;0
/dr/	drip	_____	dress	_____	drive	_____	4;0
/fr/	frog	_____	fry	_____	frame	_____	5;0
/θr/	three	_____	throw	_____	thrive	_____	7;0
/kr/	crop	_____	cream	_____	cry	_____	4;0
/gr/	gray	_____	grass	_____	grin	_____	5;0
/st/	stop	_____	stick	_____	stay	_____	4;0
/sp/	spot	_____	speak	_____	spine	_____	4;0
/sk/	scoop	_____	scout	_____	scone	_____	4;0
/sn/	snake	_____	snow	_____	sniff	_____	4;0

/sm/	smile	_____	smog		smash		4;0
/nj/	new	_____	newt		news		—
/fj/	few	_____	fume		fuel		—
/kj/	cute	_____	cuba		cube		—
/mj/	muse	_____	music		mute		—
/ʃr/	shrine	_____	shriek		shred		7;0
/str/	straw	_____	stray		street		5;0
/skw/	squat	_____	squeal		squint		6;0
/spl/	splint	_____	splash		split		7;0
/spr/	spray	_____	sprig		spree		7;0
/skr/	scram	_____	scream		scrap		7;0

Final Clusters

/mp/	lamp	_____	ramp	_____	jump	_____	4;0
/nt/	hint	_____	ant	_____	count	_____	6;0
/nd/	hand	_____	bend	_____	fond	_____	6;0
/ns/	wince	_____	mince	_____	fence	_____	—
/rd/	hard	_____	lard	_____	gourd	_____	5;0
/nz/	lens	_____	buns	_____	beans	_____	—
/ks/	likes	_____	lacks	_____	wakes	_____	4;0
/st/	past	_____	test	_____	most	_____	7;0
/kt/	act	_____	fact	_____	locked	_____	8;0
/ld/	held	_____	mold	_____	fold	_____	—
/rt/	art	_____	cart	_____	sort	_____	4;0
/ts/	bets	_____	mats	_____	mitts	_____	—
/rn/	torn	_____	warn	_____	barn	_____	5;0
/rm/	arm	_____	farm	_____	dorm	_____	4;0
/lp/	pulp	_____	help	_____	gulp	_____	4;0
/lt/	malt	_____	halt	_____	belt	_____	4;0
/lf/	self	_____	golf	_____	elf	_____	5;0

(continues)

Consonant Clusters Inventory Protocol (continued)

/lk/	elk	_____	bulk	_____	milk	_____	6;0
/zd/	buzzed	_____	dazed	_____	raised	_____	—
/rk/	park	_____	fork	_____	mark	_____	4;0
/mz/	arms	_____	aims	_____	stems	_____	—
/lz/	balls	_____	malls	_____	sells	_____	—
/gz/	bugs	_____	pigs	_____	begs	_____	—
/pt/	opt	_____	kept	_____	swept	_____	4;0
/ft/	left	_____	soft	_____	lift	_____	4;0
/rf/	scarf	_____	wharf	_____	morph	_____	5;0
/rv/	starve	_____	carve	_____	swerve	_____	—
/mpt/	bumped	_____	stamped	_____	jumped	_____	4;0
/mps/	lamps	_____	ramps	_____	bumps	_____	4;0
/nts/	ants	_____	pants	_____	rants	_____	—
/ŋz/	sings	_____	gongs	_____	kings	_____	—
/ŋk/	thank	_____	bank	_____	junk	_____	4;0
/ndz/	hands	_____	lends	_____	bends	_____	—

Comments: _____

_____

Speech Sound Assessment Protocol 6
Phonologic Pattern Protocol

Child's Name _____ DOB _____ Date _____ Clinician _____

Individualize this protocol on the CD and print it for your use.

Pattern	Definition/Examples	Examples/Child's Speech	Disappears
Reduplication	Repetition of a syllable of a target word. Sometimes called doubling. "ba-ba" for *bottle*; "ca-ca" for *car*		by 2 ½
Diminutization	Addition of /i/ or a consonant + /i/ to the target word. "cuppy" for *cup*; "fofee" for *finger*		by 3
Final consonant deletion	Omission of final consonants. "ha" for *hat* "mo" for *mom* "coa" for *coat*		by 3
Assimilation	A sound in a word changes to become more like another sound in the word. "mom" for *mop*; "cook" for *took* "boab" for *boat*; "tot" for *toss* "den" for *ten*; "pick" for *pig*		by 3
Velar fronting	Replacement of velars /k/, /g/, /ŋ/ with sounds made more anteriorly, particularly alveolars /t/, /d/, /n/. "pat" for *pack*; "doat" for *goat*; "rin" for *ring*		by 3½
Deaffrication	Replacement of an affricate with a stop or fricative. "tair" for *chair*; "sop" for *chop*; "dump" for *jump*		by 4
Syllable deletion	Omission of one or more syllables from a multisyllable word. "mato" for *tomato*; "nana" for *banana*; "key" for *monkey*		by 4

(continues)

Phonologic Pattern Protocol (continued)

Pattern	Definition/Examples	Examples/Child's Speech	Disappears
Cluster reduction	Deletion or substitution of some or all parts of a cluster. "pay" for *play*; "ack" for *black*; "gween" for *green*; "op" for *stop*		by 5
Stopping	Substitution of stops for fricatives and affricates. "pish" for *fish*; "toap" for *soap*; "dis" for *this*		by 5
Depalatalization	Substitution of an alveolar fricative or affricate for a palatal affricate. "seck" for *check*; "matses" for *matches*; "dudz" for *judge*; "Shen" for *Jen*		by 5
Gliding	Substitution of liquids /l/, /r/, by glides /w/, /y/. "wed" for *red*; "cawot" for *carrot*; "yamb" for *lamb*		beyond 5
Vocalization	Substitution of a vowel for a syllabic liquid, syllabic "-er," or postvocalic liquid. "simpo" for *simple*; "papo" for *paper*; "ca" for *car*		beyond 5
Backing	Replacement of alveolars and palatals /t/, /d/, /s/, /z/, /n/, /ʃ/, /tʃ/, /dʒ/ by posterior sounds /k/, /g/, /ŋ/. "cop" for *top*; "bike" for *bite*; "kip" for *ship*		—
Additional or unique Patterns observed in the child's speech			

Summary of phonological Patterns evident in the child's speech:

_____

_____

_____

_____

Speech Sound Assessment Protocol 7
Speech Sound Stimulability Assessment Protocol

Child's Name _____ DOB _____ Date _____ Clinician _____

Individualize this protocol on the CD and print it for your use.

- Model the phoneme in isolation or in a C-V syllable. Ask the child to watch and listen carefully, and to do what you do. If the child imitates the sound or syllable correctly, mark a "+" in the sound-syllable column. If the child does not produce the sound correctly, mark a "–" in the column.

- Model the phoneme in the initial position of words. If the child imitates it correctly, mark a "+" in the word level (initial) column, and go on to model it in the medial and final positions of words. Mark the corresponding column with a "+" or "–" as appropriate. If the child is successful at the word level, attempt simple phrases. Model the targets and document the results in the same manner. Several target words and phrases have been provided for each phoneme.

- Make a note in the "Comments" area if you provided the child with any type of instruction or cuing other than simple modeling.

Consonant Stimulability

Phoneme	Sound-Syllable Level	Word Level			Phrase Level		
		initial	*medial*	*final*	*initial*	*medial*	*final*
/p/	_____	_____	_____	_____	_____	_____	_____

pan, pie, pipe, pack, happy, apple, open, puppy, cup, deep, soup, pick up toys, eat pie, open the door, red apple, deep water, cup of soup

Comments:

Phoneme	Sound-Syllable Level	Word Level			Phrase Level		
/b/	_____	_____	_____	_____	_____	_____	_____

ball, bee, bed, boat, bubble, maybe, baby, tub, web, cub, cab, mob, ball is red, row the boat, pop the bubble, obey mom, in the tub, see the web

Comments:

(continues)

Speech Sound Stimulability Assessment Protocol (continued)

Phoneme	Sound-Syllable Level	Word Level			Phrase Level		
		initial	*medial*	*final*	*initial*	*medial*	*final*
/t/	_____	_____	_____	_____	_____	_____	_____

ten, tea, two, time, potato, tomato, plenty, eat, late, hot, boat, want, I see two, what time is it, hot potato, sail the boat, eat lunch

Comments:

/d/	_____	_____	_____	_____	_____	_____	_____

do, dog, day, dime, body, soda, ladder, bed, good, head, dad, big dog, do it, my dime, drink soda, use a ladder, time for bed, good buy

Comments:

/k/	_____	_____	_____	_____	_____	_____	_____

cup, cat, coat, king, cookie, bacon, lucky, sick, bake, book pet the cat, cup of milk, eat a cookie, lucky day, read a book, bake bread

Comments:

/g/	_____	_____	_____	_____	_____	_____	_____

go, gum, gate, gift, foggy, bigger, *Eggo*, leg, rug, pig, bag, go home, chew the gum, a foggy night, eat *Eggos*, a big pig, bag of candy

Comments:

/f/	_____	_____	_____	_____	_____	_____	_____

four, fan, five, phone, muffin, after, café, cough, loaf, beef, five cents, on the phone, after dinner, eat muffins, a bad cough, eat beef

Comments:

Phoneme	Sound-Syllable Level	Word Level			Phrase Level		
		initial	*medial*	*final*	*initial*	*medial*	*final*
/v/	_____	_____	_____	_____	_____	_____	_____

vine, vase, vest, over, movie, eleven, love, wave, dive, grape vine, wear a vest, movie time, over the hill, I love you, wave bye-bye

Comments:

/s/	_____	_____	_____	_____	_____	_____	_____

sit, soap, see, sail, messy, basic, aces, bus, toss, face, house, sit here, wash with soap, messy face, four aces, toss a ball, in the house

Comments:

/z/	_____	_____	_____	_____	_____	_____	_____

zoo, zipper, zero, dozen, easy, busy, keys, maze, boys, zoo keeper, long zipper, a dozen eggs, busy boy, use the keys, boys play ball

Comments:

/θ/	_____	_____	_____	_____	_____	_____	_____

third, thin, thanks, bathtub, author, bath, tooth, both, math, thank you, very thin, full bathtub, book author, take a bath, loose tooth

Comments:

/ð/	_____	_____	_____	_____	_____	_____	_____

the, them, that, they, mother, father, bathe, smooth, the ball, get that toy, my mother, bird feather, bathe a dog, smooth skin

Comments:

(continues)

Speech Sound Stimulability Assessment Protocol (continued)

Phoneme	Sound-Syllable Level	Word Level			Phrase Level		
		initial	*medial*	*final*	*initial*	*medial*	*final*
/ʃ/	_____	_____	_____	_____	_____	_____	_____

ship, shoe, shark, dishes, ocean, ashes, fish, wash, push, tie the shoe, shark bite, wash dishes, in the ocean, a big fish, push the door

Comments:

/ʒ/	_____	_____	_____	_____	_____	_____	_____

vision, treasure, beige, massage, big treasure, my vision, a beige hat, nice massage

Comments:

/h/	_____	_____	_____	_____	_____	_____	_____

hop, home, hat, house, behind, ahead, hop up, in the house, in the hall, go ahead

Comments:

/tʃ/	_____	_____	_____	_____	_____	_____	_____

chair, chop, chin, pitcher, matches, watch, catch, beach, on a chair, chop it up, full pitcher, no matches, watch TV, on the beach

Comments:

/dʒ/	_____	_____	_____	_____	_____	_____	_____

job, joke, jail, cages, magic, edges, page, edge, lodge, jail bird, funny joke, a magic hat, rough edges, turn the page, old lodge

Comments:

Phoneme	Sound-Syllable Level	Word Level			Phrase Level		
		initial	*medial*	*final*	*initial*	*medial*	*final*
/w/	———	———	———	———	———	———	———

we, wait, wipe, wet, away, beware, kiwi, wait for me, all wet, beware of
dog, eat kiwi

Comments:

Phoneme	Sound-Syllable Level	Word Level			Phrase Level		
/j/	———	———	———	———	———	———	———

you, yes, year, yawn, yo-yo, kayak, beyond, yes I am, what year is it, my
yo-yo, beyond time

Comments:

Phoneme	Sound-Syllable Level	Word Level			Phrase Level		
/l/	———	———	———	———	———	———	———

lamb, lie, log, leap, ally, below, chili, ball, fill, seal, whale, little lamb, big
lie, leap frog, hot chili, in the alley, fill it up, bouncy ball

Comments:

Phoneme	Sound-Syllable Level	Word Level			Phrase Level		
/r/	———	———	———	———	———	———	———

ride, rat, run, rope, rock, carrot, berry, arrow, car, hair, ear, door, more,
ride a bike, big rat, run away, orange carrot, berry pie, in the car

Comments:

Phoneme	Sound-Syllable Level	Word Level			Phrase Level		
/m/	———	———	———	———	———	———	———

man, mop, more, me, my, summer, tummy, camel, home, game, time,
more money, mop it up, for me, summer time, my tummy, time to go

Comments:

(continues)

Speech Sound Stimulability Assessment Protocol (continued)

Phoneme	Sound-Syllable Level	Word Level initial	medial	final	Phrase Level initial	medial	final
/n/	———	———	———	———	———	———	———

no, name, night, nap, knee, pony, honey, tunnel, fan, one, rain, line, no more, take a nap, bent knee, a nice pony, honey oats, one more

Comments:

| /ŋ/ | ——— | ——— | ——— | ——— | ——— | ——— | ——— |

jungle, finger, king, song, bang, jungle king, hurt finger, sing a song, bang a drum

Comments:

Vowel Stimulability

Phoneme	Sound Level	Word Level	Phrase Level
/a/	———	———	———

on, hot, dog, offer, stop, father, eat hot dogs, stop the car

Comments:

| /i/ | ——— | ——— | ——— |

me, eat, feet, keep, leaf, bean, eat the bean, feel your feet

Comments:

| /ɪ/ | ——— | ——— | ——— |

in, pin, pick, fit, lip, pickle, in a pickle, clip the pin

Comments:

Phoneme	Sound Level	Word Level	Phrase Level
/ɛ/	_____	_____	_____

end, pen, enter, best, step, better, enter the pet store, step to the west

Comments:

/e/	_____	_____	_____

lake, maybe, wait, delay, vacation, vacation at the lake, maybe I will wait

Comments:

/æ/	_____	_____	_____

at, cat, ran, pack, after, cabin, family, at the cabin, ran after the cat

Comments:

/ə/	_____	_____	_____

hiccup, begun, enough, untie, untie the rope, enough hiccups

Comments:

/ʌ/	_____	_____	_____

up, cup, under, fun, love, tough, butter, come up here, under the butter

Comments:

/u/	_____	_____	_____

you, shoe, boot, cool, new, new shoes and boots, you are cool

Comments:

(continues)

Speech Sound Stimulability Assessment Protocol (continued)

Phoneme	Sound Level	Word Level	Phrase Level
/ʊ/	_____	_____	_____
book, put, hook, pull, bullet, cookie, put the book away, pull the hook			
Comments:			
/o/	_____	_____	_____
no, nose, go, bone, hope, boat, don't go home, I hope the boat floats			
Comments:			
/ɔ/	_____	_____	_____
caught, bought, fawn, fought, he bought it, she caught the fawn			
Comments:			
/ɝ/	_____	_____	_____
her, girl, bird, turtle, shirt, purple, her bird is a girl, a purple shirt			
Comments:			
/ɚ/	_____	_____	_____
better, hotter, enter, bother, mother, color, the burger was hotter, mother and father are better			
Comments:			

Speech Sound Assessment Protocol 8
Childhood Apraxia of Speech Assessment Protocol

Child's Name _____ DOB _____ Date _____ Clinician _____

Individualize this protocol on the CD and print it for your use.

This list contains common features of childhood apraxia of speech. Use the results of the orofacial examination, diadochokinetic tasks, speech sample, and standardized tests to identify any or all of the features listed. Take note of features you find in a child that are not listed here. The presence of several of these characteristics would support the diagnosis of childhood apraxia of speech.

☐ significantly reduced speech intelligibility

☐ inconsistent errors

   • correct production of sounds in some contexts but not in others

   • speech sound production and intelligibility at the word level much better than in spontaneous speech

☐ articulation breaks down with increases in the length and complexity of utterances

☐ sound or syllable transpositions

☐ prolongations, distortions, additions, or repetitions of sounds or syllables

☐ addition of syllables to polysyllabic words, omissions of syllables, or revisions

☐ numerous and varied off target attempts at producing a word or utterance

☐ marked difficulty initiating speech

☐ abnormal prosodic features: slower than normal speech rate, abnormal stress patterns, unusual pauses

☐ automatic speech acts less effortful and with fewer speech errors than purposeful speech

☐ groping or searching behaviors noted during the orofacial examination or during attempts to produce purposeful speech

   • normal automatic oral movements (i.e., a spontaneous smile or licking the lips)

   • absence of the same movements when *asked* to perform (possible oral apraxia)

☐ receptive language skills better than expressive language skills

Speech Sound Assessment Protocol 9
Dysarthric Speech Assessment Protocol

Child's Name _____ DOB _____ Date _____ Clinician _____

Individualize this protocol on the CD and print it for your use.

Use the results of the case history, orofacial examination, speech sample, standardized tests, and child voice evaluation to identify any or all of the characteristics listed below. Take note of features you find in a child that are not listed here. The presence of a number of these characteristics would support the diagnosis of dysarthric speech in a child.

☐ The child has been diagnosed with a neurologic disease or disorder. What is the diagnosis?

☐ The child has been diagnosed with Cerebral Palsy. (circle)

    spastic   athetoid   ataxic   rigid   mixed

☐ muscle weakness or incoordination noted during the orofacial examination

☐ imprecise articulation resulting in "slurred speech"

☐ articulation errors noted during standardized tests and the speech sample

☐ speech errors are more noticeable in connected speech than in single-word productions

☐ a predominance of omissions over substitutions or distortions

☐ phonological processes noted: (circle)

    cluster reduction   stopping   depalatalization   fronting   gliding

☐ respiration problems noted: (circle)

    decreased phonation time secondary to air wastage   poor breath support

☐ abnormal prosody noted: (circle)

    monotone   monoloudness   general dysprosody

☐ voice problems noted: (circle)

    weak voice   reduced intensity   poor loudness control   breathiness
    excessive high pitch   strained

☐ resonance problems noted: (circle)

    hypernasality   nasal emission   assimilation nasality

Selected Multicultural Assessment Protocols

Most typical assessment procedures, including the case history, orofacial examination, hearing screening, and collection of a speech-language sample are necessary to assess all children, including those who are ethnoculturally diverse. However, if the child belongs to an ethnocultural minority group, it is essential to take into consideration the child and the family's cultural and linguistic background during assessment. The interview will concentrate on the family's cultural and linguistic variables that affect the child's communication patterns. The child's bilingual status, if any, will be determined. Standardized tests may or may not be administered; but the speech sample will be analyzed strictly in the context of the child's first language or the child's unique English dialect (e.g., the African American English). See Chapter 4 for more information on assessing children of ethnocultural diversity.

On the following pages, three protocols are provided for assessing speech sound production skills in African American children, Asian American children, and Hispanic children. If a child assessed belongs to one of these minority ethnocultural group, the clinician may select the appropriate protocol, complete it, and attach it to the rest of the assessment protocols used, the case history form completed, and the assessment report.

Speech Sound Assessment Protocol 10
African American English: Speech Sound Assessment Protocol

Child's Name _____ DOB _____ Date _____ Clinician _____

Individualize this protocol on the CD and print it for your use.

Analyze the child's recorded speech-language sample. Check *Yes* if the African American English feature is observed; write phonetically transcribed examples in the column provided. Take note of unique features not listed in the protocol.

AAE Speech Characteristics		If *Yes*, Give Examples from the Child's Speech
Vowel changes	Reduction of the diphthong /aʊ/ to single vowel (e.g., "at" for *out*)	☐ Yes ☐ No
	Reduction of /ɔɪ/ to single vowel in (e.g., "all" for *oil*)	☐ Yes ☐ No
	Reduction of /aɪ/ to single vowel in (e.g., "ass" for *ice*)	☐ Yes ☐ No
Omission or weak production of consonants	Final /l/ (e.g., "too" for *tool*) Medial /l/ (e.g., "a'ways" for *always*)	☐ Yes ☐ No
	Final /d/ (e.g., "ba" for *bad* and "goo" for *good*)	☐ Yes ☐ No
	Final /r/ (e.g., "doah" for *door* or "mudah" for *mother*)	☐ Yes ☐ No
	Final /m/ (e.g., "hæ" for *ham*)	☐ Yes ☐ No
	Other consonant omissions or weak productions noted; give examples (likely omissions: /b/, /p/, /g/, /k/, /n/, and /v/)	☐ Yes ☐ No
Substitution of consonants	/d/ for initial and medial /ð/ (e.g., "dis" for *this*; "broder" for *brother*)	☐ Yes ☐ No
	/v/ for final /ð/ (e.g., "smoov" for *smooth*)	☐ Yes ☐ No
	/t/ for initial /θ/ (e.g., "tin" for *thin*) or /f/ for final /θ/ "teef" for *teeth*)	☐ Yes ☐ No
	/b/ for initial /v/ (e.g., "balentine" for *valentine*)	☐ Yes ☐ No
	/n/ for final /ŋ/ in unstressed syllables (e.g., "son" for *song*)	☐ Yes ☐ No

AAE Speech Characteristics		If *Yes*, Give Examples from the Child's Speech	
Consonant cluster reduction	-sk reduced to /s/ (e.g., "des" for *desk)*	☐ Yes	☐ No
	-ft reduced to /f/ (e.g., "lef" for *left)*	☐ Yes	☐ No
	-st reduced to /s/ (e.g., "tes" for *test)*	☐ Yes	☐ No
	-kst reduced to *ks* (e.g., "neks" for *next)*	☐ Yes	☐ No
	-ʃr reduced to a non-English cluster sr (e.g., "srink" for *shrink)*	☐ Yes	☐ No
	-θr-/ reduced to /θ/ (e.g., "thow" for *throw)*	☐ Yes	☐ No
	-nθ reduced to either nf or nt e.g., "tenf" or "tent" for *tenth)*	☐ Yes	☐ No
	-mf reduced to *mp* (e.g., "triump" for *triumph)*	☐ Yes	☐ No
	-nd reduced to /n/ (e.g., "lan" for *land)*	☐ Yes	☐ No
	-ls reduced to /s/ (e.g., "fas" for *false)*	☐ Yes	☐ No
	Other cluster reductions noted; give examples; likely reductions in -lm, -lp, -ld, -lt, -lk, -nd, -kt, and -sp clusters	☐ Yes	☐ No
Unstressed syllable reduction or deletion	Deletion of unstressed vowels (e.g., "way" for *away* or "bout" for *about)*	☐ Yes	☐ No
	Deletion of an unstressed syllable in a preposition or conjunction (e.g., "hind" for *behind* or "cause" for *because)*	☐ Yes	☐ No
Other Features	Sound reversal (e.g., "aks" for *ask)*	☐ Yes	☐ No
	Varied stress patterns (e.g., "**po**lice" instead of *police* or "**De**troit" for *Detroit)*	☐ Yes	☐ No
	Relatively low fundamental frequency of voice	☐ Yes	☐ No

(continues)

African American English: Speech Sound Assessment Protocol (continued)

AAE Speech Characteristics		If *Yes*, Give Examples from the Child's Speech	
Other Features *(continued)*	Relatively high pitch variations	☐ Yes	☐ No
	Rising pitch contours	☐ Yes	☐ No
	Falling pitch contours on questions	☐ Yes	☐ No

Diagnostic Criteria: African American English features observed in the child's speech are not a basis to diagnose an articulation or phonological disorder. Deviations must be observed in features *not typical of AAE* to justify the diagnosis.

Speech Sound Assessment Protocol 11
Asian American English: Speech Sound Assessment Protocol

Child's Name _____ DOB _____ Date _____ Clinician _____

Individualize this protocol on the CD and print it for your use.

Analyze the child's recorded speech-language sample. Check *Yes* if the Asian American English feature is observed; write phonetically transcribed examples in the column provided. Take note of unique features not listed in the protocol.

Asian American Speech Characteristics		If *Yes*, Give Examples from the Child's Speech
Vowel changes	Deletion of syllables in polysyllabic words (e.g., "Ephant" for *elephant*)	☐ Yes ☐ No
	Truncated vowels (causing choppiness of speech)	☐ Yes ☐ No
	/ɑ/ for /æ/ (e.g., "block" for *black*)	☐ Yes ☐ No
	/i/ for /ʌ/ (e.g., "evin" for *even*)	☐ Yes ☐ No
	/ɑ/ for /ɔ/ (e.g., "ail" for *oil*)	☐ Yes ☐ No
Omission of sounds	Many final consonants. (e.g., "sha" for *shop* or "be" for *bet*)	☐ Yes ☐ No
	Initial /h/ (e.g., "Ouse" for *house*)	☐ Yes ☐ No
	/r/ in clusters (e.g., "gull" for *girl* or "tone" for *torn*)	☐ Yes ☐ No
Substitution of sounds	/l/ for /r/ (e.g., "lize" for *rise*)	☐ Yes ☐ No
	/r/ for /l/ (e.g., "raundry" for *laundry*)	☐ Yes ☐ No
	/ʃ/ for /tʃ/ (e.g., "sheep" for *cheap*)	☐ Yes ☐ No
	/s/ for /ʃ/ (e.g., "sine" for *shine*)	☐ Yes ☐ No
	/b/ for /v/ (e.g., "base" for *vase*)	☐ Yes ☐ No

(continues)

Asian American English: Speech Sound Assessment Protocol (continued)

Asian American Speech Characteristics		If *Yes*, Give Examples from the Child's Speech
Substitution of sounds (continued)	/v/ for /w/ (e.g., "vater" for *water*)	☐ Yes ☐ No
	/p/ for /f/ (e.g., "pall" for *fall*)	☐ Yes ☐ No
	/a/ for /æ/ (e.g., "block" for *black*)	☐ Yes ☐ No
	/d/ for /ð/ (e.g., "dose" for *those*)	☐ Yes ☐ No
	/t/ for /θ / (e.g., "tin" for *thin*)	☐ Yes ☐ No
	/dʒ/ for /z/ (e.g., "jipper" for *zipper*)	☐ Yes ☐ No
	A non-English retroflex for /l/ (e.g., a retroflex for /l/ in *Paul*)	☐ Yes ☐ No
	Voiceless cognates for voiced sounds (e.g., "Fresno" for *Frezno*)	☐ Yes ☐ No
Addition	Insertion of schwa within a cluster (e.g., "səpoon" for spoon)	☐ Yes ☐ No

Diagnostic Criteria: These and other speech characteristics are not a basis to diagnose an articulation or phonological disorder in bilingual Asian American children. To diagnose a disorder in English, children should exhibit deviations other than what is typical of bilingual-Asian American children. Because of variations in Asian languages, each child's particular phonological characteristics need to be understood.

Speech Sound Assessment Protocol 12
Spanish-Influenced English: Speech Sound Assessment Protocol

Child's Name _____ DOB _____ Date _____ Clinician _____

Individualize this protocol on the CD and print it for your use.

Analyze the child's recorded speech-language sample. Check *Yes* if the Spanish-influenced English feature is observed; write phonetically transcribed examples in the column provided. Take note of unique features not listed in the protocol.

Spanish-Influenced English Characteristics		If *Yes*, Give Examples from the Child's Speech
Vowel Changes	/i/ for /ɪ/ (e.g., "peeg" for *pig*)	☐ Yes ☐ No
	/ɛ/ for /æ/ (e.g., "pet" for *Pat*)	☐ Yes ☐ No
	ah for /æ/ (e.g., "Cahn" for *can*)	☐ Yes ☐ No
Substitutions of consonants	/b/ for /v/ (e.g., "Boice" for *voice*)	☐ Yes ☐ No
	/tʃ/ for /ʃ/ (e.g., "Cheep" for *sheep*)	☐ Yes ☐ No
	/d/ for /ð/ (e.g., "Dose" for *those*)	☐ Yes ☐ No
	/z/ for /ð/ (e.g., "Zat" for *that*)	☐ Yes ☐ No
	/t/ for /θ/ (e.g., "Tin" for *thin*)	☐ Yes ☐ No
	/j/ for /dʒ/ (e.g., "Yune" for *June*)	☐ Yes ☐ No
	/ŋ/ for /n/ (e.g., "Tang" for *tan*)	☐ Yes ☐ No
	Voiceless finals for voiced finals (e.g., "mase" for *maze*)	☐ Yes ☐ No

(continues)

Spanish-Influenced English: Speech Sound Assessment Protocol (continued)

Spanish-Influenced English Characteristics		If *Yes*, Give Examples from the Child's Speech
Omission of sounds	Many final consonants except for /a/, /e/, /i/, /o/, /u/, /l/, /r/, /n/, /s/, and /d/ that end words in Spanish.	☐ Yes ☐ No
	Omission of /h/ in the initial positions (e.g., "ouse" for *house*)	☐ Yes ☐ No
Different manner of productions	More frontal production of /s/ (lisp-like)	☐ Yes ☐ No
	Dentalized production of /t/, /d/, and /n/	☐ Yes ☐ No
	Deaspiration of stops (causing weak productions)	☐ Yes ☐ No
	Trilled production of /r/	☐ Yes ☐ No
Addition of sound	Insertion of a schwa at the beginning of initial consonant clusters (e.g., "ʌschool" for *school*)	☐ Yes ☐ No
	Trapped or trilled /r/	☐ Yes ☐ No
	Silent /h/ in initial positions (e.g., "old" for *hold* or "it" for *hit*)	☐ Yes ☐ No

Diagnostic Criteria: These and other speech characteristics are not a basis to diagnose in articulation or phonological disorder in children whose English is influenced by their Spanish. To diagnose such a disorder, the child's speech should deviate in other respects. Because a variety of Spanish dialects influence English, it is essential to understand the particular variety that affects the speech of a Spanish-English bilingual child.

PART III

Assessment of Language Skills in Children

CHAPTER 8

Assessment of Language Skills in Children: Resources

- Overview of Language
- Overview of Verbal Behavior
- Prevalence of Child Language Disorders
- Overview of Child Language Disorders
- Clinical Conditions Associated with Language Disorders
- Specific Language Impairment
- Factors Related to Language Disorders
- Overview of Assessment of Child Language Disorders
- Screening for Language Disorders
- Language Sampling
- Integrating Alternative Assessment Techniques
- Assessment of Language Understanding
- Assessment of Other Aspects of Communication
- Standardized Language Diagnostic Tests
- Assessment of Language Skills in Ethnoculturally Diverse Children
- Analysis and Integration of Assessment Results
- Differential Diagnosis of Child Language Disorders
- Postassessment Counseling

Assessment and treatment of language disorders in children are a major responsibility of speech-language pathologists working in most professional settings. To make an adequate assessment that serves as a basis for treatment planning and execution, clinicians need a good understanding of not only what language disorders are, but also of the concept of language or verbal behavior, its normal course of acquisition, and its functional analysis. It is only by assessing all aspects of this verbal skill that a speech-language pathologist can determine whether a child has a language disorder (Hegde & Maul, 2006).

Ethnocultural considerations are especially important in assessing verbal skills in children. Whether the child is bilingual and speaks English as a second language will influence the selection of assessment instruments and analysis of results. A bilingual child's primary language is important to consider, as it may influence the acquisition and production of English (or any other second language). Similarly, whether the child speaks another form of English (e.g., African American English), another dialect of English (e.g., Southern, Eastern, or Appalachian) needs to be considered as well. Many standardized tests used to evaluate mainstream children may not be valid for assessing verbal skills of ethnoculturally diverse children. In assessing such children, the clinician needs to use alternative approaches (see Chapters 4 and 5) that are more valid and lead to ethnoculturally appropriate clinical decisions.

In this chapter, we offer an overview of language and verbal behavior, the different skills that need to be assessed, and disorders of language in children. The chapter also describes the various assessment approaches, including several alternatives to the commonly used standardized test-based approach. We also present an integrated assessment model that draws on the strengths of the traditional and some newer, alternative approaches. In the next chapter, we provide the necessary assessment protocols that the clinicians may use to evaluate and diagnose language disorders in children.

Overview of Language

Linguistics defines **language** as an arbitrary system of codes and symbols that people use to express thoughts, ideas, and experiences. Across cultures and societies, languages are thought to have different sets of symbols or codes that represent external events and objects and internal (subjective) ideas, emotions, and other kinds of experiences. Selection of these symbols or codes is thought to be arbitrary because the same object, event, or experience is represented by different sets of symbols (words, in a simple sense) in different languages (McLaughlin, 2006; Owens, 2012; Pence & Justice, 2012).

In each language, symbols or codes, are organized and sequenced. Linguists derive rules from these patterns of organization and sequence found in each language. *Phonetic* or *phonemic rules* help sequence sounds to create words; *morphologic rules* help modify the meaning of words by adding other elements to them (e.g., inflections, prefixes, and suffixes); *syntactic rules* dictate how words may be arranged into phrases and sentences; and *pragmatic rules* govern the social conventions of language expression (Gerken, 2009; McLaughlin, 2006). Although rules that help combine elements of language into socially acceptable forms of expression exist in all languages, specific rules that govern phonetic sequences, word order, and sentence structure may be unique to each language. Therefore, it is important to understand the specific rules of a given language that is being assessed in a child. To assess a bilingual child or a child who speaks another form of English, the clinicians needs a knowledge of rules and social conventions of different languages or different forms of the same language the child speaks.

Within the linguistic approach, language is divided into *phonologic, semantic, syntactic, morphologic,* and *pragmatic* components or aspects (Huilit, Howard, & Fahey, 2011; McLaughlin, 2006). From a clinical and academic standpoint, the components may be considered different sets of language skills. A skill-oriented description of language (especially the behavioral analysis of language described in a later section) is especially useful to teachers and clinicians who teach *language* to children. Skills are observable, measurable, and teachable. A component of a language is not directly observed, measured, and taught; it comprises a theoretically static view of language.

In addition to the different components of language, speech-language pathologists, perhaps more so than linguists, also describe language in terms of two main *modalities,* which are the manners in which language is experienced: *production* and *comprehension.* We describe the distinction in a later section.

Speech Production Skills

Language is a broader concept that includes the speech sound production skills. The linguistic study of patterns of speech sound production is known as *phonology.* As noted before and similar to other aspects of language, linguists have derived rules from phonologic regularities found in children's and adults' speech production (Peña-Brooks & Hegde, 2007).

Although technically, normal speech sound production skills (and their disorders by implication) are a part of language and language disorders, clinicians assess and treat speech sound disorders and language disorders separately, mainly because of clinical convenience and analytic practicality. In assessment and treatment, it is convenient to concentrate on speech sound disorders (including articulation and phonological disorders) or language disorders, even when they coexist in a child. Therefore, we have addressed the resources and protocols for assessing speech production skills and speech sound disorders in Chapters 6 and 7. In this chapter, we concentrate on semantic, morphologic, syntactic, and pragmatic language skills of children and disorders therein that need to be assessed.

Semantic Skills

Semantics is the study of meaning (Berko, Gleason & Ratner, 2009; McLaughlin, 2006). Words and word meanings are a basic unit of the *semantic component* of language. Clinicians assess or estimate the number of words (*lexicon* or *vocabulary)* a child produces and understands. Words and word meanings in most languages may be categorized as *simple (concrete), complex, multiple, abstract,* or *figurative.* Children master the more concrete and simple meanings of words before they master the multiple, complex, and figurative meanings. Children with severe language disorders may fail to acquire even the simple and concrete words. Most children with language disorders tend to have difficulty understanding and producing the complex and the abstract meaning of words, phrases, and sentences. Difficulty with abstract and metaphoric language may be a prominent characteristic of older children and adolescents who have a language disorder (Nippold, 2007).

The different kinds of meanings children seem to learn are described as **semantic relations**, which are contrasting units of meaning that are expressed in different forms of words, phrases, and sentences. Table 8–1 lists semantic relations found in two-word utterances of 2-year-old children.

In assessing the semantic skills in children, clinicians sample the kinds of words the child produces, the different kinds of semantic relations that become evident in the child's language sample, and whether the child can understand and produce utterances that signal different kinds of meaning. Two classic studies (Benedict, 1979; Nelson, 1973) have offered some data on the initial 50 or more words that children typically produce. According to these two studies, the initial words children produce belong to the following categories (the range reflects the difference between the two studies):

- General nominals: 51 to 51%
- Specific nominals: 11 to 14%
- Action words: 14 to 19%

Table 8–1. Semantic Relations and Children's Two-Word Utterances

Semantic Relation	Linguistic Structures	Example of Two-Word Utterance	Meaning, Suggested by Context
Nomination	Demonstrative + Noun	*That baby!*	*That is a baby.*
Nonexistence	Negative + Noun	*No kitty*	*There is no kitty here.*
Agent-object	Noun + Noun	*Doggie food*	*The dog is eating his food.*
Agent-action	Noun + Verb	*Daddy sleep*	*Daddy is sleeping.*
Action-object	Verb + Noun	*Kick ball*	*Let's kick the ball!*
Action-indirect object	Verb + Noun	*Drink baby*	*Give baby a drink.*
Action-locative	Verb + Noun *or* Verb + Locative	*Go home* *Jump here!*	*Let's go home.* *Jump right here!*
Possessor-possession	Noun + Noun	*Mommy hat*	*That is Mommy's hat.*
Entity-locative	Noun + Noun *or* Noun + Locative	*Horsie barn* *Granma here!*	*The horse is in the barn.* *Grandma is here!*
Entity-attribution	Noun + Adjective *or* Adjective + Noun	*Dolly pretty* *Pretty dolly*	*The dolly is pretty.*
Recurrence	Adjective (*more or another*) + Noun	*More milk!*	*I want more milk!*
Rejection	Negative + Noun	*No milk!*	*I don't want milk!*
Conjunction	Noun + Noun	*Shoes socks!*	*I need my shoes and socks.*

Source: Compiled from Bloom (1970), Bloom and Lahey (1978), Brown (1973), and Schlesinger (1971).]

- Modifiers: 9 to 10%
- Personal-social: 9 to 10%

The two studies (Benedict, 1979; Nelson, 1973) generally agree on the categories and their percentages in the total vocabulary. However, the clinicians need to interpret these data with caution as the young children of the 21st century may have a different distribution of words and the child from ethnoculturally different backgrounds may differ still more. With these caveats in perspective, the clinician may use the *Task-Specific Assessment Protocol for Basic Vocabulary* given in Chapter 9 to evaluate the first few functional words a child does or does not produce. It would be interesting if the clinician wrote down words not on the protocol to understand differences among children and from the classic study results.

In assessing the semantic skills of older children and adolescents, the clinician targets additional skills that include comprehension and production of figurative language, abstract academic language, and advanced discourse and discussion skills (Nippold, 2007). Some of the standardized tests of language described in a later section are useful in assessing these skills.

Morphologic Skills

Assessment of morphologic skills is especially important because deficiencies in those skills are a diagnostic marker of language disorders in children. A part of grammar, **morphology** is the study of different word structures that signal differences in meaning. A *morpheme* is the smallest element of grammar and meaning. Morphemes may be words or such smaller grammatic units as prefixes, suffixes, inflections, and such other elements as articles, prepositions, the present progressive-*ing*, and so forth. Morphemes that are smaller than words are sometimes referred to as *grammatic morphemes*. Bound morphemes (prefixes and suffixes) are attached to free morphemes (words). Table 8–2 presents a list of most common grammatic morphemes, their rank order of acquisition, and the age of mastery.

There is a rough sequence in which most children seem to acquire the various morphologic features. The sequence presented in Table 8–2 is based mostly on Brown's (1973) longitudinal study of early language acquisition in three children. Additional data from deVilliers and deVilliers (1973) had shown some differences in rank ordering of morphologic acquisition. The ranking should not be taken too literally; they are only broad guidelines, and individual differences will be marked.

An assessment of morphologic production in children is completed with an analysis of the *mean length of utterance.* As an index of language development in children, it is more useful with younger children than with older children. A language sample may be used to calculate the mean length of utterance by counting the number of morphemes in a language sample, the clinician should follow the rules given in Table 8–3.

The results may be compared against norms, presented in Table 8–4. The clinicians should exercise caution in such comparisons as the normative data are obtained on small samples and most likely do not apply to children of ethnocultural diversity.

Morphologic skills may be assessed through standardized tests described in a later section. The clinicians also may use the *Task-Specific Assessment Protocol for Grammatic Morphemes* given in Chapter 9.

Table 8–2. Rank Order of Acquisition and the Typical Age of Mastery of Selected Grammatic Morphemes

Rank Order	Morpheme/Example	Age of Mastery in Months
1	Present progressive -ing walking, talking	19–28
2/3	Prepositions in and on Cookie in bag; Kitty on table	27–30
4	Regular plural allomorphs My books; Give me dolls	27–33
5	Irregular past tense My car is broke; he went	25–46
6	Possessive allomorphs Daddy's hat; Jenny's car	26–40
7	Copula (uncontractible) He is; This was	27–39
8	Articles a and the I see a kitty; Give me the pen	28–46
9	Regular past tense allomorphs I walked; she pulled me; he painted	26–48
10	Third person, present tense regular Daddy walks, he shows	26–46
11	Third persons, present tense irregular He does it; she has it	28–50
12	Auxiliary (uncontractible) He is!; She was	29–48
13	Copula (contractible) She's nice; She is nice	29–49
14	Auxiliary (contractible) Mommy's cooking; Mommy is cooking	30–50

Note: The ranking is mainly from Brown's (1973) study; note that ranked morphemes overlap in the age of mastery and the mastery is achieved over a wide range of months, suggesting significant individual differences; Be cautious about predicting the age of mastery for any morphemes in an individual child.

Syntactic Skills

Syntax is a collection of rules that specify how word combinations and sentences may be formed in a language. A basic syntactic rule, for example, is that a complete sentence must include a *noun* (or *subject*) and a *verb*. All languages have syntactic rules, although some may be unique to given languages (Chomsky, 1957, 1965).

Table 8–3. Rules for Counting Morphemes in Language Samples

Do count:

- each free morpheme (a word with no prefixes, suffixes, or grammatic markers) as **one**
- each bound morpheme (e.g., *-ing,-ed*, plural *s*, possessive s) as **one**
- contracted words as **two** (the word counts as one and the contractive morpheme as one, so a word such as *you're* is counted as two morphemes)
- compound words as **one** (e.g., sidewalk, outdoors, birthday)
- *catenatives* such as *gonna, wanna, hafta* as **one**
- irregular plural forms as **one** (e.g., *feet, mice*)
- irregular verb forms as **one** (e.g., *ate, threw, went*)
- gerunds (verb forms that function as nouns, e.g., ***Running** is my favorite exercise!*) as **one**
- names of persons, places, or titles of books or movies as **one** (e.g., *Aunt Mary, Goldilocks and the Three Bears, Peter Piper's Pizza Place*)
- words that are ritualistically repeated as **one** (e.g., *bye-bye* is counted as one)

Don't count:

- frequently used interjections such as "you know" or "um"
- words used in false starts leading to revisions ("**I went to the**—Mom took me to the store")
- words that are repeated as dysfluencies; count only the final production (e.g., "I-I-I-I go to school" is counted as four, not seven)
- utterances that are unintelligible
- utterances that are imitations of adult models
- utterances that are incomplete
- rote utterances (e.g., recited nursery rhymes, dialogue from T.V. commercials)

Source: Compiled from Brown (1973) and Owens (2004).

The terms *syntax* and *grammar* should be distinguished. Being a broader term, grammar includes syntax as well as morphologic features of language. Syntactic rules help formulate acceptable sentences by creatively combining words whereas morphologic rules help modulate meanings of words, phrases, and sentences.

Assessment of language disorders in children requires an analysis of their syntactic skills. In fact, deficiencies in syntactic and morphologic skills are a hallmark of language disorders. Clinicians who evaluate bilingual or bidialectal children need to make the analysis in light of the specific rules of the child's language, languages, or dialects. See Chapters 4 and 5 for additional information on assessing children of ethnocultural diversity who often tend to be bilingual or bidialectal.

Table 8–4. Normative Data on Mean Length of Utterance

Age in Months	Range of MLU
18	1.0–1.6
21	1.1–2.1
24	1.5–2.2
27	1.9–2.4
30	2.0–3.1
33	2.2–3.5
36	2.5–3.9
39	2.7–4.2
42	3.0–4.6
45	3.2–5.0
48	3.5–5.3
51	3.7–5.7
54	3.8–6.1
57	3.9–6.5
60	4.0–6.8

Source: Data based on studies by Brown (1973), Miller (1981), and Miller and Chapman (1981).]

Cautionary note: These data should not be used to predict or evaluate the MLU of a given child; the data are based on extremely small, nonrepresentative, samples; for some age groups, speech may have been sampled from fewer than 10 children. Data probably do not apply to children of different ethnocultural backgrounds. MLU norms are not discriminative after age 3 years.

Children acquire most of the syntactic rules of their native language by the time they enter the first grade (McLaughlin, 2006; Owens, 2012). Table 8–5 presents some of the available normative data on the acquisition of major syntactic structures.

Clinicians may assess syntactic skills through language samples, standardized tests, or selected alternative approaches that have ethnocultural validity. The *Language Sample Analysis Protocol: Syntactic, Morphologic, and Pragmatic Skills*, included in Chapter 9, allows for a comprehensive analysis of language skills, including syntactic skills. Syntactic skills also may be assessed through standardized language tests described in a later section.

Pragmatic Skills

Language is a form of social behavior and social communication is the essence of it. The study of language as produced in social contexts is called **pragmatics**. Pragmatic language skills include all the skills associated with social interactions, including narration

Table 8–5. Acquisition of Major Syntactic Structures Within Brown's Stages of Language Acquisition

Stages and Skills	Age and MLU
I (Early) Declarative forms agent + action; agent + object Negative *no, all gone,* and *gone; negative* + X Interrogative *what* and *where; yes/no* with rising intonation Naming in a series, but without a conjunction Requests with *more, want, mine*	12–22 months 1–1.5 MLU
I (Late) Declarative forms subject + verb + object Negative *no* and *not* used interchangeably Interrogative that + X; *what* + noun + verb; *where* + noun + verb Preposition *in* and *on* Conjunction *and*	22–26 months 1.5–2 MLU
II (Early) Declarative forms subject + copula + complement or adjective	27–28 months 2–2.25 MLU
II (Late) Declarative forms subject + verb + object used more frequently and by most children Negative forms *no, not, don't,* and *can't* used interchangeably Interrogative *what* or *where* + subject + predicate; *what* or *where* + copula + subject Embedded *gonna, wanna, gotta*	28–30 months 2.25–2.5 MLU
III (Early) Declarative forms subject + auxiliary + verb + object; auxiliary *can, do, have, will,* and *be* Conjunctions *but, so, or,* and *if*	31–32 months 2.5–2.75 MLU
III (Late) Declarative forms subject + auxiliary + copula + X Negative *won't* Interrogative *do, can,* and *will* in questions; inversion of subject and auxiliary verb in *yes/no* questions	33–34 months 2.75–3 MLU
IV (Early) Negative form subject + auxiliary + negative + verb Interrogative wh-questions with inversion of auxiliary verb and subject; embedded wh-questions Embedded object-noun phrase complements with *think, guess,* and *show* Conjunction *because;* possibly, clausal conjoining with *and*	35–37 months 3–3.5 (MLU)
IV (Late) Declarative double auxiliary forms auxiliary + auxiliary + verb + X Negative *isn't, aren't, doesn't,* and *didn't* Interrogatives *when* and *how;* inverted copula and subject in *yes/no* questions; addition of *do* to *yes/no* questions Embedded infinite phrases at the end of sentences	38–40 months 3.5–3.75 (MLU)

(continues)

Table 8–5. *(continued)*

Stages and Skills	Age and MLU

V
    Declarative form subject + auxiliary + verb + indirect object
    Negative *wasn't, couldn't,* and *shouldn't*; subject + copula + negative
    Interrogative modals; more frequent production of inverted auxiliary; tag-questions
    Embedded relative clauses in object position; multiple embedding toward the end of the stage
    Conjunction *if* and three-clause declaratives
	41–46 months
	3.75–4.5 MLU

Post-V
    Negative indefinite forms *nobody, no one, none,* and *nothing*; problems with double negatives
    Negative interrogatives after age 5
    Embedded gerunds, relative clauses attached to the subject, embedding and conjoining within the same sentence when MLU reaches or exceeds 5
    Causal conjunction *because* with *when, but,* and *so* after the MLU exceeds 5
	47 + months
	4.5 + MLU

Note: Unless specified otherwise, the norms refer to the age at which a syntactic form is thought to be observed for the first time or initially produced by about 50% of children. There may be overlaps in skill acquisition across stages. Individual differences are known to be significant. Therefore, the stages and ages of skill acquisition may only be gross approximations and cannot always predict skill acquisition in individual children.

and conversation. Pragmatic skills, because they refer to interactions between two or more individuals in social contexts, are different from the semantic, syntactic, and morphologic skills. Though still structurally oriented with no particular regard for functional (cause-effect) units of language, the pragmatic view avoids an analysis of language as a mental system in an idealized speaker: a basic weakness of Chomskyan syntactic view of language.

Generally, *verbal pragmatic skills* are those that help initiate and sustain conversation and narration and include:

- Topic initiation (initiating conversational exchanges)

- Turn-taking (playing the alternating roles of speaker and listener during conversation)

- Topic maintenance (sustaining conversation on an initiated topic for socially appropriate durations; avoiding abrupt or inappropriate shifts in topics of discourse)

- Topic shifts (changing the topic of conversation at appropriate times; avoiding abnormal persistence of a topic that may lead to loss of communication)

- Conversational repair (making various kinds of requests that help get an unclear message clarified or making helpful modifications in one's own speech when someone fails to understand what is being said)

- Social appropriateness of language (producing language that is appropriate to context and situation)

- Narration (telling stories and describing experiences and events in a coherent, logical, and temporally consistent manner, offering sufficient details and substance)

- Listener-appropriate speech (modifying speech style to suit the listener; for example, speech appropriate to a child may not be appropriate to an adult).

Nonverbal pragmatic language skills are various physical, emotional, and gestural aspects of communication that supplement, expand, or even contradict what is said in words; popularly called "body language," they include:

- Maintenance of eye contact

- Acceptable physical distance maintained during communication (*proxemics*)

- Gestures and facial expressions.

Pragmatic language skills are heavily influenced by cultural factors. Maintenance of eye contact, physical distance between speakers, and the amount and intensity of gestures and facial expressions vary across cultures. Therefore, in assessing an ethnoculturally diverse child, clinicians should first investigate what is accepted or not in the child's culture before making diagnostic decisions.

Although such advanced pragmatic language skills as narration and storytelling are mastered during later childhood years (school-age), even infants and preschoolers exhibit various social communication skills. For instance, an infant turns toward the direction from which the mother's voice is heard; establishes eye contact, and nonverbally evokes speech by smiles and other gestures. As the child's language skills improve, conversational skills, including topic initiation through verbal means, topic maintenance, turn-taking, conversational repair, and other skills are also learned and mastered (McLaughlin, 2006; Owens, 2012). Table 8–6 presents a summary of pragmatic language learning in children.

Clinicians may assess pragmatic language skills through some of the standardized tests described in a later section. The clinicians also may use the *Task-Specific Assessment Protocol for Conversational Skills* given in Chapter 9.

Comprehension and Production

Often described as two modalities of speech, *comprehension* is also known as *receptive language* and production as *expressive language*. **Comprehension** is evident when the responses to verbal stimuli are appropriate; it is inferred from the listener's verbal and nonverbal behavior because it is not as directly observed as production of language. A lack of comprehension is inferred when a verbal stimulus evokes a wrong verbal response, a wrong gesture, or an inappropriate behavior.

Typically, adults who speak a language can understand it, but children on occasion produce utterances they do not understand (McLaughlin, 2006). Generally, young children who are still learning their language comprehend more than they produce; they can give appropriate nonverbal responses to verbal stimuli that they themselves cannot produce.

Table 8–6. Acquisition of Pragmatic Language Skills

Pragmatic Language Skill	Age
Most pragmatic skills are difficult for the very young preschooler; many preschoolers introduce topics but their narratives are simple and brief; may take two or more conversational turns; may show better turn-taking with mothers; may repeat when the listener fails to understand or to maintain a topic; may request clarification nonverbally (e.g., confused look) or just by "what?"; difficulty with contingent and connected speech; utterances may be unrelated to conversational partners' previous utterance. Boys tend to say *no* to prohibit some one's action, and girls to deny or reject. Four-year-olds can assume roles and talk in different registers (e.g., talking like the mother; louder voice for male roles and softer voice for female roles).	Preschoolers
About 50% of 5-year olds introduce topics and sustain conversation through 10 or 12 turns; produce mostly personal narratives; sequences of narratives improve, but may lack character or main theme; may begin to produce different forms of narratives (e.g., personal, descriptive, fictional) by age 6. In response to request for clarification, repetition still common, but 6-year-olds begin to elaborate. Makes mostly direct requests and commands, but indirect requests may be on the increase by age 6.	5–6 years
Narrates stories with a beginning, a middle plot, an end, and a resolution; maintains conversation on concrete topics; some children understand speakers' intentions; may begin to understand nonliteral meanings in indirect requests; Understands indirect requests and hints; correctly produces most deictic words (e.g., *here, there, this,* and *that*).	7–8 years
Better initiation of topics; much improved conversational turn-taking; may maintain topics through several conversational turns; narratives include major elements of story grammar; senses conversational breakdowns and makes repairs.	9–10 years
Sustains conversation on abstract topics; may begin most narrative sentences with the conjunction *and*.	11–12 years
Understands jokes that involve syntactic ambiguities.	13–15 years
Understands and produces expressions of sarcasm and double meaning; produces metaphors; understands that the conversational partner may have a different perspective than one's own.	16–18 years

Note: Normative age specifications for pragmatic language skills, which are more reliably produced after the preschool years, tend to be less specific than those for morphologic productions; individual differences and cultural influences may be even more marked on the acquisition of pragmatic language skills.

Language comprehension is assessed by the number of correct verbal or nonverbal responses a child gives to commands or during conversation. Comprehension of single words may also be measured by having the child point to picture stimuli the clinician names.

Assessment of Overall Language Development in Children

Case history, interview, and direct observation of the child during the assessment session help assess the overall language development. A concise description of major milestones of language development helps clinicians get a general idea of the child's semantic, syntactic, morphologic, and pragmatic communication skills and their deficits.

To facilitate a quick survey of child's language skills, Chapter 9 offers a *Normal Language Assessment Protocol* that allows the clinician to record the child's major language milestones on a structured form. The form is structured according to different age levels. The clinician can gather information by starting at a level below the child's chronologic age and move down if necessary and move up the age levels to complete the form.

Overview of Verbal Behavior

Concepts of language are linguistic, and those of verbal behavior are behavioral. While linguistics emphasizes structure of communication, behavioral science emphasizes the causal or functional analysis of verbal skills. Speech-language pathologists (SLPs) have traditionally adopted the linguistic view of language. Nonetheless, they use the behavioral methods to treat not only language disorders, but almost all disorders of communication (Barbera, 2007; Cordes & Ingham, 1998; Duffy, 2005; Hegde, 1998; Hegde & Maul, 2006; Onslow, Packman, & Harrison, 2003; Peña-Brooks & Hegde, 2007; Rosenbek, LaPointe, & Wertz, 1989).

The verbal behavior approach, including applied and experimental analysis of behavior, has been marshaling evidence to show that not only behavioral treatment methods, but also the concepts of verbal behavior, offer technical and conceptual advantages to speech-language pathologists. Therefore, it is useful for SLPs to gain a balanced understanding of both the linguistic and behavioral views of language.

Skinner's (1957) description of verbal behavior does not ignore the forms of language, but it emphasizes a causal analysis of what speakers say. As described in greater detail in Chapter 5, a preoccupation with structural units in linguistics has precluded an analysis of the conditions under which people behave verbally and the consequences that maintain those behaviors. When attention is paid to why children and adults say what they say, structures of what they say seem less important in organizing language; the traditional linguistic terms (words, phrases, grammatic or syntactic structures) do not serve well in a causal analysis. Consequently, Skinner invented new terms to describe verbal behaviors.

As described in Chapter 5, a causal analysis results in more efficient classes of primary and secondary verbal behaviors that may be assessed in children. Essentially, primary verbal behaviors include *mands* caused by a state of motivation within the speaker; *tacts* evoked by an environmental event or a more specific stimulus; *echoics* evoked by another person's verbal responses (although there may be self-echoics); and *intraverbals,* evoked by one's own or another person's verbal responses. Secondary verbal behaviors are *autoclitics,* which include the traditional syntactic arrangements and grammatic morphemes. Skinner's analysis includes the audience control, which addresses the role of the listener who evokes speech (Hegde, 2010).

See *Behavioral Assessment* in Chapter 5 for more on verbal operants, their relevance to speech-language pathology, and to understand how they better bridge the gap between the concepts and treatment procedures. In the next chapter, we present a Behavioral Assessment Protocol to evaluate the verbal operants of children with language disorders.

Prevalence of Child Language Disorders

Precise prevalence rates of language disorders in children have been difficult to establish, mostly because of the diverse children in whom they are found. Rates would vary greatly depending on various subgroups that are either included or excluded from a cross-sectional study on prevalence. For instance, a study that includes children with many genetic syndromes, intellectual disabilities, hearing impairment, autism spectrum disorders, certain psychiatric conditions, cerebral palsy and other neurologic impairments, cleft palate and other craniofacial anomalies, and children with specific language impairment can be expected to report a higher prevalence rate than those that exclude some or most of these subgroups. Different studies have looked at different combination of subgroups, resulting in varied estimates of the prevalence of language disorders in children (Hegde & Maul, 2006).

Evaluating clinical records in public schools and other clinical facilities for the number of children receiving services for language disorders has been a standard method of estimating the prevalence of those disorders (Portney & Watkins, 2000; Rothman & Greenland, 1998). According to some available evidence, language disorders are prevalent in 12 to 13% of children. A Canadian study of 1,655 5-year-old children reported a prevalence rate of 12.6% and 4.56% of them also had speech disorders (Beitchman, Nair, Clegg, & Patel, 1986). A U.S. study of 1,502 kindergarten children reported a prevalence rat of 13.58% (Tomblin, Records, & Zhang, 1996). Considering the heterogeneity of children who exhibit language disorders, the reported prevalence rates across the two countries is surprisingly similar.

Prevalence rates of specific language impairment (SLI), a type of language disorder in children who have no other complicating clinical conditions (described in a later section), also are relatively consistent. In one study, SLI was observed in 7.4% of 7, 218 monolingual English-speaking kindergarten children (Tomblin et al., 1996). The differential prevalence of SLI in boys and girls was, respectively, 8% and 6%. Another study also reported an SLI prevalence of 7.5% in kindergarten children (Ruben, 2000). Finally, a study by the National Institutes of Health reported a prevalence rate of 7.6% among 5-year-old children (Ervin, 2001). Therefore, it is generally thought that 7 to 8% of children may have SLI.

If children who have other clinical conditions also are sampled, it is likely that the overall prevalence of language disorders in children will be much higher than either 7 to 8% reported for SLI or 12 to 13% reported for unselected children. No comprehensive figures for all subgroups combined are available.

Overview of Child Language Disorders

The complexity and diversity of language disorders in children have prompted varied definitions of language disorders in children; each has certain limitations. American Speech-language-Hearing Association Ad Hoc Committee on Service Delivery in the

Schools (1993) states that a language disorder is an impairment in understanding and speaking language and in reading and writing as well.

Impairment in understanding spoken language is typically described as either a language comprehension or receptive language problem. Impairment in speaking one's own language is described as an expressive language disorder. Many children with a language disorder tend to have difficulty in both expressive and receptive language (DSM-IV-TR, 2000).

As verbal behavior, language is a means to affect the behavior of others. Therefore, expressive language disorders may also be thought of as ineffective social repertoire; limited language skills fail to affect the behaviors of other persons in social, educational, and occupational milieu. Receptive language disorders may be thought of as a failure to get affected by the verbal behaviors of other persons (Hegde & Maul, 2006). From the standpoint of assessment, a description of the skills that are impaired is essential.

Description of Language Disorders in Children

To assess and treat language disorders in children, most definitions of language disorders need to be translated into a set of observable skills that are lacking in children (Hegde & Maul, 2006). Therefore, a description of the following kind may be more useful than a definition of language disorders:

- *Limited amount of language:* Language disorders almost always imply a limited quantity of language learned, produced, and perhaps comprehended as well. Sparse verbal repertoire is a general feature of language disorders. Early signs of a language disorder include no or limited infant vocalizations, smaller vocabulary, and a slower rate of new-word learning. Later, due to their limited amount of language skills, descriptions of events and personal experiences will be poor, inadequate, or sparse. As the child grows older, limitations in producing and understanding academic and abstract language will be evident, along with deficient literacy skills.

- *Deficient grammar:* Difficulty in learning, comprehending, and producing language with adequate grammatic elements is a crucial diagnostic feature of language disorders in children. Even the child who has learned a sufficient number of words to form word combinations, may fail to do so. Telegraphic speech that omits the grammatic elements and shorter and simpler sentences lacking in variety are among the most easily recognized features of language disorders in children.

- *Inadequate or inappropriate social communication:* Language disorders are further characterized by a lack of social communication skills and inappropriate production of what they have acquired. Significant features of these *pragmatic language problems* include social communication that may be inappropriate to the time, place, person, and topic of conversation. Even if they have some verbal skills, children with language disorders may fail to initiate and maintain conversation on a given topic, may interrupt the speaker, or avoid eye contact during social interactions. These children may fail to take steps to restore broken communication by requesting clarifications from the speaker and modifying one's own expressions to help their listener understand what they say.

- *Deficient nonverbal communication skills:* Verbal language disorders may be associated with limited nonverbal communication skills, including deficiencies in producing and comprehending gestures and other nonverbal means of communication. Their limited verbal communication may lack support from nonverbal expressions.

- *Deficient literacy skills:* Limited or deficient language skills are likely to affect the children's reading and writing skills, which are language based. The children's difficulty with abstract and academic language is bound to limit their academic achievement.

Limited language skills, of the kind just described, may or may not be associated with additional problems. We briefly review these two varieties of language disorders.

Clinical Conditions Associated with Language Disorders

Not all children with language disorders have associated clinical conditions that are serious enough to render a dual diagnosis. Those who do present a more complex clinical picture, require a dual diagnosis of a language disorder and another diagnosis. Space does not permit a detailed description of clinical conditions associated with language disorders; therefore, we offer a brief overview of some of the main conditions:

Intellectual Disabilities

Language disorders are found in children who also have intellectual disabilities; generally, the lower the IQ, the greater the severity of language disorders. Language disorders, however, are found in children whose IQs fall within the normal range; therefore, deficient intelligence is not a cause of, or a necessary condition associated with, language disorders. Nonetheless, the presence of significant intellectual disability almost always implies limited language skills (Hegde & Maul, 2006; Long, 2005a).

Children with intellectual disabilities tend to have both a speech sound and a language disorder. They may have significant difficulty in correctly producing the speech sounds. Language problems of these children are similar to the description provided previously, including significant language comprehension deficiencies.

Autism Spectrum Disorders

This spectrum, also known as *pervasive developmental disorders*, includes autism, Asperger's disorder (syndrome), Rett's disorder, and childhood disintegrative disorder (CDD). A uniquely impaired language is a diagnostic criterion of both autism and Asperger's syndrome. Significant emotional and behavioral problems, lack of appropriate emotional responses, stereotypic interests and activities, and stereotypic and repetitive movements and play activities characterize autism. Social inappropriateness (with otherwise acceptable language skills), insensitivity to others' feelings and viewpoints, and intense and highly knowledgeable interest in odd topics characterizes Asperger's syndrome (Hegde & Maul, 2006; Long, 2005b).

Although children with autism generally have IQs below 71, those with Asperger's syndrome have IQs within the normal or even superior range. Whereas both bizarre and limited language skills may characterize autism, normal or even superior verbal skills may characterize the Asperger's. Nonetheless, significant social communication problems, which generally include tactless and inappropriate expressions, distinguish Asperger's syndrome. Although children with autism show no or little interest in social communication, those with Asperger's syndrome have great interest in telling others (not conversing with them) about their highly specialized interests (e.g., memorized train or airplane schedules).

Rett's disorder and the CDD are less common than autism and both have an initial period of 2 or more years of normal development before the symptoms appear. Rett's disorder almost exclusively affects female children, and CDD primarily affects the male; the former is associated with a mutation of the MeCP2 gene on the long arm of the X-chromosome whereas the genetic basis of the latter is unclear. Repetitive hand movements, a gradual loss of purposeful hand movements, gait disturbances, decelerated head growth, and loss of (and further limited) language skills characterize Rett's disorder. Children with CDD show a sudden and serious regression in language, self-help, social, and motor skills. The impairments are profound and the child may be mute.

Assessment of children with an autism spectrum disorder requires an examination of behavior disorders as well as communication disorders. It is the responsibility of speech-language pathologists to assess the communication impairments and serve on the team that makes a final diagnosis.

Hearing Loss

Children with hearing loss have difficulty learning oral language in the usual manner because of reduced or absent auditory awareness of speech and reduced auditory feedback of one's own speech attempts. Hearing loss varies on a continuum, and the extent of the effects depends on the degree of loss. Children who are *hard of hearing* are aware of spoken speech, can learn oral language, perhaps with the help of amplification (hearing aids), and have a hearing loss that does not exceed 70 dB HL. Generally, children who are hard of hearing experience less severe effects than those who are deaf. The *deaf* are unaware of spoken speech, their residual hearing does not support oral language acquisition, and generally have a hearing loss that exceeds 71 dB HL.

Assessment of hearing is the responsibility of audiologist. Speech-language pathologists may assess the oral communication skills of children with hearing loss. In the United States, the deaf typically tend to acquire the American Sign Language (ASL) in which they gain excellent proficiency. The educators of the deaf may formally teach not only ASL, but all academic subjects in ASL. Children who are hard of hearing, who learn significant oral language skills may require the services of a speech-language pathologist. Depending on the level of hearing loss, the child's oral speech and language skills may be deficient. Speech sound and language disorders, along with voice and prosodic disorders, are associated with significant hearing loss. Oral language fluency also may be significantly limited in children with hearing loss.

Language disorders associated with hearing loss include a generally slower rate of language learning, limited vocabulary, limited comprehension of spoken language, absence of many grammatic morphemes, a marked difficulty in learning the verb forms, limited syntactic skills, and somewhat limited pragmatic language. Reading and writing problems are commonly associated with hearing loss (Hegde & Maul, 2006).

Genetic Syndromes

Various genetic syndromes—too numerous to describe here—are associated with language disorders (Hegde, 2008a; Jones, 2005; Shprintzen, 2000; Weidemann & Kunze, 1997). Most genetic syndromes affect physical, behavioral, and communication skills; many are associated with intellectual disability, cleft palate and other craniofacial abnormalities, and hearing loss, all of which produce their own negative effects on speech and language learning. Depending on the presence or absence of such conditions and the severity of the syndromic expression, the child's speech and language skills may be more or less limited. Some of the syndromes that speech-language pathologists more commonly encounter include:

- *Down syndrome,* which is due to one of the most commonly occurring chromosomal abnormality; the child is born with an extra chromosome (47, rather than the normal 46). Children with Down syndrome are prone to conductive hearing loss that affects language learning. Both speech and language disorders may be observed.

- *Fetal alcohol syndrome,* a congenital (not inherited) syndrome, which is due to maternal alcoholism during pregnancy; associated with craniofacial anomalies (including cleft lip and palate), growth retardation, heart and kidney problems, and intellectual disabilities. Children with fetal alcohol syndrome exhibit deficiencies in all aspects of language, especially with significant intellectual disability.

- *Fragile X syndrome,* a sex-linked genetic syndrome due to an abnormality on the long arm of the X-chromosome; associated with significant language problems including jargon, echolalia, telegraphic speech (omission of grammatic features), perseverative speech, self-talking, and inappropriate and irrelevant language. Gestures and other nonverbal communication features may be absent and speech sound and voice disorders may be observed.

- *Prader-Willi syndrome,* a genetic syndrome caused by a deletion in the region of the paternal long arm of chromosome 15; associated with intellectual disabilities; characterized by initially slow but subsequently somewhat accelerated language learning; the severity of language disorders will depend on the degree of intellectual disabilities.

- *Tourette's syndrome,* a syndrome thought to be genetic, although no specific gene abnormality has been identified; a predominant symptom is uncontrollable tics and facial grimaces; a notable feature is vocal tics which may include grunting, humming, yelling, and screaming; abnormal language behaviors include coprolalia (compulsive swearing, uttering obscenities); palilalia (repetition of one's own utterances), and echolalia; frequently associated with stuttering.

Assessment of children with genetic syndromes is the responsibility of a multidisciplinary team that includes medical and nonmedical specialists. The speech-language pathologist makes a thorough assessment of speech, voice, language, and fluency.

Other Associated Clinical Conditions

Language (and speech sound) disorders may be associated with many other clinical conditions, including *cerebral palsy, traumatic brain injury,* and *cleft palate.* As described in Chapter 6, the main effect of cerebral palsy is on speech because of the neuromotor disorders that characterize this congenital condition. However, some children also may exhibit delayed language acquisition and deficient language skills. Standard language assessment procedures also are useful in diagnosing language disorders in children with cerebral palsy.

Traumatic brain injury (TBI) affects all aspects of communication. However, the effects of TBI may be more evident on general communicative behaviors than on specific semantic, syntactic, morphologic aspects. Most likely affected are pragmatic aspects of communication. Initially, the child may be mute, but may gradually recover some or most of the communication skills. The child may be impulsive or uninhibited, inattentive, incoherent, and inappropriate in giving verbal responses. Most of the communication problems may be a function of the child's lack of attention, fatigue, and lack of control over one's own behavior. In addition to these difficulties, children with TBI tend to exhibit dysarthria—a speech disorder associated with neuromotor impairment (Hegde, 2006).

Children with cleft palate also tend to have more serious speech disorders than language disorders. However, if the cleft is surgically closed early in life, as it is the case in most countries, the effect on speech and language may be minimal. If the surgical treatment is delayed, or if the child has additional problems including intellectual deficiencies or hearing loss, then the effects on the oral communication skills may be significant. Language problems of children with cleft may be assessed with the same general procedures clinicians use.

Specific Language Impairment

A language problem that is isolated and is not accompanied by a serious and obvious clinical condition is called **specific language impairment (SLI).** As the term implies, the problem is *specific* to language; there is only *one* impairment, limited to language; and the disorder exists in a child who is otherwise comparable to normally developing children. When this definition of SLI was offered and generally accepted, there was no evidence of any other difficulty associated with it. In recent years, however, there have been some and somewhat controversial evidence that children who have SLI may have subtle cognitive and motoric difficulties (see Hegde & Maul, 2006; Leonard, 1998, for review of conflicting evidence). Nonetheless, the term SLI continues to be used with its original definition, or with some qualification.

Signs of SLI may be observed in infants and toddlers. Some infants and toddlers who show such signs are "late bloomers"—they catch up with their normally talking peers.

Therefore, SLI is diagnosed only after age 4 (Rescorla, 1989). The late bloomers' language problem is characterized by a failure to acquire 50 single words and two-word productions by 2 years of age; this temporary problem is sometimes called slow early language development (SELD). But of the 15% estimated late blooming preschool children, roughly half eventually catch up with their normal language learning peers and the other half continue to have language difficulties. It is in these 7 to 8% of preschool and school-age children who have language problems but no other obvious and serious problems that SLI is diagnosed (Leonard, 1991, 1998). Nonetheless, children with SLI may have academic difficulties due largely to their limited language skills.

Children with SLI learn language skills at a slower rate, but their pattern of acquisition is not grossly abnormal or deviant. Therefore, compared to children without language disorders, children with SLI exhibit lower language skills at each age or grade level. Also, children with SLI may exhibit a pattern of language development that is asynchronous; some of their language skills may be more advanced than other skills. Pragmatic language skills, for example, are often less impaired than are syntactic and morphologic skills. In general, children with SLI exhibit various combinations of phonologic, semantic, morphologic, syntactic, and pragmatic problems.

In assessing children with SLI, the clinician needs to look for the following salient features:

- *Errors of speech sound production.* Up to 40% of children with SLI may have speech sound disorders (Rescorla & Lee, 2001). Omission of phonemes, often observed in these children, may contribute to the language disorder. For instance, a child who omits /t/, /d/, /s/, or /z/ will not produce such morphologic features as the regular past tense *t* or *d* (e.g., *walked* or *begged*), the third person singular present tense (e.g., *walks*), the possessive morpheme (e.g., *Mommy's*), and the regular plural words (e.g., *hats* or *bags*).

- *Semantic problems.* Difficulty learning words and their meanings is an early sign of SLI. Children with SLI are slow to acquire their first few words and fail to show the typical explosive increase in the acquisition of new words between the ages of 18 and 24 months. Compared to 200 words of normally developing children at age 2, those that are likely to be later diagnosed with SLI may produce only about 20 words (Rescorla, Roberts, & Dahlsgaard, 1997). In addition, children with SLI may continue to *overextend* (e.g., calling all adults as *Daddy*) or *underextend* (e.g., calling only the family dog as *dog*, but not any other dog) word meanings beyond the age of 3 years.

- *Delayed word combinations.* Children with SLI may be slower in learning such two-word combinations that signal different meanings as *noun + verb* combinations, possession ("My kitty"), disappearance ("Kitty gone"), or rejection ("No kitty!").

- *Naming errors.* School-age children with SLI make errors in naming pictures of common objects.

- *Difficulty with abstract and figurative language.* Older and adolescent students who have had SLI continue to exhibit problems with abstract words, proverbs, idioms, similes, and such other figurative language; this difficulty will negatively affect their academic performance; their speech and writing may be full of such nonspecific words as *this, that, thing,* and *stuff.*

- *Significant morphologic problems.* Difficulty in producing morphologic features of language is a diagnostic feature of SLI. They tend to omit or misuse most of the grammatic morphemes described previously.

- *Limited syntactic structure and variety.* Simpler sentence forms; lack of syntactic variety; absence of complex, compound, embedded, and passive sentence forms; and difficulty in transforming one type of sentence (e.g., active declarative) to another form (e.g., a question) all characterize the language skills of children with SLI.

- *Controversial pragmatic language problems.* Some studies suggest that pragmatic language problems are not prominent in children with SLI whereas others suggest the opposite (see Hegde & Maul, 2006 and Leonard, 1998 for review of studies). Possibly, topic initiation and maintenance, turn-taking skills, and conversational repair strategies will be less impaired than joint attention, detailed and sophisticated narration of stories or personal experiences, group interactions and discussions, and discussion of advanced academic topics. Because of the controversial nature of evidence, clinicians should assess all pragmatic language skills in children with SLI.

As noted earlier, it is possible that children with SLI have additional, though subtle problems, including memory and attentional deficits, complex reasoning difficulties, hyperactivity, and so forth. To what extent these should be assessed depends on the clinician's theoretical orientation (Hegde & Maul, 2006; Leonard, 1998). It may be practical to concentrate on assessing speech and language skills because they are most productively targeted in treatment.

Factors Related to Language Disorders

In assessing children with language disorders, the clinician needs to consider all factors that may be related to, or correlated with, language impairment. Even if the diagnosis is likely to be SLI, the clinician cannot ignore the prenatal, perinatal, and postnatal factors that may have contributed to the disorder. In assessing these factors, case history and medical information of the mother and the child are especially important. During the interview, the clinician should explore the potential factors that are known to be associated with language disorders in children.

Obviously, some of the listed factors will be absent if the child has an SLI, but to make that diagnosis the clinician should rule them out; hence, the need to obtain information on such factors as the following in all cases of a potential language disorder (Hegde & Maul, 2006; Reed, 2012):

- *Genetic factors.* Language disorders, including SLI, may be related to genetic factors. Family history of SLI is known to be higher than that in the general population. Therefore, the clinician should obtain detailed information on the familial prevalence of language disorders.

- *Other clinical conditions.* As noted previously, such other clinical conditions as hearing loss, intellectual disabilities, autism spectrum disorders, traumatic brain injury, and various genetic syndromes may be associated with language disorders not diagnosed as SLI. The clinician should assess these additional problems in detail to rule them out to establish SLI as the diagnosis.

- *Prenatal risk factors.* Lack of prenatal care, maternal drug and alcohol abuse, infections that affect the fetal growth, maternal age at delivery (under 16 or over 36), multiple gestations, kidney failure, premature rupture of the membrane, fetal distress, premature birth, and other conditions need to be explored though the case history and interview.

- *Perinatal risk factors.* Abnormally long labor, uncontrolled or precipitated delivery, abnormal fetal presentation, fetal distress, placental abnormalities, and so forth need to be documented or ruled out.

- *Neonatal risk factors.* Negative factors that affect the infant's growth during the first 28 days after the birth (the neonatal period) include very low or very high birth weight, jaundice, feeding problems, infections, congenital anomalies, craniofacial abnormalities (e.g., cleft palate, hydrocephaly, macrocephaly, microcephaly), and so forth.

- *Variations in parent-child interactions.* Even though they may be effects, not causes of language disorders in children, unusual parent-child interactions have been noted. Parents may reduce their interaction with a child who has a language disorder, give direct commands and instructions, use simpler language, ask fewer questions, and so forth (Hegde & Maul, 2006). Because these parental behaviors need to be modified during treatment, the clinician should explore these patterns of interactions during the interview.

- *Home literacy environment.* Inadequate home literacy environment may be an additional risk factor for learning reading and writing, if not for limited oral language skills. Because literacy skills are language skills, it is essential to find out if the parents read stories to the child and provide literacy role models (themselves reading and writing at home) and whether the home environment supports reading and writing (e.g., availability of books, facilities to write).

An additional important factor that is not necessarily a risk factor for language disorders that still needs to be investigated in assessing language disorders is the *ethnocultural variables* and *bilingualism.* It will be important to find out if the child speaks a different English dialect (e.g., African American English or another U.S. English dialect) or has learned English as a second language. See Chapter 4 for issues to be considered in assessing children of ethnocultural diversity.

Overview of Assessment of Child Language Disorders

Assessment of language disorders in children includes both standard and special procedures. Most of these typical and standard procedures of assessment are adapted to concentrate on the child's language skills. The standard procedures include:

- **Case history:** Most clinicians use a standard case history form; use the *Case History Protocol* given in Chapter 2.

- **Interview:** The clinician structures the interview to get more specific information on the child's language development and potential risk factors the child may have been exposed to. If the child belongs to an ethnocultural minority group, the standard interview schedule may be further modified to seek information on the dialectal, bilingual, and bicultural status of the child and the family; use the *Interview Protocol* given in Chapter 9.

- **Hearing screening and orofacial examination:** Standard procedures; use the protocol given in Chapter 2.

- **Language sampling:** A procedure commonly used in assessing various communication disorders, language sampling will be especially structured to maximize opportunities for the child to produce various morphologic, syntactic, and pragmatic skills in the case of a child with a language disorder. To assess the literacy skills, the clinician may get a reading and writing sample from the child. Use the suggestions offered in this chapter and the *Language Sample Transcription Protocol* and *Language Sample Analysis Protocol* given in Chapter 9.

- **Administration of standardized tests:** If considered appropriate for the child, the clinician may select a suitable language test and administer it; see standardized assessment tools in a later section in this chapter and consider the issues related to tests addressed in Chapter 3.

- **Assessment of overall language development:** Use the *Normal Language Assessment Protocol* given in Chapter 9 to record the child's major language milestones on a structured form.

- **Administration of alternatives assessment procedures:** The clinician may make a functional behavioral assessment, devise client-specific or criterion-referenced procedures (e.g., tell a story the child retells, ask the child to narrate a personal experience, read his or her favorite book, or give a brief client-specific or criterion-referenced test of morphologic features); may select reading and writing samples or other academic work samples to be included in the report; see Chapter 5 for additional information on alternative procedures and how to integrate them with the traditional procedures. Use the *Task-Specific Assessment Protocols* given in Chapter 9 to assess a child's basic vocabulary, grammatic morphemes, and conversational skills. When warranted, use an appropriate *Multicultural Assessment Protocol* given in Chapter 9.

- **Postassessment counseling:** The clinician counsels the parents about the assessment results, suggests a tentative diagnosis, discusses prognosis for improvement, makes recommendations, and answers questions about language disorders and treatment options.

- **Data analysis in relation to the child's unique ethnocultural background:** The clinician analyzes the assessment data in relation to the child and the family's cultural and linguistic background to help make clinical decisions.

- **Report writing:** The clinician writes a report that is shared with the parents and other concerned professionals; see Chapter 2 for a basic assessment outline that may be used to generate a report.

The goal of child language assessment is a reliable description of the child's language repertoire, including literacy skills when appropriate, along with the family communication patterns. Parent interview, carefully structured language sampling, appropriately selected standardized assessment tools, and alternative means of assessment of language skills will provide much of the needed information to evaluate the child's language strengths and weaknesses.

Screening for Language Disorders

Clinicians in public schools may regularly screen for language disorders in children. Screening helps establish that some children's communication skills are within normal limits, and therefore, do not need a diagnostic assessment, whereas a few other children need it. A *pass* on a screening test means that the child's communication skills are within the normal limits. A *fail* will suggest a need for diagnostic assessment.

There are various standardized language screening tools. Table 8–7 lists some of the commonly used screening tests. Clinicians may find additional screening tests on ASHA's Web site (http://www.asha.org/assessments.aspx). Any screening test selected should meet the standards of reliability, validity, and appropriateness for the particular child on whom the screening test will be administered.

Language Sampling

A **language sample** is typically an audio record of a child's conversation or naturalistic verbal interaction. The clinician, one or more family members, or both the clinician and family members may help evoke naturalistic language production from the child. The verbal interaction involved in language sampling may not be entirely spontaneous or naturalistic because the clinician designs and guides the interaction to make specific observations. Nonetheless, it is more naturalistic than assessing language skills through standardized test administration.

A language sample is the most important aspect of assessing a child's language skills to diagnose a language disorder. A reliable language sample is a more valid means of assessing language skills than standardized tests. Unlike tests, language samples may be flexibly structured to suit the individual child and the family. Comprehensive samples also help assess language and other communication skills in a more naturalistic setting.

Naturalistic language sampling is desirable in assessing all children, but the method is especially valuable in assessing language in ethnoculturally diverse children. The clinician can select stimulus materials that are especially relevant to a given child. Depending on the child, there is also the possibility that stimuli can be largely avoided in favor of a naturalistic conversation. Furthermore, the clinician can explore skills that are not included in specific standardized tests. Parents or other family members can assist in evok-

Table 8–7. Child Language Screening Tests

Screening Instrument	Age Range	Language Skills Assessed (administration time)
CSBS DP Infant-Toddler Checklist and Easy-Score (Wetherby & Prizant, 2003)	6 months to 24 months	Gestures, sounds, words, eye gaze, object use, other nonverbal communicative behaviors (5–10 minutes)
CELF-4 Screening Test (Semel, Wiig, & Secord, 2004)	5 years to 21 years	Expressive and receptive language: vocabulary and syntax (15 minutes)
Fluharty-2: Fluharty Preschool Speech and Language Screening Test (Fluharty, 2000)	3 years to 6;11 years	Expressive and receptive language: repeating sentences, answering questions, following directions, describing actions, sequencing events; also screens articulation (10 minutes)
Joliet 3-Minute Preschool Speech and Language Screen (Kinzler & Johnson, 1993)	2 years to 4 years	Expressive and receptive language: syntax and vocabulary; also screens articulation (3–5 minutes)
Joliet 3-Minute Speech and Language Screen (Revised) (Kinzler & Johnson, 1992)	K, 2nd, and 5th graders	Expressive and receptive language: syntax and vocabulary; also screens articulation (3–5 minutes)
Kindergarten Language Screening Test-Second Edition (KLST-S) (Gauthier & Madison, 1998)	3–6 years to 6;11 years	Expressive and receptive language: following directions, repeating sentences, making comparisons between common objects (5 minutes)
Speech-Ease Screening Inventory (K-1) (Speech-Ease, 1985)	K through 1st grade	Expressive and receptive language: vocabulary, associations, auditory recall, basic concepts (7–10 minutes)

ing a representative sample from the child, something a standardized test will not allow. Because of its inherent flexibility and suitability to children of all ethnocultural backgrounds (including mainstream children), language sampling helps overcome some of the limitations of standardized, norm-referenced testing. It is indeed the main method of language assessment; standardized tests only supplement naturalistic language sampling.

Language samples are more efficient than standardized tests. At best, a standardized test of language somewhat inadequately samples only a specific aspect of language. For instance, a test may sample only vocabulary, semantic features, limited and selected morphologic features, few syntactic structures, or specific pragmatic language skills. To make a thorough analysis of all aspects of language skills, the clinician may need to use multiple tests of language. Even then, language tests will not help reliably assess fluency and dysfluencies, voice characteristics, and phonologic skills. A carefully structured and minimally directed language sample can help assess not only all aspects of language, but also all other aspects of communication including fluency and dysfluencies, voice characteristics, resonance problems, prosodic variations, and phonologic skills (Hegde & Maul, 2005).

In recording a reliable and valid language sample, the clinician should strike a balance between some structure and direction needed to evoke important language skills from the child on the one hand and the need to keep it as naturalistic as possible on the other. Without a minimal amount of structure and direction, the sample may be empty of relevant productions or incomplete because of missing aspects of language. With too rigid a structure and too frequent directions issued to the child, the sample may be more contrived than naturalistic. Generally, following a few directions will help achieve a balance between these two constraints (Hegde & Maul, 2006).

- *Structure the language sampling session, but only minimally.* Minimize the formality of language sampling to keep it as naturalistic as possible. Use only a few necessary concrete stimulus materials. Do not limit language sampling to evoking isolated productions by showing pictures the child names or while playing with toys.

- *Record a meaningful and naturalistic language sample.* The main clinical task is to obtain a representative, naturalistic language sample from the child; this can be accomplished only by engaging the child in conversational speech. Following the principles of authentic assessment described in Chapter 5 (Stockman, 1996b; Udvari & Thousand, 1995), evoke a conversational speech with topics that are relevant, meaningful, and naturalistic. Do not be the clinician who cannot talk to a child but always needs pictures or toys to evoke noncommunicative productions. Let the child talk about topics that he or she is interested in.

- *Select the few needed stimuli carefully.* A few carefully selected stimuli may be useful in getting the child started. Select them from storybooks that prompt the child to narrate a story instead of simple, concrete pictures that prompt naming responses. Based on the interview and case history information, select stimuli that are familiar and relevant to the child. If practical, have the parents bring the child's favorite books or a few toys to the assessment session. Limit the use of toys that promote silent play; some children get absorbed in play activity when presented with such materials as play dough.

- *Talk with the child.* Evoke conversation, not just single word responses. Add concrete stimuli as needed and only to evoke conversational speech. For instance, while showing a complex picture that depicts a farm scene, ask about the child's experiences with a farm, farm animals, and farm products, instead of simply asking the child to describe what is seen. Perhaps the child has visited a farm or has lived on one. If the child is talkative, this kind of conversation is often all that is necessary to gather an adequate language sample.

- *Use stimuli to evoke extended language production.* Ask open-ended questions, instead of asking too many questions the child will answer with a *yes* or *no*. For example, ask, "What do you see here?" instead of, "Do you see a horse here?" Prefer questions that prompt descriptions to those that prompt naming. For example, ask such questions as, "What is happening in this picture?" instead of "What is this?" Make requests instead of asking one questions after another. For example, such requests as, "Tell me about everything you see in this picture" may be more effective in evoking continuous speech than a question, "What do you see here?" Use close-ended question only as a prelude to asking more open-ended questions. For example, "Did you go to Disney Land during the break?" may be a good question, if the child answers "yes" and you follow up with such open-ended questions as, "Oh, good! tell me all about it!" "Who took you there?" And, "Tell me about all the rides you took there."

- *Use stimuli to introduce conversational topics.* When the child is describing a stimulus picture, introduce a topic of conversation. For example, when the child is describing a circus or a zoo scene, ask the child whether he or she has seen a circus or visited a zoo. Prompt the child to talk about what he or she saw there.

- *Introduce various conversational topics that might interest the child.* Depending on the information gathered through parent interview, ask questions about the child's interests and hobbies. Prompt the child to talk about them. Use such other topics as the child's school, friends and teachers in school, favorite academic subjects, leisure activities, favorite television shows, playmates in the neighborhood, birthday parties, vacations, siblings, grandparents, and so forth. This technique may be especially useful in recording meaningful, naturalistic language from school-age children.

- *Narrate a brief story and ask the child to retell it.* This task will be helpful not only in analyzing the production of varied words, sentences, and morphologic features, but also in assessing such narrative skills as story description with details and correct chronologic order. Prompt the child to say more or give more details. In assessing all narrative tasks, ask questions about characters in the story and events and their sequences. If necessary, give hints about missing details and wrong sequence of events being narrated.

- *Ask the child to tell a story.* Most children can tell a brief story. Let the parents prompt a story they believe the child knows. Ask such questions as, "What happened then?" and "Who did what?" This task also will help assess semantic, grammatic, and pragmatic language skills.

- *Have the child silently read a brief story and retell it.* This task is useful when the child can read and fails to spontaneously tell a story. Select a story that is appropriate for the child's academic level and ethnocultural background. Let the child read the story and retell it. Prompt the child to say more or give more details.

- *Ask attending siblings or parents to engage the child in conversation on a topic.* Parents or siblings may help evoke more naturalistic language. Toddlers and preschoolers who may not talk much to strangers may need this strategy more so than school-age children. This task also will help assess the family communication patterns. For example, the clinician may observe that some parents or older siblings interrupt and direct the child's speech whereas others more patiently listen and offer only indirect suggestions. The clinician may find that an older sibling hardly gives a chance for the child to talk.

- *Vary the activities.* To maintain the child's interest, use different kinds of activities, including conversation, play activity designed to evoke further language, a brief game activity that prompts the child to ask questions, reading and telling a short story, retelling a story narrated, a topic on which the child speaks in a monologue, and so forth.

- *Take notes on the context of utterances.* Take written notes on the context of the child's utterances. Without such notes, problems with some utterances may be indiscernible on the audio-record. For example, the utterance, "I see book" on an audiotape may not reveal the missing plural morpheme without the contextual knowledge that the child's response was to several books. The fact that the child wants the toy car will not be evident from the statement "car" recorded on the audiotape.

- *Arrange interaction to evoke conversational (pragmatic) skills.* Use the narrative tasks and naturalistic conversation to assess conversational skills.
  - Trigger *topic initiation* by showing pictures, mentioning a story, or within induced conversations. Draw the child's attention to a stimulus item and then wait for the child to initiate conversation about that item. Initiation of brief conversational episodes is sufficient evidence of the skill.
  - Evoke *topic maintenance* by having the child select topics of interest for talking. Prompt and suggest topics if necessary, let the child talk about the selected topic. Make such comments as, "I see!" "That's funny!," "I like your story!," "Tell me more," "What happened next?," and so forth to have the child sustain conversation on the same topic. Start and stop a stopwatch to measure the duration (seconds or minutes) for which the child maintained the same topic of conversation. Measure topic maintenance for at least three topics.
  - Observe *conversational turn-taking* during the entire assessment session. Take note of the frequency of the child's interruptions when you are talking. Note whether the child begins to talk when you pause for the child to take a turn talking.
  - Evoke *requests for clarification* by making ambiguous statements that require such requests. For example, say, "Show me the toy" when the picture depicts several toys. Say, "Give me the car" when several toy cars are displayed in front of the child. Say something too softly for the child to hear. Use some complex words the child may not understand. Take note of the frequency with which the child requests clarification (e.g., "What do you mean?") when something is not clear.
  - Evoke *clarification of one's statements*, by pretending not to understand the child's statements. Ask the child to repeat or say "I don't understand" or "What do you mean?" In addition, negate a child's utterance so the child will clarify by assertion (e.g., "You're not 2 years old, are you?;" the child might answer, "No! I'm 4 years old!").
  - Observe *eye contact* during the entire period of assessment and conversation with the child. Use the interview information about ethnocultural variability in eye contact.

- Evoke *narrative skills* as described before. In addition to previously suggested tactics, tell a story with the help of pictures, and then ask the child to retell it while looking at the pictures. Also, ask the child to describe such everyday routines as grocery shopping, eating in a restaurant, organizing birthday parties, baking a cake, planning a camping trip, and so forth.

- *Obtain at least one language sample in an extraclinical situation.* A fully naturalistic, meaningful, and representative language sample may be recorded only in a nonclinical setting, such as the child's home. While recording such a sample, the child should be talking to a friend, a sibling, a parent, the babysitter, or other familiar caregiver. When requested and supported with information on how to do it, most parents will submit a home language sample. If this is not practical in a school setting, the clinician may record a brief sample in the classroom, in the cafeteria during lunch time, or on the playground. As needed, the clinician may obtain assistance from the teacher and other school personnel.

Integrating Alternative Assessment Techniques

As discussed in Chapter 5, available alternative assessment techniques are not just for assessing language skills of ethnoculturally diverse children. Many features of most alternative approaches are relevant for assessing language skills of all children, including those from mainstream social strata. We have already suggested that consistent with the principles of authentic assessment, the language sample should be naturalistic and meaningful. In addition, the clinician may take the following steps to integrate useful features of alternative assessment into standard (not necessarily *standardized*) assessment:

- *Make a skill-specific, criterion-referenced, or client-specific assessment.* Even in an extended sampling time, a child may fail to produce many verbal skills for lack of opportunities (contexts). Therefore, throughout the sampling period, observe the skills produced and take note of those that are not produced. For instance, you may notice that the child did not produce the present progressive *-ing*, the possessive morpheme, a particular pronoun, the copula, the passive sentence, or the adverbial suffix *-ly*; did not maintain eye contact; or never requested clarification when you made ambiguous statements. In such situations, use task-specific procedures that tend to be both criterion-referenced and client-specific. Task-specific procedures are designed to increase the probability of certain kinds of verbal behaviors; see selected Task-Specific Assessment Protocols in Chapter 9. A few examples will illustrate the strategy:
  - To evoke the production of the present progressive *-ing*, demonstrate actions (e.g., take a few steps, gesture drinking from a cup), and ask the child to tell what you are doing or you did.
  - To evoke the production of *possessive morphemes*, direct conversation in which the child would talk about things that belong to people and animals; the child may talk about *daddy's car, mommy's hat, brother's books,* or *dog's bowl.* When the child is describing a picture scene with an elephant, you might say, "Look! Here is a huge trunk! Whose trunk is that?" to evoke, "The elephant's."

- To evoke the production of the *pronoun he*, ask the child to talk about a male person; for example, ask the child to talk about his or her *brother, father, a male teacher,* and so forth to increase the probability that the child on occasion will produce the pronoun instead of the noun. Similar strategies will work for other missing pronouns.

- To evoke the production of the *copula is* in sentences (e.g., *she is nice, it is small*) induce conversation on qualities or characteristics of people, animals, or things. Direct conversation to include adjectives (*nice, big, small, smooth, rough, tall,* etc.) that require the use of the copula is (or copula *are*, as in *people are big*).

- To evoke the passive sentences, use the sentence completion format. For instance, show the picture of a boy kicking a ball, and say, "This boy just kicked the ball. If you want to say it differently, you could say the ball was . . ." to see if the child would complete it; note that this is more contrived than natural. During more naturalistic conversation, you might ask the child to rephrase an active declarative sentence just produced into a passive sentence, by giving an example or two.

- To evoke the *adverbial suffix -ly,* demonstrate such actions as talking too softly and then too loudly, or writing something on a piece of paper too quickly and then too slowly. At the end of each demonstration, ask the child to describe the action (e.g., "How am I talking?" or "How am I writing?).

- To make sure that the child indeed does not *maintain eye contact* during conversation, once or twice during conversation, ask the child to look at your face when talking; do not repeat the instruction too frequently, as this might teach the child to maintain eye contact; if a few reminders do not improve eye contact, perhaps the child lacks this skill; be cautious in interpreting the absence of this skill as it may be cultural.

- To evoke requests for *clarification*, make several ambiguous statements; follow the suggestions offered earlier.

- *Model the missing language skills.* If task-specific directions and procedures are ineffective, periodically model skills to see if the child would begin to produce them. To avoid teaching the skill during assessment, *do not*: (a) model too frequently, (b) require imitation from the child, and (c) reinforce the child for correct productions of the missing skill. Recall that in the *dynamic assessment procedure* described in Chapter 4, the clinician spends extended time to teach a skill within a test-teach-test format. We are not necessarily recommending this extended strategy that requires additional sessions to teach before making a diagnosis. Nonetheless, the strategy of modeling the missing skills during assessment is consistent with dynamic assessment philosophy (Gutierrez-Clellen & Peña, 2006; Olswang, Bain, & Johnson, 1992; Peña, 1996; Ukrainetz, Harpell, Walsh, & Coyle, 2000).

- *Prompt the missing language skills.* Once again, prompt infrequently. Such statements, made periodically through the assessment session, will serve as prompts: "I think it is the dog's bowl;" "Do you keep your things neatly in your room?;" "At home, I keep my books *on* my table;" "Instead of saying *my brother* all the time, you could sometimes say *he*;" "Instead of saying *boy walking* or *Mom talking*, you might say *the boy is walking* or *my Mom was talking*;" and so forth.

- *Expand the assessment database.* Following the recommendations stemming from portfolio assessment described in Chapter 4, seek data that are not typically sought in completing child language assessment (DeFina, 1992; Kratcoski, 1998). The portfolio assessment approach advocates that the clinician include not only the traditional pieces of assessment evidence (e.g., the results of standardized tests, language samples, orofacial examination) but also other kinds of evidence including the child's writing samples, pieces of drawing or painting, teacher's comments about the child's speech and language skills, observational notes on the child's communication skills in classrooms or other nonclinical settings; any audio- or videotapes of child's communication patterns recorded at home, results of teacher's assessment of language and literacy skills, and so forth. Obviously, such an expanded database is a continuous process, will not be completed during the initial assessment, but may begin at that time. For instance, an audiotaped home language sample; the child's writing, drawing, or painting samples; teacher's or other professional's comments that may have been included in the referral letter, among others, may be made a part of the initial assessment. Subsequently, additional materials, including interviews with the teachers, siblings, or peers in the school about the child's previous and current language skills may be included in the portfolio.

- *Make a behavioral assessment.* Consider the advantages of the behavioral assessment as described in Chapter 5. Assessment of functional verbal behaviors will better inform language treatment targets than an assessment of linguistic structures. Furthermore, functional behavioral treatment targets are in tune with the commonly used behavioral treatment procedures, including modeling, prompting, and offering precise consequences for appropriate and inappropriate client behaviors. Using the Behavioral Assessment Protocol given in Chapter 9, find out the frequency with which the child produces such verbal behaviors as echoics, mands, tacts, intraverbals, autoclitics, and textuals.

The clinicians in all professional settings are under time pressure to complete the assessment as quickly as possible. Behavioral, portfolio, and dynamic assessment approaches are especially demanding of clinician's time and effort. Nonetheless, clinicians need to make a thorough and valid assessment to bridge the gap between knowing what the child can and cannot do and specifying the target skills that need to be taught.

Assessment of Language Understanding

Although much assessment time is devoted to children's language production skills, it is essential to make a basic assessment of responses to spoken language, which is typically described as *comprehension*. Generally, children with language disorders have difficulty responding verbally to language spoken to them; however, they may respond nonverbally, suggesting that they understand more than they produce. From a treatment standpoint, it is preferable to teach production than comprehension because once production of language responses is taught under appropriate and varied stimulus conditions, comprehension problems seem to disappear. Unless the clinician finds that the child may have more serious problems in comprehension than what the production problems suggest, it is not essential to spend much time assessing comprehension.

Language *comprehension* is not directly observed, and hence it is of limited validity; it is inferred from appropriate verbal and nonverbal responses given to verbal stimuli. Therefore, comprehension may be assessed throughout the assessment session by taking note of any irrelevant or incorrect responses to verbal stimuli. Taking note of the child's performance when the clinician gives various comments and directions during assessment is adequate to assess responses to verbal stimuli (presumed comprehension) at a simple level. For instance, typical assessment tasks include pointing to correct pictures or objects in a stimulus array, as well as responding to complex, multistep commands (e.g., "First pick up the pencil, point to the block with it, and then to the comb;" "Point to the big red ball and the small blue car"). These tasks help observe breakdowns in nonverbal responses to verbal stimuli. Because the nonverbal responses given to verbal stimuli cannot be effectively scored from audiotapes, the clinician should take notes on such behaviors during assessment. Recorded dialogue may reveal misstatements that are suggestive of misunderstanding, however.

Evaluation of reading comprehension may be an important part of language assessment in school-age children. The child may be asked to silently read a story from his or her grade book or a familiar book. The child may then be asked to retell what was read.

Assessment of Other Aspects of Communication

A complete assessment of children with language disorders requires at least a quick screen of other forms of communication disorder. In some children with language disorders, speech sound disorders may be more common than other problems, but the clinician needs to keep all other communication disorders in perspective. Case history and interview of the parent and the child (if appropriate) will have suggested the main and additional problems for which help is sought. By the end of a language sample, clinicians would know whether to spend additional time on assessing these other problems.

While recording the language sample and throughout assessment, the clinician should take note of speech sound errors, dysfluencies, any tension associated with speech, motor behaviors associated with dysfluencies, mismanagement of airflow during speech, and voice quality deviations (e.g., harsh, horse, or nasal speech). An extended language and conversational speech sample is often adequate to rule out fluency, voice, and speech sound disorders. If warranted, the child may be scheduled for a specific speech, fluency, or voice assessment at a later time. If the child being assessed is nonverbal or minimally verbal, the targets of assessment will be gestures, pointing, grabbing the clinician's hand to get something, sign language, and other forms of nonverbal communication. The clinician in such cases may use the procedures described in Chapters 14 and 15.

Finally, assessment of language disorders in children requires that the clinician pay attention to literacy skills in children. Aspects of literacy assessment may be integrated into language assessment. The *Behavioral Assessment Protocol* in the next chapter includes procedures to assess basic textual responses (reading skills). If a more extensive literacy assessment is needed, the clinician may use the detailed information given in Chapter 16.

Standardized Language Diagnostic Tests

Tests are commonly used in assessing language skills of mainstream children. However, as pointed out in Chapter 3, standardized tests have their limitations regardless of the standardization sample. Even when a test is standardized on a particular ethnocultural group, some of the serious limitations of that test (e.g., limited sampling of the skill or questionable reliability) remain. As suggested in Chapter 3, a prudent use of a norm-reference test is to consider it as supplemental to other procedures, including a naturalistic language sample, a home language sample, a criterion-referenced assessment tool, a child-specific skill-oriented assessment tool, and so forth. Such alternative procedures, when combined with a naturalistically recorded language sample, will provide more valid data than a standardized test when used as the primary source of information.

Before selecting standardized language assessment tests, the clinician should review Chapters 3 and 4 that describe the strengths and limitations of tests and factors to consider in selecting tests for both mainstream and ethnoculturally diverse children. Several standardized tests are commercially available to assess language skills in children. Table 8–8 lists some of the commonly used standardized tests from which the clinician can select one or more to be administered to a child. American Speech-Language-Hearing Association lists many more tests the clinician can select from (http://www.asha.org/assessments .aspx). It is the clinician's responsibility to select tests that are reliable, valid, and appropriate for the individual child for whom the test is meant to be administered.

Assessment of Language Skills in Ethnoculturally Diverse Children

Verbal skills, being social skills, are a part of the larger cultural practices of a community. Therefore, assessment of language skills is always a culturally sensitive enterprise. It is true for all children, the mainstream as well as the ethnoculturally diverse. Most of the assessment instruments, especially standardized language tests, have been developed in the context of the mainstream culture, although in recent years, test developers have sampled ethnic and linguistic minority children in their test standardization or revision. Most tests take into consideration, as they should, the mainstream cultural practices and patterns of communication. However, when the same instruments are used in assessing children of ethnoculturally diverse children, there may be a dissonance between the instruments and the culturally based communication patterns the instruments are geared to assess. Therefore, the clinicians need to consider issues of culture and communication patterns, along with any bilingual status, in assessing ethnoculturally diverse children.

Table 8–8. Standardized Tests of Child Language Skills

Assessment Instrument	Age Range	Language Skills Tested
Assessment of Literacy and Language (ALL) (Lombardino, Lieberman, & Brown, 2005)	Preschool to Grade 1	spoken and written language skills, including comprehension and early literacy skills
Bankson Language Test (Bankson, 1990)	4 years to 8 years	production of semantic, syntactic, and morphologic skills
Boehm Test of Basic Concepts (Boehm, 2001)	3 years to 7;11 years	comprehension of basic semantic concepts
Clinical Evaluation of Language Fundamentals-Fourth Edition (CELF-4) (Semel, Wiig, & Secord, 2003)	5 years to 21years	expressive and receptive language: vocabulary and syntax
CELF-Preschool- Second Edition (Semel, Secord, & Wiig, 2004)	3 years to 6 years	expressive and receptive language: includes pragmatic language skills
Comprehensive Receptive and Expressive Vocabulary Test-2 (CREVT-2) (Wallace & Hammill, 2002)	4 years to 17;11 years	expressive and receptive language: defining words and pointing to pictures
Evaluating Communicative Competence (Simon, 1986)	9 years to 17 years	comprehension and production of pragmatic skills
Expressive One-Word Picture Vocabulary Test-Fourth Edition (EOWPVT-4) (Brownell, 2011)	2;0 years to 80; 11 years	expressive and receptive vocabulary: one-word naming of pictured stimuli
Expressive Vocabulary Test (EVT) (Williams, 1997)	2;6 years to adult	expressive language: labeling and synonyms
Peabody Picture Vocabulary Test (3rd edition) (Dunn & Dunn, 1997)	2;6 years to adult	receptive language: point-to-picture task
Preschool Language Scale, Fourth Edition (PLS-4) (Zimmerman, Steiner, & Evatt-Pond, 2002b)	Birth to 6;11 years	expressive and receptive language: vocabulary, basic concepts, morphology, syntax
Receptive One-Word Picture Vocabulary Test-Fourth Edition (ROWPVT-4) (Brownell, 2011)	2;11 years to 12 years	receptive language: point-to-picture task

Table 8–8. *(continued)*

Assessment Instrument	Age Range	Language Skills Tested
Sequenced Inventory of Communication Development-Revised (SIDC-R) (Hedrick, Prather, & Tobin, 1995)	4 months to 4 years	comprehension and production of communication skills
Structured Photographic Expressive Language Test 3 (SPELT-3) (Dawson & Stout, 2003)	4 years to 9;11 years	expressive language: morphologic and syntactical forms (includes alternative responses for African American dialects)
Test for Auditory Comprehension of Language-3 (TACL-3) (Carrow-Woolfolk, 1999)	3 years to 9;11 years	receptive language: vocabulary, grammatic morphemes, elaborated phrases and sentences
Test for Examining Expressive Morphology (Shipley, Stone, & Sue, 1983)	3 years to 8;11 years	production of morphologic skills
Test of Early Language Development- Third Edition (TELD) (Hresko, Reid, & Hammill, 1999)	2;0 years to 7;11 years	spoken language as well as receptive and expressive language skills
Test of Language Development-Primary (TOLD-P:4) (Newcomer & Hammill, 2008a)	4 years to 8;11 years	receptive and expressive language: vocabulary, syntax, sentence imitation
Test of Language Development-Intermediate (TOLD-I:4) (Newcomer & Hammill, 2008b)	8;0 years to 17;11 years	sentence combining, vocabulary, syntax, abstract language, multiple meanings
Test of Narrative Language (Gillam & Pearson, 2004)	5;0 years to 11;0 years	narrative language skills
Test of Pragmatic Language-Second Edition (Phelphs-Terasaki & Phelps-Gunn, 2007)	6;0 years to 18;11 years	social communication skills including abstract language
Test of Semantic Skills-Primary (TOSS-P) (Bowers, Huisingh, LaGiudice, & Orman, 2002)	4 years to 8;11 years	expressive and expressive language: labels, categories, attributes, functions, definitions

(continues)

Table 8–8. *(continued)*

Assessment Instrument	Age Range	Language Skills Tested
Test of Semantic Skills-Intermediate (Huisingh, Bowers, LaGiudice, & Orman, 2003)	9 years to 13;11 years	receptive language: temporal and spatial concepts
Test of Word Finding (German, 2000)	6;6 years to 12;11 years	single-word retrieval skills
Test of Word Finding in Discourse (German, 1991)	6;6 years to 12;11 years	word retrieval deficits in conversation
Token Test for Children-Second Edition (DiSimoni, 2007)	3 years to 12;11 years	receptive understanding of temporal and spatial concepts
Utah Test of Language Development–3 (Mecham, 2003)	3 years to 9;11 years	language production and comprehension
Wiig Criterion-Referenced Inventory of Language (Wiig, 1990)	4 years to 13 years	criterion referenced assessment of semantic, syntactic, morphologic, and pragmatic skills

We do not go into the details of assessment of ethnoculturally diverse children in this chapter because they are offered in Chapter 4. We summarize here a few main points that are specific to language assessment:

- Tailor the interview questions designed to find out specific information about the child's and the family's cultural and linguistic background; use the *Interview Protocol* given in Chapter 9 and modify it to suit the individual child and the family.

- Find out if the child and the family members speak African American English (AAE), and if so, to what extent; ask whether the child speaks both mainstream English and AAE and whether the parents are concerned about the child's academic performance in school and whether they want their child gain proficiency in mainstream English as well.

- Find out if the child speaks English as a second language, and if so, what is the primary language; ask questions about the child's and the family members' proficiency in either or both the languages; question parents about the child's academic performance and the need to gain proficiency in English. It is essential to ask parents whether they can read and write English because if they do not, the child may not be receiving the needed support for English academic and literacy learning at home.

- Design the rest of the assessment procedures in light of the child's and the family members' ethnocultural and linguistic background; follow the guidelines offered in Chapter 4 and Chapter 5; essentially:
  - Complete the standard/common procedures, including the case history, hearing screening and orofacial examination; as mentioned before, tailor the interview questions to suit the child and the family.
  - Use the most useful and practical elements of alternative assessment procedures; use only those tests that have been standardized on a sample drawn from the child's ethnocultural group; if such tests are not available, use only the alternative methods.
  - Obtain the language sample with stimuli and storybooks that are relevant to the child's background; if possible, arrange for parents to bring the child's favorite books to the assessment session.
  - Analyze the assessment data in the context of the child's language features; see, Chapter 4 for the language features of AAE, Spanish-influenced English, Asian language-influenced English, and English influenced by a Native American English.
- Use one of the multicultural assessment protocols given in Chapter 9 to assess an African America child, an Asian American child, or a Hispanic child.
- Diagnose a language disorder in an ethnoculturally diverse child (or in a child that speaks a different dialect of American English) only when:
  - The child's language pattern (a) deviates from the child's own dialect (for example, the language pattern of a Southern U.S. child deviates from Southern dialect)
  - The child's language pattern deviates from the pattern of AAE when the child speaks AAE or when the child's language pattern deviates from the expected patterns of mainstream English, but the deviations are not due to the influence of AAE
  - The language pattern of a second language deviates from the normal pattern of the child's primary language (e.g., Spanish or an Asian language)
  - The child's language pattern deviates from mainstream English, but the deviations are not due to the influence of the child's primary language

If an ethnoculturally diverse child also has a speech sound, fluency, or a voice disorder, the clinician should follow the guidelines given in respective chapters on those disorders. In addition, the clinician should follow the general guidelines given in Chapters 4 and 5.

Analysis and Integration of Assessment Results

To confirm the initial diagnosis of a language disorder, the clinician should analyze the assessment data and integrate them with the case history and interview information, along with any reports received from other professionals. Several steps may be taken to achieve an integrated analysis of all information.

Transcribe and Analyze the Language Sample

The first step in analyzing assessment data is to transcribe the language sample. Each intelligible utterance should be transcribed on a separate line, with written notes on the context of utterances. The number of unintelligible utterances should be noted as well. The transcription is necessary to measure the frequency of language skills to be evaluated. Production of words, sentence types, morphologic features, and various conversational skills may all be scored from the transcript. More specifically, the following kinds of analysis may be made from the transcript.

- The *mean length of utterance.* As discussed previously, the mean length of utterance may be calculated with procedures outlined in Table 8–3 and the child's mean length of utterance may be compared against the normative data given in Table 8–4.

- *Word productions.* The different kinds of words the child produced, including naming pictures, objects, and toys; naming objects by category (e.g., *food, toys, clothes*); naming objects within a category (e.g., naming as many animals as possible); and naming actions (verb productions)

- *Word combinations.* Presence and the frequency of word combinations including noun phrases (e.g., *pretty ball, my pink shoes*); verb phrases without the auxiliary *is* (e.g., *he walking*)

- *The type-token ratio (TTR).* A measure of *different* words a child produces, the TTR is calculated by counting each different word in the sample. A word repeated in the sample is counted only once. The TTR is typically about .45 to .50 for children ages 3 to 8 (Templin, 1957). It means that about half the number of total words spoken is different and the other half is repeated. A significantly lower than .5 TTR suggests limited expressive vocabulary. The ratio is calculated by the following formula:

$$\frac{\text{Total number of different words produced}}{\text{Total number of words produced}}$$

  - *Sentence structures and types.* The frequency measure with which different kinds of sentences are used is a useful measure. Clinicians may note the production of:
  - *Simple sentences*; an independent clause without a subordinate clause (e.g., *I laughed.*)
  - *Declarative sentences*; most descriptive statements (e.g., *This is my cat.*)
  - *Compound sentences;* a sentence with at least two independent clauses joined by a comma and a conjunction or with a semicolon; containing no subordinate clauses (e.g., *I went to the store, and then I went home*)
  - *Complex sentences*; a sentence with one independent clause and one or more subordinate clauses (e.g., *I played with my doll while Mommy washed dishes*)
  - *Questions* of various kinds (e.g., *What do you mean? Who is this? Where is it?*); different forms of *requests* (e.g., *Please help me, Tell me more*); imperatives that require a yes/no answer (e.g., *Is this a boy? Is that a balloon?*); and *direct commands* (e.g., *Sit down! Give me that!*)

- *Negative sentences*; sentences that reject or deny an affirmation (e.g., *That's not his ball; She is not here*)
- *Prepositional phrases* (e.g., *The dog is in the house*)
- *The Subject-verb-direct object constructions* (e.g., *He hit the ball*).

- *Grammatic morphemes.* Each morpheme may be counted for its frequency. See Table 8–2 for examples of some major grammatic morphemes. Counting the number of correct productions of a morpheme and the number of obligatory contexts in which the morpheme should have been used but was not, the clinician may calculate the percent correct production, specially for the bound morphemes (such as the regular plural and possessive inflections, the present progressive, and the regular past tense inflections); the following formula is used:

$$\frac{\text{The number of correct production}}{\text{The number of obligatory contexts}} \times 100$$

- *Conversational (pragmatic) language skills.* Various conversational skills that may be measured, depending on the level of language skill the child exhibits, include:
- *Topic initiation:* The frequency of new topic initiation during conversation
- *Topic maintenance:* The duration for which the child sustained conversation on a single topic
- *Conversational turn-taking:* The frequency with which the child took turns talking and listening; the number of interruptions the child made when expected to be listening
- *Conversational repair:* The frequency of requests for clarification and the frequency of appropriate responses to requests for clarification
- *Eye contact:* The frequency or durations for which the child maintained eye contact during conversation
- *Narrative skills:* Storytelling or retelling with adequate details, appropriate characterization, correct temporal sequencing, and with good beginning and ending
- *Eye contact as noted during the entire assessment session* (not scored from the transcript).

Evaluate the Language Sample for Other Disorders

The clinician may assess several other aspects of language production directly from the recorded audiotapes. Most clinicians will have concluded that the child does or does not have other communication disorders during the assessment session itself. If in doubt or to confirm the initial impressions, the clinician may listen to the sample for additional disorders and make appropriate judgments. If additional disorders are evident, the clinician schedules the child for further evaluation. Listening to the child's language samples, the clinician may assess:

- *The presence of other speech disorders.* The clinician will take note of any speech sound and fluency disorders heard on the audiotape. Any evidence of childhood apraxia of speech and dysarthria also will be noted.

- *The presence of voice and resonance disorders.* Whether the child has hoarseness, harshness, breathiness, hyper- or hyponasality, too high or a too low pitch or intensity may be noted while listening to the language sample.

Differential Diagnosis of Child Language Disorders

Most children who are routinely assessed and treated for language disorders may have specific language impairment (SLI). Other children may have associated clinical conditions as described previously (e.g., hearing impairment, autism spectrum disorders, intellectual or neurologic disabilities). Genetic syndromes may complicate language assessment and diagnosis. Generally, whether an associated clinical condition exists or not, the language disorders are diagnosed solely on the basis of limited language skills. Therefore, for the speech-language pathologist, the parameters of language are what are crucially important in diagnosing language disorders in children (Hegde & Maul, 2006).

Associated clinical conditions produce at least two differential diagnostic consequences. The first is the *severity* of the disorder. Although SLI also varies in severity, it is an associated clinical condition, such as severe intellectual disability, an extreme condition of autism, or profound hearing loss that produces the most severe language disorder.

The second is the *more complicated clinical picture.* The child with such associated clinical conditions almost always presents additional features and disabilities in nonverbal skills; certain unique verbal problems also may be evident. For instance, the child with intellectual disabilities may have deficient motor skills, impaired daily living skills, and more serious academic problems than a child with SLI. Depending on the severity of the disorder, the child's language skills, including basic vocabulary, may be extremely limited. A child who is deaf may have even more limited oral language skills than the one with SLI, but may have acquired an efficient sign language system (e.g., American Sign Language). A deaf child may also present serious and persistent voice and resonance problems that may not be prominent in children with SLI. A child who has an extreme case of autism may present such additional problems as emotional detachment and stereotypic and idiosyncratic responses.

The third is that an assessment and diagnosis of children with associated clinical conditions is a *team effort,* to which the speech-language pathologist contributes. Other specialists (e.g., psychologists, audiologists, geneticists, neurologists) help diagnose the additional problems associated with speech and language disorders. Whereas, the assessment and diagnosis of children who have SLI is the *sole responsibility* of speech-language pathologists, although there may be reasons to make a referral to other specialists.

The differential diagnostic guidelines that follow should be interpreted flexibly. They are guidelines and not rules, and even rules can have too many exceptions in a clinical science. All diagnostic categories may have additional features that should not be overlooked. For instance, speech disorders in SLI, stuttering in a child with Down syndrome, craniofacial anomalies, and hearing loss in children with certain genetic syndromes, should be assessed along with language skills.

Diagnose SLI if the child:

- Does have significant language problems in the context of normal or near-normal general development. Although all aspects of language may be affected, the impairment may be more pronounced in morphologic and syntactic aspects of language than in basic vocabulary and rudimentary pragmatic skills.

- Does not present significant intellectual, sensory, neurologic, and emotional disabilities, even though the child may have (controversially) subtle problems in certain intellectual functions as noted previously

Diagnose **language disorders associated with other clinical conditions** as follows:

- *Language disorders associated with hearing loss.* Make a complete assessment of language, speech, fluency, and voice; base your diagnosis on the impaired language features associated with hearing impairment as discussed in a previous section, but only when *supported by an audiologist's diagnosis of hearing loss.* Additional support may come from an otologist's diagnosis of auditory pathology.

- *Language disorders associated with autism spectrum disorders.* Diagnose a language disorder associated with autism, Asperger's syndrome, Rett's syndrome, and childhood disintegrative disorder with their unusual, stereotypic, persistent, and idiosyncratic production that characterize the spectrum; make differential diagnosis within the spectrum based on the unique characteristics; support the diagnosis with the primary diagnosis of an autism spectrum disorder by a psychologist or psychiatrist.

- *Language disorders associated with intellectual disabilities.* Diagnose a language disorder based on limited language skills, including a significantly limited vocabulary: a feature that might help contrast children with SLI to some extent. Support the diagnosis with a psychologist's independent assessment and diagnosis of intellectual disability. Take note of any genetic condition that may be associated with intellectual disabilities and seek additional diagnostic information as found necessary from a geneticist or physician.

- *Language disorders associated with genetic syndromes.* Unique language features that distinguish the various genetic syndromes are few. Therefore, diagnose language disorders based on limited language skills and support the diagnosis of an associated condition by a medical geneticist's independent diagnosis of the syndrome. Take note of any craniofacial anomalies that are often associated with genetic syndromes with their own consequences on speech and voice.

- *Language disorders associated with neurologic impairments.* Make a diagnosis based primarily on the impaired language features, but support the diagnosis with additional observations of neuromotor impairments, attention deficits, impulsive actions, irrelevant speech, disorientation, and so forth. Support the diagnosis also with an independent diagnosis of the neurologic impairment (e.g., cerebral palsy, traumatic brain injury) from a medical specialist.

Postassessment Counseling

During the final segment of the assessment session, the clinician counsels the parents or others who accompany the child. Depending on the age, the child may be part of this postassessment counseling. Although the results of the assessment will not have been fully analyzed, the clinician will have gained clinical impressions that are valid enough to summarize the results, make a tentative diagnosis, offer recommendations, describe treatment options, suggest a prognosis, and answer the most frequently asked questions.

Make a Tentative Diagnosis

Summarize your observations and clinical impressions gained from the observations. To the extent the observations justify, make as clear a diagnosis as possible. For example, you can say that according to the assessment data, the child has a language disorder, and it is called *specific language impairment*. Describe the main features of the child's language disorder that justifies your diagnosis. You might point out the limited vocabulary and deficient syntactic and morphologic skills observed and assessed through various means.

If the child's language disorder is associated with other clinical conditions, point out their typical association. For example, you might say that children with autism typically have language problems or those with Down syndrome are known to have difficulties in learning and producing language. Avoid any implication that one clinical condition the child has is the cause of another clinical condition when both coexist in a child. For instance, do not imply that autism is the cause of the child's language problem.

Make Recommendations

There is little or no controversy about recommending treatment to a child with a language disorder. If the diagnosis is firm, recommend language intervention. Treatment may be postponed only if the diagnosis is uncertain. In such cases, additional assessment sessions or home language samples may be necessary to confirm or rule out a language disorder.

Suggest Prognosis

Prognosis for improved language skills is good for SLI if effective treatment is offered as early as possible. Generally, the younger the age at which treatment is started, the better the prognosis for greatly improved or even near-normal language skills.

Limited prognosis is often a result of several factors, including ineffective, inefficient, or improperly administered treatment; the presence of multiple handicapping conditions as in severely expressed genetic conditions; deafness; profound intellectual disabilities; and severe neurologic impairments. Even then, language treatment is recommended, at least on an experimental basis, because children with the same severe conditions vastly differ in their response to treatment.

Answer Frequently Asked Questions

Most parents of children with language disorder ask clinicians questions about language disorders and its treatment. The clinician should give answers that are scientifically justifiable. Some commonly encountered questions and their answers follow; you may need to modify the terms you use to suit the age, education, and general judged sophistication of families in formulating your answers.

What Causes Language Disorders in Children?

Although we know about several potential causes of language disorders, it is difficult to say what caused it in a given child. Some children develop normally in all other respects, and yet have difficulty learning their language. This kind of difficulty is called *specific language impairment* or *SLI*. It is often not clear what causes it, although there may be some genetic influence. However, no specific gene has been identified for SLI. [*Give more details on SLI if the child has it.*] In other children, language disorder may be a part of other problems. Autism, hearing loss, intellectual disabilities, traumatic brain injury, genetic syndromes may all be associated with language disorders. [*Give more details if the child has one of these conditions in addition to language disorders.*]

How Long Does It Take to Treat Language Disorders Effectively?

It depends on several factors. The sooner the treatment is started, the more sustained and systematic the treatment, the faster the progress. If parents work with their children at home, following suggestions given, the progress is faster. Generally, the more severe the disorder, the greater the length of treatment. [*Address the child's specific severity of the disorder and make comments on potential duration of treatment.*] It usually takes one or more years to teach all aspects of language that the child may have to learn. In later years, the child may need some help with understanding and producing advanced and abstract language skills, including proverbs, metaphor, similes, and so forth.

What Are Some of the Treatment Options?

There are many well-researched treatment options. Both individual and group teaching techniques are available, but individual, one-on-one teaching is the most effective in the initial stages. Later, teaching in a group context may promote better social interactions. In almost all teaching methods, we select specific and useful language skills, model them for the child, and praise the child for correct responses. We may give some corrective feedback when the child gives incorrect responses. We use prompts, hints, and other devices that help avoid mistakes and learn the skills faster.

Also, in almost all procedures, we typically start with simpler skills the child lacks and add more complex skills as the child masters the simpler ones. For most children, a set of useful words and the small elements of grammar: the plural *-s*, the present progressive *-ing*, the pronouns, prepositions, the past tense *–ed*, and so forth are good initial skills to teach. We then move on to different kinds of sentences and conversational skills.

When Do We Start Treatment?

We recommend that we start treatment sooner rather than later for better and lasting outcome. We can set up a date now or you can call me or the clinic office later to begin treatment. [*Depending on the service setting, the clinician offers additional information on when and how to begin a treatment program for the child.*]

CHAPTER 9

Assessment of Language Skills: Protocols

- Note on Common Protocols
- Note on Specific Protocols
- Interview Protocol
- Normal Language Assessment Protocol
- Language Sample Transcription Protocol
- Language Sample Analysis Protocol: Syntactic, Morphologic, and Pragmatic Skills
- Task-Specific Assessment Protocol for Basic Vocabulary
- Task-Specific Assessment Protocol for Grammatic Morphemes
- Task-Specific Assessment Protocol for Conversational Skills
- Behavioral Assessment Protocol
- Selected Multicultural Assessment Protocols
- African American English (AAE): Language Assessment Protocol
- Asian American English: Language Assessment Protocol
- Spanish-Influenced English: Language Assessment Protocol

Note on Common Protocols

In completing a language assessment, the clinician may use the common protocols given in Chapter 2, also available on the CD. To make a comprehensive assessment of language disorders in children, the clinician may modify as needed and print for use the following common protocols from the CD:

The Child Case History Form

Orofacial Examination and Hearing Screening Protocol

Use this protocol along with the *Instructions for Conducting the Orofacial Examination: Observations and Implications.* If the preliminary findings of the orofacial examination suggests the possibility of velopharyngeal inadequacy or incompetence, use the *Resonance and Velopharyngeal Function Assessment* protocol in Chapter 13.

Assessment Report Outline

Expand the language section in the outline to include all relevant information gathered through the case history, interview, assessment, and reports from other professionals.

Note on Specific Protocols

This chapter contains a collection of protocols that can be used individually or combined in a variety of ways to facilitate the evaluation of a child's language skills. Each of these protocols is also available on the CD.

The protocols on the CD may be individualized and printed out as a group and used for a complete language assessment. Also, one or more protocols may be selectively printed out and used as needed. In assessing children with multiple disorders of communication, the clinician may combine these language assessment protocols with protocols from other chapters. For example, the clinician may combine language assessment protocols with speech assessment protocols (Chapter 7), fluency assessment protocols (Chapter 11), or voice assessment protocols (Chapter 13).

Language Assessment Protocol 1
Interview Protocol

Child's Name _____ DOB _____ Date _____ Clinician _____

Note that your interview of the parents or caregivers and the child (if appropriate) is mainly concerned with getting additional information on the child's language and general behavioral development, current language skills, associated clinical conditions, and current academic concerns including literacy problems.

Individualize this protocol on the CD and print it for your use.

Preparation

☐ Review the "interview guidelines" presented in Chapter 1.

☐ Make sure the setting is comfortable with adequate seating and lighting.

☐ Record the interview whenever possible.

☐ Find out if the parent is comfortable having the child in the same room during the interview. If so, have something for the child to do (toys, books, etc.). If not, make arrangements for someone else to supervise the child in a different room during the interview.

☐ Review the case history ahead of time, noting areas you want to review or obtain more information about.

Introduction

☐ Introduce yourself. Briefly review your assessment plan for the day and give an estimate of the duration of assessment.
to take.

    Example: "Hello Mr. /Mrs. [*the parent's name*]. My name is [*your name*] and I am the speech-language pathologist who will be assessing _____ [*the child's name*] today. I would like to start by reviewing the case history and asking you a few questions. Once we are finished talking, I will work with _____ [*child's name*]. Today's assessment should take about _____ [*estimate the amount of time you plan to spend*]."

Interview Questions

Ask the following kinds of questions to get clarifications or additional information. Skip or rephrase questions as found appropriate. Some parents need to be questioned in greater detail about the kinds of language problem the child exhibits because they only describe the problem in general terms; others give more specific descriptions. Note that many answers the parents give to the initial question may require additional follow-up questions not specified in the outline. During the interview, replace the term "he" or the phrases "your child," and "your son" with the child's name. Although the outline shows the questions that need to be asked and answered, avoid relentless questioning. Frequently, paraphrase what the informants say by way of answers to your questions. Ask about the informants' views, thoughts, or feelings. If appropriate, express approval of what they say. Note that it is not just the clinician who asks questions; parents or other informants, too, will have questions that the clinician needs to answer. If they have questions about the typical features of language disorders, causes of the problem, treatment options, and so forth, answer briefly and promise more detailed information later.

- ☐ What is your primary concern regarding your son's [or daughter's] language skills?
- ☐ Can you describe the problem?
- ☐ Do you think his language was delayed compared to other children? [Did your other child say the first words sooner?]
- ☐ Did you or the attending physicians notice anything unusual when your son was born? [*Ask follow-up questions if the answer is "yes;" ask questions about genetic syndromes, physical abnormalities, and so forth*]
- ☐ As an infant, was he responsive to your [mother's] speech and voice? Do you remember him turning in the direction of your [mother's] voice?
- ☐ How old was he when he began to babble sounds that were similar to *aa* or *uu* and so forth?
- ☐ So you think your son's language skills are not as expected. How old was he when he said his first few words? Like *Mommy* or *Daddy*.
- ☐ When he was about 2 years of age, how many words did he say?
- ☐ In your rough estimate, how many words does he use now? How many words does he seem to understand?
- ☐ How old was your son when he began to combine words into phrases? Phrases like, *More milk* or *Where Daddy?*
- ☐ Did he always seem to understand speech better than produce speech?
- ☐ Did you find it necessary to repeat what you say to him?
- ☐ Did you ever notice him being unresponsive to your speech, commands, requests, and so forth?
- ☐ Does he use gestures instead of speech to let you know that he wants something? For example, does he point to something he wants, instead of asking for it by name? [Did he do that when he was younger?]
- ☐ Does he often take your hand and lead you to something he wants? [Did he do that when he was younger?]
- ☐ Have you ever noticed him cry or fuss when he wanted something? This may be quite natural for a child who cannot request verbally.
- ☐ Does he have the usual kinds of facial expressions and gestures when he talks?
- ☐ Do you have to sometimes speak for him? [Do any of your other children speak for him, maybe because he does not answer?]
- ☐ Is it easy to understand what he says? Do people ask for him to repeat?

☐ Does he have difficulty pronouncing the sounds of English?

☐ What sounds does he pronounce correctly? What sounds does he still have problems with?

☐ What about putting sentences together? Was there a delay in doing that?

☐ Typically, how many words does he use in a sentence? Are you concerned that his sentences are not long enough and complex enough for his age?

☐ Can you give some examples of his typical sentences?

☐ How about striking a conversation with you? Can he start by saying, "Mom, I want to talk about—"?

☐ Can he continue to talk on a given topic, without getting distracted by other topics or comments?

☐ Does he typically look at you when he talks?

☐ What does he do when he doesn't understand what you tell him? Does he normally ask, "What do you mean?" or "Say it again." Or may be he will show that he does not understand by his facial expressions.

☐ What does he do when you tell him that you don't understand what he is saying? Does he say it differently?

☐ Can he strike a conversation with strangers you introduce to him?

☐ I think what you have described is typical of most children who have a language problem. They start babbling late, say their first words later than other children, and learn new words slowly. They take more time to begin combining words and have difficulty with sentence structures. Difficulty with small elements of grammar, like the plural -s, the possessive -s, the present progressive -ing, and past tense inflections are especially difficult for them. Striking and maintaining a conversation also could be difficult. Beyond these, some children may say things that are socially inappropriate. Does your son do that? [*Ask follow-up questions if the child is inappropriate in social situations.*]

☐ Have you recently seen any acceleration on learning language or has his progress been the same over the years?

☐ Is your son generally sociable or somewhat reluctant to talk?

☐ Does he play well with other children? [With his brothers and sisters?]

☐ Do you feel that your son's language problems are affecting his social interactions?

☐ Do you feel that your son's language difficulties are affecting his school performance?

☐ Do you think your child's reading and writing skills are fine? At what level is your son reading or writing? [*Ask this question when appropriate to the child's age; ask follow-up questions about literacy problems.*]

☐ What kind of concerns have you heard from your son's teachers? [*Ask follow-up questions about the effects language disorders have on the child's social, academic, and personal life.*]

(continues)

Interview Protocol (continued)

☐ Does your child have any other communication problems that you are concerned with?

☐ What do you think of his voice? Does his voice sound normal to you? [*Ask follow-up questions about other communication disorders the child may have.*]

☐ What is your first language? What is it your [husband's, wife's] first language?

☐ Is English your son's first language? If not, what other language or languages does he speak? Also, what language is routinely spoken at home?

☐ Does he speak the two languages equally well? If not, which language is stronger?

☐ Who reads stories to your son, talks more, and spends more play time with him? You or your [husband, wife]? Maybe both of you do to the same extent. [*Ask follow-up questions about the family's ethnocultural background, bilingual status, and family communication patterns.*]

☐ Are you aware of any family history of language problems? On either side of the family? [*Ask follow-up questions on the family history of language disorders*]

☐ Why do you think your son had difficulty learning his language? Do you have any thoughts about the causes of your son's language problems?

☐ Do you think your son hears normally?

☐ Did your son have ear infections in the past? Does he have any ear infections now?

☐ Has your child ever had a hearing test? If yes, when and where? What were the results?

☐ Has your child seen any other specialists for his stuttering? If so, who and when? What were their recommendations? How have you followed up on this?

☐ Has your child received language therapy? When and where?

☐ What did they work on in therapy? Can you describe the types of activities that were used? How did your child respond? Do you feel the therapy was helpful? Why or why not?

☐ Did your child receive any other kind of speech therapy? Maybe articulation therapy for correcting speech sound errors? [*Ask follow-up questions about previous treatment for speech, language or any other communication disorder and the nature and effects of such treatment.*]

☐ Have you taken your child to a psychologist for any kind of testing? [*Ask follow-up questions on any assessment done and diagnoses made*]

☐ Are there any other kinds of concerns you have about your child that you wish to let me know? [*Ask follow-up questions about any other problem the informants may mention; may include behavior problems, autism, intellectual disabilities, neuromotor problems, academic difficulties, vision problems, and so forth.*]

Before concluding the interview, review the case history and follow up with any additional questions you need to ask. Fill in any "blanks" in the medical, developmental, social, and educational histories.

Close the Interview

Before you close the initial interview, summarize the major points you have learned from the interview, allowing the parent or the caregiver an opportunity to interrupt or correct information. Close the interview with the following:

☐ You have given me sufficient information to begin my assessment. I know that your child has limited language skills that you are mostly concerned about. Now, do you have any questions for me at this point?

☐ Thank you very much for you input. The information has been very helpful.

☐ Now, I will work with [the child's name]. When we are finished, we will discuss the findings. I will also answer your questions about language difficulties and its treatment.

Language Assessment Protocol 2
Normal Language Assessment Protocol

Child's Name _____ DOB _____ Date _____ Clinician _____

Use the case history information, interview, and your direct observations to fill out the form. Place a check mark to indicate the presence of the skill; begin at a level that is 6 to 12 months below the child's chronological age; move up or down as found necessary.

Individualize this protocol on the CD and print it for your use.

Birth to 3 Months
☐ Startle responses to loud sound
☐ Visual tracking of the source of sound ☐ Turning toward sound source
☐ Attending to and turning head toward human voice
☐ Reflexive smiles ☐ Quiets when picked up
☐ Ceasessation of activity or cooing back when talked to (by 2 months)

4–6 Months
☐ Beginning of marginal babbling ☐ Production of double syllables (e.g., "baba") ☐ Putting lips together for /m/
☐ Moving or looking toward family members when they are named (e.g., "Where's Daddy?").
☐ Vocal play (e.g., growling and squealing) ☐ Production of adultlike vowels
☐ Arm-raising when the caregiver says, "Come here," or reaches toward child (by 6 months)

7–9 Months
☐ Looking at named common objects ☐ Comprehension of "no" ☐ Inflected vocal play
☐ Beginning of gestures ☐ Playing pat-a-cake or peek-a-boo ☐ Shaking head for "no"
☐ Production of sound combinations ☐ Imitation of heard intonation and speech sounds
☐ Variegated babbling (e.g., "mabamaba") ☐ Uncovering hidden toys (object permanence)

10–12 Months
☐ Comprehension of up to 10 words (e.g., *no, bye-bye, pat-a-cake, hot*)   ☐ Comprehension of one simple direction like "sit down" (accompanied by gesture)
☐ Relating tp symbol and object   ☐ Production of first true word
☐ Response to requests (e.g., giving a toy upon request)   ☐ Imitation of gestures and actions
☐ Looking in correct place for hidden toys   ☐ Head turning when name is called
☐ Gesturing or vocalizing to indicate needs   ☐ Joint reference   ☐ Loud jabbers
☐ Production of a variety of sounds and intonations   ☐ Vocal pitch variations
☐ Consonants and vowel production in vocal play   ☐ Production of meaningful words
1–2 Years
☐ One-word sentence productions (e.g., "up" may mean "Pick me up")
☐ Production of emphatic or imperative statement (e.g., "Car!" may mean "look at the car")
☐ Rising intonation to signal questions   ☐ Noun productions (approximately 51%)
☐ Single-word declarative statements (e.g., "Car" may mean *it is a car*)   ☐ Asks for "more"
☐ Word combinations (at around 18 months)   ☐ Three- or four-word responses (at 2 years)
☐ Production of 10–50 words around 18 months   ☐ Understanding about 200 words
☐ Overextensions (e.g., all women may be "Mommy")
☐ Correct response to "What's this?"   ☐ Nodding or shaking to yes/no questions
☐ Following one-step commands   ☐ Following simple directions accompanied by gestures (e.g., "Give Mommy the spoon.")
☐ Following directions involving one or two prepositions (e.g., *in* or *on* between 19–24 months)
☐ Pointing to one to five body parts on command   ☐ Pointing to recognized objects
☐ Listening to simple stories   ☐ Listening to repeated stories between 19–24 months
☐ Self-reference with pronoun and name (e.g., "Me Johnny" between 19–24 months)
☐ Verbalizations of immediate experiences (e.g., "Bath hot!")

(continues)

Normal Language Assessment Protocol (continued)

☐ Beginning production of verbs and adjectives.

☐ Beginning production of presuppositions

☐ Listening when spoken to

☐ Beginning of question asking (e.g., "why?" or "what that?")

☐ Giving directions to others (e.g., "Give me that")

☐ Production of words that describe experiences (e.g., "yummy" while licking a lollipop)

☐ Expression of wants (e.g., "I want ball.")

☐ Verbal interactions (e.g., "Hi, Daddy.")

2–3 Years

☐ Telegraphic speech (e.g., "doggy sit")   ☐ Verb-object (e.g., "push Barbie")

☐ Word combinations (at 36 months)

☐ Sentences with 3–4 words (subject-verb-object format; e.g., "Daddy throw ball")

☐ Production of *wh*-questions (e.g., "What's that?")   ☐ *Yes-no* questions

☐ Negation by adding "no" or "not" in front of verbs

☐ Comprehension of up to 2,400 words at 30 months   ☐ 3,600 words at 36 months

☐ Production of 200–600 words (average of 425 words at 30 months)

☐ Production of words related to objects, events, actions, adjectives, adverbs, spatial concepts, and temporal (time)

☐ Production of the first pronouns *I* and *me*

☐ Answering simple *wh*-questions (e.g., "What runs?")

☐ Understanding most questions   ☐ Asking *wh*-questions at 30 months)

☐ Identification of body parts   ☐ Carrying out one- and two-part commands

☐ Giving simple account of experiences or brief stories (36 months).

☐ Accelerated morphologic learning   ☐ Present progressive *ing*

☐ Prepositions *in* and *on*   ☐ Regular plurals   ☐ Possessives   ☐ Articles

☐ Pronouns   ☐ Irregular past   ☐ Forms of copula (e.g., *is, are*)

☐ Regular past-tense inflections (e.g., *walked, bended*)

☐ Overgeneralization of past-tense inflections (e.g., *goed, throwed*)

☐ Overgeneralization of regular plural morphemes (e.g., *feets, mousse*)

☐ Production of contractions (e.g., *don't, can't, it's, that's*)

☐ Topic maintenance in about 20% of the time (age 3)

☐ Making criticism, commands, requests, and threats

☐ Asking questions ☐ Gives answers

3–4 Years

☐ Comprehension of up to 4,200 words (42 months)

☐ Up to 5,600 words (48 months) ☐ Production of 800–1,500 words

☐ Production of conjunctions *and* and *because* in sentences

☐ Beginning production of complex verb phrases (e.g., "I should have been able to do it")

☐ Modal verbs (e.g., *could, should*)

☐ Tag questions (e.g., "You want to go, don't you?") ☐ Embedded forms

☐ Passive voice (e.g., "She's been bitten by a dog")

☐ Production of sentences averaging 5–5½ words per utterance (48 months)

☐ Beginning production of *do*-insertions (e.g., "Does the kitty run around?")

☐ Negation (e.g., "Timmy can't swim")

☐ Beginning production of complex and compound sentences

☐ Asking *how, why,* and *when* questions

☐ Answering questions involving *which, where,* and *what* (42 months)

☐ Labeling most things in the environment ☐ Relating experiences

☐ Describing activities in sequential order

☐ Understanding preschool stories (48 months)

☐ Reciting a poem from memory ☐ Singing a song

☐ Several nursery rhymes

☐ Knowing one's own full name, name of street

☐ Understanding some opposites (e.g., *day–night, little–big*)

☐ Understanding such concepts as *heavy–light, empty–full* (42 months)

☐ Understanding agent-action (e.g., "Tell me what flies, swims, bites")

☐ Production of pronouns *you, they, us, them, I,* and *me*

☐ Answering "what if" questions (e.g., "What would you do if you fell down?"

☐ Completion of incomplete sentences (e.g., "The apple is on the .")

☐ Completion of opposite analogies such as "Daddy is a man; Mommy is a ."

☐ Production of the irregular plural words (e.g., *children*) ☐ Third-person singular

☐ Present tense (e.g., "he runs") ☐ Regular past and present progressives

☐ Regular plurals (e.g., *boys, houses, lights*) ☐ Possessive morphemes

☐ Contracted forms of modals (e.g., *can't, won't*) ☐ Reflexive pronoun *myself*

☐ Negatives ☐ *is, are,* and *am* in sentences ☐ *is* at beginning of questions

(continues)

Normal Language Assessment Protocol (continued)

- ☐ Topic maintenance
- ☐ Beginning of speech modification speech to suit the age of listener
- ☐ Making requests   ☐ Expression of agreement   ☐ Denial
- ☐ Compliance   ☐ Refusal

- ☐ Early expressions of social conventions or routines (e.g., saying *hi, bye)*
- ☐ Calling out (e.g., "Hey, Mommy!")   ☐ Saying *please* and *thanks*
- ☐ Protesting and objecting   ☐ Making claims (e.g., as "I'm first!")
- ☐ Giving warnings (e.g. "Look out or you'll fall!")
- ☐ Teasing others (e.g., "You can't have this!")

4–5 Years

- ☐ Production of 6–6.5 words per sentence (by 5 years)
- ☐ A range of 1,500 to 2,000 words
- ☐ Speaking mostly in complete sentences   ☐ Producing complex sentences
- ☐ Future tenses (e.g., "he will do it"   ☐ Conjunction *if* and the adverb
- ☐ Conjunction *so*   ☐ Beginning production of passive sentences
- ☐ Production of *why-* and *how*-questions
- ☐ Production of most pronouns including the possessive forms
- ☐ Category naming (e.g., animals)   ☐ Asking word meanings
- ☐ Production of comparatives (e.g., *bigger, nicer,)*, modal verbs *could* and *would* in sentences
- ☐ Production of some irregular plurals (e.g., *mice, teeth)*

- ☐ Comprehension of about 5,600 words (48 months)
- ☐ Comprehension of about 6, 500 words (54 months)
- ☐ Comprehension of about 9,600 words (60 months)
- ☐ Understanding time concepts (*morning, tomorrow, before, after)*

- ☐ Answering *when-, how often-,* and *how long*-questions
- ☐ Demanding explanations by asking *why*

- ☐ Definition of common words by age 5
- ☐ Pointing to objects by use and function (e.g., "Show me what tells time," "Show me which one gives us milk")
- ☐ Picture identification of past and future verbs ("Show me who kicked the ball," "Who will kick the ball?")
- ☐ Judging grammatical correctness of sentences

- ☐ Telling longer stories accurately ☐ Modifying the age of listeners
- ☐ Telling jokes and riddles (around age 5)

5–6 Years

☐ Language that approximates the adult model with present, past, and future tenses

☐ Stringing of words with conjunctions ☐ Asking *how*-questions

☐ Production of the auxiliary *have* and conjunction *if* in sentences

☐ Answering "What happens if?" type of questions

☐ Understanding passive sentences

☐ Understanding and producing all prepositions

☐ Comprehension of 13,000–15,000 words by age 6

☐ Distinguishing *alike, same,* and *different*

☐ Telling left from right in self (not in others) ☐ Object definitions by use

☐ Understanding and producing common opposites (e.g., hard—soft, fat—thin)

☐ Giving complete address ☐ Telling longer stories

☐ Understanding such concepts as yesterday—tomorrow, more—less, some—many, several—few, most—least, before—after, now—later

☐ Stating similarities and differences between objects

☐ Naming position of objects: first, second, third

☐ Naming days of week in order

☐ Production of indefinite pronouns (e.g., *any, anything, every, both, few, many*)

☐ Production of superlative *-est* (e.g., *smartest*)

☐ Production of some adverbial word endings (e.g., *-ly*)

☐ Making conversational repairs ☐ Making polite and indirect requests

☐ Addressing people formally (e.g., Mr., Mrs.)

☐ Saying "thank you" and "I'm sorry"

☐ Asking permission to use objects belonging to others

☐ Participation in adult conversation

6–7 Years

☐ Correct production of most morphologic features

☐ Production of reflexive pronouns (e.g., *himself, myself*)

☐ Beginning production of perfect tense forms (e.g., *have, had*)

☐ Increased embedded sentences (e.g., *"The girl who bought the dress went to the party."*)

☐ More correct production of irregular comparatives (*good, better, best*)

☐ Beginning production of gerunds (adding *-ing* to a verb infinitive, e.g., *fish, fishing*)

☐ Early derivational morpheme productions\ (e.g., changing verbs into nouns, as in *catch—catcher*).

(continues)

Normal Language Assessment Protocol (continued)

☐ Comprehension of 20,000–26,000 words

☐ Tells what one does in each seasons of the year

☐ Left-to-right letter formation with few reversals and inversions

☐ Copying alphabet and numerals from printed models

☐ Reciting the alphabet sequentially

☐ Naming capital letters   ☐ Matching lower to upper case letters

☐ Rote counting to 100.

7–8 Years

☐ More frequent production of complex sentences

☐ Literal interpretation of jokes and riddles

☐ Anticipation of story endings   ☐ Better details in description

☐ initiation of conversation suggested by pictures

☐ Enjoying storytelling   ☐ Retelling a story, keeping main ideas in correct sequence

☐ Production of some figurative language

☐ Production of most irregular verb forms (some mistakes in irregular past tense)

☐ More consistent production of superlatives (*biggest, prettiest*) and adverbs

☐ Small group conversation initiation and maintenance

☐ Role-playing and taking the listener's point of view

☐ Talking in appropriate discourse codes and styles (e.g., informal with friends, formal with adults)

☐ Appropriate nonverbal behaviors (e.g., postures and gestures)

☐ Announcing topic shifts

☐ Sustaining concrete conversational topics through several turns (by 8 years)

☐ Sustaining abstract conversational topics (by age 11 years)

Language Assessment Protocol 3
Language Sample Transcription Protocol

Child's Name _____ DOB _____ Date _____ Clinician _____

Individualize this protocol on the CD and print it for your use.

Instructions

1. Collect a minimum of 50 utterances.
2. Write out each utterance, transcribing any words that contain articulation errors.
3. Use a dash (—) to represent unintelligible words.
4. Count the number of words and the number of morphemes
5. To complete your language analysis task:
    a. generate a list of correctly produced and missing *grammatic morphemes*
    b. generate a list of correctly produced *syntactic forms*
    c. generate a list of observed and missing *conversational (pragmatic) skills*
    d. generate a list of observed and missing *receptive language skills*
    e. calculate the mean length of utterance
6. To complete your speech analysis:
    a. generate a *list of phonemic errors*
    b. calculate *% intelligibility*

Record the Utterances and Score the Language Skills on this Form

1. _____

2. _____

3. _____

4. _____

5. _____

6. _____

7. _____

8. _____

9. _____

10. _____

11. _____

(continues)

Language Sample Transcription Protocol (continued)

12. _____

13. _____

14. _____

15. _____

16. _____

17. _____

18. _____

19. _____

20. _____

21. _____

22. _____

23. _____

24. _____

25. _____

26. _____

27. _____

28. _____

29. _____

30. _____

31. _____

32. _____

33. _____

34. _____

35. _____

36. _____

37. _____

38. _____

39. _____

40. _____

41. _____

42. _____

43. _____

44. _____

45. _____

46. _____

47. _____

48. _____

49. _____

50. _____

(add additional lines for any sample over 50 utterances)

Information needed to Calculate the Mean Length of Utterances (MLU):

Total Number of Utterances = _____

Total Number of Words = _____

Total Number of Morphemes = _____

Calculations:

MLU for words $= \dfrac{\text{total \# of words}}{\text{total \# of utterances}} =$ _____ words per utterance

MLU for morphemes $= \dfrac{\text{total \# of morphemes}}{\text{total \# of utterances}} =$ _____ morphemes per utterance

Calculate Speech Intelligibility:

Total Number of Utterances = _____

Number of Intelligible Utterances = _____ (Note: For this figure, if any part of an utterance is unintelligible, then the whole utterance is unintelligible.)

Total Number of Words = _____

Number of Intelligible Words = _____

(continues)

Language Sample Transcription Protocol (continued)

% Intelligibility on a Word-by-Word Basis:

$$\frac{\text{\# of intelligible words}}{\text{total \# of words}} = \underline{\hspace{1.5cm}} \times 100 = \underline{\hspace{1.5cm}}\%$$

> **Example:** Intelligibility on a word-by-word basis:
>
> # of intelligible words = <u>25</u>   # of words = 50;   <u>.50</u> × 100 = <u>50%</u> intelligibility

% Intelligibility on an Utterance-by-Utterance Basis:

$$\frac{\text{\# of intelligible utterances}}{\text{total \# of utterances}} = \underline{\hspace{1.5cm}} \times 100 = \underline{\hspace{1.5cm}}\%$$

> **Example:** Intelligibility on an utterance-by-utterance basis:
>
> # of intelligible utterances = <u>40</u>
>
> # of total utterances = 50;   <u>.80</u> × 100 = <u>80%</u> intelligibility

Language Assessment Protocol 4
Language Sample Analysis Protocol: Syntactic, Morphologic, and Pragmatic Skills

Child's Name _____ DOB _____ Date _____ Clinician _____

Individualize this protocol on the CD and print it for your use.

Syntactic Forms		Morphologic Features		Conversational Skills	
Produced	Missing	Produced	Missing	Produced	Missing
Score Syntactic Forms: Telegraphic Simple active declarative Complex sentences Compound sentences Compound/complex *Wh*-questions *Yes-No* questions Negative forms Passive forms Requests Other forms:		*Score Morphologic Features:* Present progressive *ing* Plurals (regular/irregular) Past tense (regular/ irregular) Possessives Prepositions Auxiliary *(is, are, was, were)* Copula *(is, are, was, were)* Pronouns Articles Conjunctions Comparatives/superlatives Third person singular Other features:		*Score Conversational Skills:* Topic initiation Topic maintenance Turn-taking Requests for clarification Correct response to requests for clarification Narrative skill Eye contact Other skills:	
Phonemes in error	Initial:		Medial:		Final:
Percent Intelligibility	Word-by-word:			Utterance-by-utterance:	

See Chapter 8 for details on, and examples of, syntactic forms, morphologic features, and conversational skills.

Language Assessment Protocol 5
Task-Specific Assessment Protocol for Basic Vocabulary

Child's Name _____ DOB _____ Date _____ Clinician _____

It is unlikely that a traditional language sample will contain all of the following initial words children are thought to produce. Therefore, assess this basic vocabulary through interview with the caregivers, home samples, and additional observations during the initial treatment sessions. Place a check mark to indicate the child produces that word reliably. Add other words the child produces in each category.

Individualize this protocol on the CD and print it for your use.

Words/Categories	Score	Words/Categories	Score
Clothing and Personal Items			
1. Belt	☐	6. Shirt	☐
2. Bib	☐	7. Shoes	☐
3. Boots	☐	8. Socks	☐
4. Hat	☐	9. Sweater	☐
5. Jacket	☐	10. Shoes	☐

Other clothing items the child names:

Food			
11. Apple	☐	24. Meat	☐
12. Banana	☐	25. Melon	☐
13. Bread	☐	26. Milk	☐
14. Cake	☐	27. Orange	☐
15. Candy	☐	28. Peach	☐
16. Cheese	☐	29. Pickle	☐
17. Chips	☐	30. Pizza	☐
18. Cookie	☐	31. Soda	☐
19. Crackers	☐	32. Soup	☐
20. Egg	☐	33. Spaghetti	☐
21. Gum	☐	34. Taco	☐
22. Hamburger	☐	35. Toast	☐
23. Juice	☐	36. Water	☐

Other food items the child names:

Words/Categories	Score	Words/Categories	Score

Toys

37. Ball	☐	45. Puzzle	☐
38. Bike	☐	46. Teddy Bear	☐
39. Baby	☐	47. Car	☐
40. Barbie	☐	48. Train	☐
41. Blocks	☐	49. Choo Choo	☐
42. Doll	☐	50. Truck	☐
43. Swing	☐	51. Plane	☐
44. House	☐		

Other toy names the child produces:

Furniture and Household Items

52. Bed	☐	58. Light	☐
53. Blanket	☐	59. Pillow	☐
54. Clock	☐	60. Telephone	☐
55. Cup	☐	61. Plate	☐
56. Crib	☐	62. Towel	☐
57. Door	☐		

Other furniture and household items the child names:

Kinship Terms

63. Mother	☐	7o. Grandmother	☐
64. Father	☐	71. Parent	☐
65. Brother	☐	72. Uncle	☐
66. Sister	☐	73. Aunt	☐
67. Son	☐	74. Cousin	☐
68. Daughter	☐	75. Niece	☐
69. Grandfather	☐	76. Nephew	☐

Names of the family members the child says:

(continues)

Task-Specific Assessment Protocol for Basic Vocabulary (continued)

Words/Categories	Score	Words/Categories	Score
Adjectives			
77. Big	☐	85. Low	☐
78. Little	☐	86. Happy	☐
79. Large	☐	87. Sad	☐
80. Small	☐	88. Red	☐
81. Tall	☐	89. Blue	☐
82. Short	☐	90. Yellow	☐
83. Long	☐	91. Green	☐
84. High	☐		

Other adjectives the child produces:

Words/Categories	Score	Words/Categories	Score
Names of Animals			
92. Dog	☐	98. Snake	☐
93. Kitty	☐	99. Hippo	☐
94. Fish	☐	100. Rhino	☐
95. Bird	☐	101. Chicken	☐
96. Lion	☐	102, Monkey	☐
97. Tiger	☐		

Other animal names or the names of pets the child says:

Language Assessment Protocol 6
Task-Specific Assessment Protocol for Grammatic Morphemes

Child's Name _____ DOB _____ Date _____ Clinician _____

Sample only those features that the child did not produce in his or her conversation with you (language sampling). Change words as needed, to suit the child's ethnocultural background. Add additional words within each category. Score a missing feature as incorrect.

Individualize this protocol on the CD and print it for your use.

Morpheme	Example	Correct	Incorrect
Present Progressive *ing*	He is *eating*.		
	She is *smiling*.		
	It is *jumping*.		
	They are *running*.		
	The cat is *sleeping*.		
	The boy is *reading*.		
	The girl is *riding* the horse.		
Regular Plural *(s, z, vz,l əz)*	Two *cats*. (*s*)		
	I see two *cups*. (*s*)		
	They are two *dogs*. (*z*)		
	My *shoes* are white. (*z*)		
	Leaves are green. (*vz*)		
	I see *wolves*. (*vz*)		
	You have two *boxes*. (*əz*)		
	I see two *houses*. (*əz*)		
Irregular Plural	I see two *women*.		
	I have two *feet*.		
	I see three *mice*.		
	They are all *men*.		
	Many *children* come to my school.		
	I have many *teeth*.		

(continues)

Task-Specific Assessment Protocol for Grammatic Morphemes (continued)

Morpheme	Example	Correct	Incorrect
Possessive (*s, z, əz*)	It is the *cat's* bowl. (*s*)		
	Elephant's trunk is long. (*s*)		
	It is my *Mommy's* bag. (*z*)		
	It is the *boy's* balloon. (*z*)		
	Santa Clause's *elves*. (*əz*)		
	It is the *horse's* tail. (*əz*)		
Prepositions (*in, on, under,* *behind*)	Car is *in* the bucket.		
	Pencil is *in* the mug.		
	The ball is *on* the table.		
	The book is *on* the floor.		
	The doll is *under* the table.		
	The coin is *under* the cup.		
	The book is *behind* the ball.		
	The cat is *behind* the box.		
Pronouns (*she, he, it, they*)	*She* bakes cookies.		
	She rides a bike.		
	He reads a book.		
	He eats a sandwich.		
	It moves slowly.		
	It licks its paw.		
	They are big trees.		
	They are eating apples.		
Conjunctions (*and, but, because*)	These are spoons *and* forks.		
	These are cups *and* plates.		
	She wants to paint, *but* there is no paint.		
	She wants to eat, *but* there is no food.		
	He is sleeping *because* he is tired.		
	She is eating *because* she is hungry.		

Morpheme	Example	Correct	Incorrect
Irregular Past Tense	I ate the candy you gave me.		
	The pencil fell from your hand.		
	I went to school yesterday.		
	This car is broke.		
Regular Past Tense (*t, d, ted, ded,*)	Mom baked cookies. (*t*)		
	She talked on phone. (*t*)		
	You moved the chair. (*d*)		
	I closed the door. (*d*)		
	I painted on this paper. (*ted*)		
	I counted to 10. (*ted*)		
	You folded the paper. (*ded*)		
	You bended your finger.(*ded*)		
Articles (*a, the*)	I see *a* dog.		
	That is *a* chair.		
	The ant is small.		
	The elephant is big.		
Auxiliary (*is, was, are, were*)	The girl *is* talking on the phone.		
	The boy *is* kicking the ball.		
	Yesterday, Daddy *was* working in his office.		
	Yesterday, I *was* playing with my brother.		
	You *are* writing.		
	They *are* watching animals.		
	Yesterday my Mom and Dad *were* working.		
	At six o' clock yesterday, we *were* eating dinner.		

(continues)

Task-Specific Assessment Protocol for Grammatic Morphemes (continued)

Morpheme	Example	Correct	Incorrect
Copula *(is, was, are, were)*	This *is* a tiny car.		
	That *is* a big book.		
	My teacher *was* nice to me yesterday.		
	Yesterday, my Mom *was* happy.		
	My friends *are* nice.		
	These trees *are* tall.		
	After the school yesterday, we *were* all hungry.		
	Animals *were* free when they were in the jungle.		

Summary of child's morphologic skills: _____

Language Assessment Protocol 7
Task-Specific Assessment Protocol for Conversational Skills

Child's Name _____ DOB _____ Date _____ Clinician _____

Individualize this protocol on the CD and print it for your use.

Pragmatic Skill	Child-Specific Strategy	Score
Topic Initiation Assess with at least three topics as suggested. Evoke additional topics if the data are unclear.	• **Topic 1.** Show a large picture of a scene within a zoo; wait a few seconds to see if the child begins to talk about something specific (e.g., animals). If the child did not initiate conversation, show another picture to see if the child does. If the child does not, prompt the child to talk about something; tell the child that something you talk about is a *topic*; prompt the child to say, "I want to talk about—." Prompt, "May be you can talk about the animals in the zoo. That is a topic." • **Topic 2.** Without a picture, evoke a conversational topic from the child, by asking "I want you to talk about another topic. Tell me what topic you are going to talk about." Prompt a topic if necessary (e.g., "My birthday party"). • **Topic 3.** Evoke another conversational topic by asking, "I want you to talk about one more topic. Tell me what topic you are going to talk about." *Do not prompt.* • Show one or two more story scenes and take note whether the child begins to talk about something specific. *Do not prompt.*	Measure the number of topics initiated with various kinds of help separately from those initiated without much help (prompts and other kinds of suggestions).

Topic Maintenance
 	
Use the same, minimally three, topics the child initiates to assess topic maintenance.
	• For **the first one or two** initiated topics with or without a prompt, encourage topic maintenance by asking the child to:
	  ○ say more
	  ○ tell what is happening? What happened? What will happen next?
	  ○ tell me about [this or that character]
	  ○ tell me about how the [character] felt
	  ○ explain events (why did it happen?)
	  ○ talk about subtopics (talking about vacations while discussing a zoo scene)
	  ○ stay on the same topic
	• For the **subsequent topics** initiated, refrain from prompts and suggestions to say more, but interact normally (e.g., express agreement, make typical comments).
		Measure the duration for which the child maintained conversation on the same topic; make judgments about the adequacy of topic maintenance. Measure durations separately for prompted topics and topics maintained in a more naturalistic manner.

(continues)

Task-Specific Assessment Protocol for Conversational Skills (continued)

Pragmatic Skill	Child-Specific Strategy	Score
Turn-Taking	• Measure the frequency of talking and listening. • Hold a conversation with the child on a shared topic (e.g., your and the child's birthday parties) to get additional data on talking and listening.	Also measure inappropriate interruptions and failure to take turns.
Requests for Clarification	• During assessment take note of (a) requests for clarification when the child did not understand you; and (b) the child's wrong responses—verbal or nonverbal—that suggest a failure to request for clarification. • Make ambiguous statements to see if the child asks "What do you mean?" or anything to that effect. • Place two or more similar objects (e.g., a yellow and a red comb) on the table and ask the child to point to one without specifying it (e.g., "Point to comb") to evaluate whether the child asks "Which one?"	Measure the total number of wrong responses attributable to a failure to request clarification and the number of times you made unclear statements and the frequency of requests for clarification.
Response to Request for Clarification	• During assessment, request clarification (e.g., "what do you mean?" "I don't understand") and count the correct or failed clarifications. • During the narrative task, request clarification and take note of the frequency with which the child modified his or her utterances to comply with your request.	Take note of the frequency with which the child adequately modified his or her productions.
Narrative Skill	• Ask the child to narrate a personal experience (e.g., birthday party, visit to the zoo or an amusement park, visit to grandparents, vacation, school experience, holiday cerebrations, hobbies, games). • Tell a short story and ask the child to retell it. • Ask the child to read a short story silently and retell it. • Ask the child to tell a story he or she knows. Prompt stories the child may know. Ask for parental suggestions and prompts, if necessary.	Evaluate the narratives for their completeness, details, chronologic sequences, characterization, appropriate beginning and end of the story, moral of the story, and so forth.
Eye Contact	• During assessment, observe eye contact during conversation. Take note of the frequency of with which the child avoids eye contact. • Ascertain whether lack of eye contact during conversation is a part of the child's ethnocultural background.	Make qualitative judgments whether the degree of eye contact is appropriate and whether lack of it is cultural.

Summary of Conversational Skills Assessment

Topic initiation: # of topics initiated: _____ .   Appropriate: ☐   Inappropriate: ☐

Topic maintenance: Average duration: _____ .   Appropriate: ☐   Inappropriate: ☐

Turn-Taking: # of turns taken: _____ .   Appropriate: ☐   Inappropriate: ☐

Request for clarification: # of requests: _____ .   Appropriate: ☐   Inappropriate: ☐

Response to request for clarification: _____ .   Appropriate: ☐   Inappropriate: ☐

Narrative skills: # of narratives: _____ .   Appropriate: ☐   Inappropriate: ☐

Eye Contact: Appropriate: ☐   Lacking: ☐   Lacking, but cultural: ☐

Comments: _____

_____

Language Assessment Protocol 8
Behavioral Assessment Protocol

Child's Name _____ DOB _____ Date _____ Clinician _____

Individualize this protocol on the CD and print it for your use.

The objective of this assessment is to establish the frequency with which each of the verbal operants a child emits during assessment.

Preparation for Behavioral Assessment

1. Review the *Behavioral Assessment* section in Chapter 5 to get refreshed on verbal operants and how they may be evoked.

2. Arrange for a special language sample structured to evoke specific verbal operants by gathering toys, puzzles, picture books, paper, crayons or pencils, and simple words printed on sheets of paper the child will be asked to name (read).

3. Prepare 10 to 12 modeling stimuli to evoke the echoics.

4. Prepare 10 to 12 brief sentence completion tasks and questions to assess intraverbals.

5. Select picture and verbal stimuli to evoke simple autoclitics (especially the basic grammatic morphemes).

6. Based on the case history and parental interview, think of a few simple topics on which to converse with the child to assess conversational skills

7. Plan the kinds of reinforcing consequences you might deliver for the different kinds of verbal operants (verbal for most, and physical or tangible for the mands).

8. Check the exemplars listed in the next section to prepare the various kinds of needed stimuli specified in this list.

Assessment of Primary Verbal Operants

Child's Name _____

Echoics

To assess echoics, model a verbal stimulus to evoke a response takes the same form as your modeled stimulus. To classify a response as an echoic, the verbal model and the response should be more or less identical; see also intraverbal for the similarity and the critical difference.

Use the *Task Specific Assessment Protocol for Basic Vocabulary (Language Assessment Protocol 5)* to evaluate the echoics. First, use that protocol to assess production of the listed words. Select only the words the child did not produce; model them to assess their imitation. Score the response or its absence by placing a check mark in the appropriate box.

Words	Echoic Responses			
	Complete	Partial	Wrong	Absent
1.				
2.				
3.				
4.				
5.				
6.				
7.				
8.				
9.				
10.				
11.				
12.				
13.				
14.				
15.				

Opening this protocol on the CD, select the words the child did not produce on *Language Assessment Protocol 5,* enter them on this page, extend the list as necessary and print it out for assessment. Model the words to evoke echoics and score the responses.

(continues)

Behavioral Assessment Protocol (continued)

Child's Name _____

Mands

To evoke mands, withhold objects the child seem to want (establishing operation); reinforce the mand by giving what is manded; check whether the response and the reinforcement matched (see the *Behavioral Assessment* section in Chapter 5). If the child does not mand verbally and spontaneously (SP) but implies it in other ways (e.g., tries to reach for the object), prompt (PR) a mand by asking such questions as, "What do you want?" "What do you want to play with?" Write down the mand; note that the mand may take any form (single words to complete sentences), and may be verbal or nonverbal. If nonverbal describe it (e.g., *pointed to the . . .*).

Mand Setup	Mand		Reinforcement	Match
Ask the child to complete a simple puzzle; withhold a piece needed to complete it	☐ SP	☐ PR	Hand the piece of puzzle to the child.	☐ Yes ☐ No
Play with a toy truck to see if the child mands it	☐ SP	☐ PR	Give the truck to the child.	☐ Yes ☐ No
Display some juice in a small transparent cup	☐ SP	☐ PR	Give the cup of juice.	☐ Yes ☐ No
Bounce a colorful ball in front of the child	☐ SP	☐ PR	Give the ball	☐ Yes ☐ No
Give a piece of paper, withhold the crayon, and ask the child to draw something.	☐ SP	☐ PR	Give the crayon	☐ No ☐ No
A toy displayed on a high shelf (specify):	☐ SP	☐ PR	Give the requested toy	☐ Yes ☐ No
A toy displayed on a high shelf (specify):	☐ SP	☐ PR	Give the requested toy	☐ Yes ☐ No
A toy displayed on a high shelf (specify):	☐ SP	☐ PR	Give the requested toy	☐ Yes ☐ No
A toy displayed on a high shelf (specify):	☐ SP	☐ PR	Give the requested toy	☐ Yes ☐ No
A toy displayed on a high shelf (specify):	☐ SP	☐ PR	Give the requested toy	☐ Yes ☐ No

Add additional items to this table on the CD, print it out, and assess 15 to 20 mands that are scored *Yes* for *Match*.

Child's Name _____

Tacts

To evoke tacts (naming, describing), use objects or pictures the child is likely to be familiar with; reinforce the tact with verbal praise; check whether the response and the reinforcement matched (see the *Behavioral Assessment* section in Chapter 5). Specify each stimulus. To evoke tacts, ask such questions as: "What is this?" "What is its name?" "Can you describe what you see?" If there is no response (SP), prompt it by describing and demonstrating the use of the object: "You write with it" "You bounce it like this." Write down the tact, which may be a single word, a sentence, or a brief description.

Stimuli for Tacts	Tact		Match	Reinforcement
1.	☐ SP	☐ PR	☐ Yes ☐ No	
2.	☐ SP	☐ PR	☐ Yes ☐ No	
3.	☐ SP	☐ PR	☐ Yes ☐ No	Offer such social reinforcement as:
4.	☐ SP	☐ PR	☐ Yes ☐ No	"You're right!"
5.	☐ SP	☐ PR	☐ Yes ☐ No	"That's correct!" "I think so, too!"
6.	☐ SP	☐ PR	☐ Yes ☐ No	"I like what you said!" "You know that!"
7.	☐ SP	☐ PR	☐ Yes ☐ No	"Great!"
8.	☐ SP	☐ PR	☐ Yes ☐ No	"Excellent!" "You are smart!"
9.	☐ SP	☐ PR	☐ Yes ☐ No	
10.	☐ SP	☐ PR	☐ Yes ☐ No	

Add additional items to this table on the CD, print it out, and assess 15 to 20 tacts that are scored *Yes* for *Match*.

(continues)

Behavioral Assessment Protocol (continued)

Child's Name _____

Intraverbals

To evoke intraverbals, you can ask the child to answer questions, name items within a category, complete partially modeled sentences, count numbers, recite the alphabet, sing a song, tell a commonly told (and typically remembered) story, and so forth. To consider a response an intraverbal, the stimulus must be verbal; it cannot be physical, a state of motivation, or a printed material. Both the echoics and intraverbals are controlled by verbal stimuli, but in the former, the response and the stimuli match, but in the latter, the two are different. Substitute the items to suit the child, and write down the responses.

Verbal Stimuli	Response	Correct	Incorrect
1. What is your name?		☐	☐
2. What color is your shirt?		☐	☐
3. What do you wear on your feet?		☐	☐
4. Can you name some fruits?		☐	☐
5. Can you name some animals?		☐	☐
6. Can you name some flowers?		☐	☐
7. Where is your bed?		☐	☐
8. Where does your mom [dad] cook?		☐	☐
9. Where do you keep your toys?		☐	☐
10. Can you say your ABCs? Okay, I will get you started. *A, B, C . . .*		☐	☐
11. Can you count the numbers? Okay, I will get you started. *One, two, . . .*		☐	☐
12. Do you know the days of the week? Okay, I will get you started. *Sunday, Monday . . .*		☐	☐
13. Do you know the *Pussy cat, pussy cat* song? Okay, I will get you started. *Pussy cat, pussy cat . . .*		☐	☐

Verbal Stimuli	Response	Correct	Incorrect
14. Can you sing *Frosty the snow man* song? Okay, I will get you started. *Frosty the snow man . . .*		☐	☐
15. Ask the child to tell a small story; if no response, read a brief story aloud and ask the child to retell it.	Score this from audiorecording. Take note of the number of elements repeated.		

Add additional items to this table on the CD to sample more intraverbals. For items 10 through 14, note down the number of intraverbal elements the child completed. For example, *counted to 4* or *completed the next line of the song,* or *the entire song.*

(continues)

Behavioral Assessment Protocol (continued)

Child's Name _____

Autoclitics

Autoclitics, the secondary verbal operants that include grammar and more, are a large category of verbal behaviors. For an initial assessment, the clinician may concentrate on morphologic features that are typically taught to children with language disorders.

Use the *Task-Specific Assessment Protocol for Grammatic Morphemes* (Language Assessment Protocol 6) to sample morphologic autoclitics. A comprehensive language sample may help assess the frequency with which the child produces the microautoclitics (grammatic morphemes added to word forms). In addition, the clinician may use the protocol for morphemes to make sure that all morphemes are adequately sampled. Summarize the results in the following table. Specify the error patterns.

Microautoclitics	Error Patterns	Percent Correct
Present progressive *ing*		
Regular plural (s, z, vz, əz)		
Irregular plural		
Possessives (s, z, əz)		
Prepositions (*in, on, under, behind*)		
Pronouns (*she, he, it, they*)		
Conjunctions (*and, but, because*)		
Irregular past tense		
Regular past tense (*t, d, ted, ded*)		
Articles (*a, the*)		
Auxiliary (*is, was, are, were*)		
Copula (*is, was, are, were*)		

Add additional items to this table on the CD, print it out and use it during assessment.

Child's Name _____

Textuals

Textuals are under the control of printed material. A child being assessed is a reader, ask the child to read few simple words and sentences. This will allow you to make a basic literacy skill assessment while doing a language evaluation. Accessing the CD, create child-specific stimulus materials that you gauge after talking with the parent and sampling the books the child is familiar with. Print the stimuli and ask the child to read each on discrete trials.

Score the responses as C for *Correct,* PC for *Partially Correct,* WR for *Wrong,* and NR for *No response*

Stimuli (specify)	C	PC	WR	NR
I. List of Words the child was asked to read				
1.				
2.				
3.				
4.				
5.				
6.				
7.				
8.				
9.				
10.				
II. List of sentences the child was asked to read				
1.				
2.				
3.				
4.				
5.				
6.				
7.				
8.				
9.				
10.				

Alternatively, request parents to bring a book the child reads at home, and ask the child to read words and sentences.

Selected Multicultural Assessment Protocols

Common assessment procedures, including the case history, orofacial examination, hearing screening, and collection of a speech-language sample are necessary to assess all children, including those who are ethnoculturally diverse. In addition, it is necessary to take into consideration the child and the family's cultural and linguistic background to assess ethnoculturally diverse children. The interview will concentrate on the family's cultural and linguistic variables that affect the child's language skills. The child's bilingual status, if any, will be determined. Standardized tests may or may not be administered; but the language sample will be analyzed in the context of the child's first language or the child's unique English dialect (e.g., African American English). See Chapter 4 for more information on assessing children of ethnocultural diversity.

On the following pages, three protocols are provided for assessing language skills in African American children, Asian American children, and Hispanic children. If a child assessed belongs to one of these ethnocultural group, the clinician may select the appropriate protocol, complete it, and attach it to the rest of the assessment protocols used, the case history form completed, and the written assessment report.

Language Assessment Protocol 9
African American English (AAE): Language Assessment Protocol

Child's Name _____ DOB _____ Date _____ Clinician _____

Analyze the child's recorded speech-language sample. Check *Yes* if the African American English feature is observed; give phonetically transcribed examples in your report. Take note of unique features not listed in the protocol. The reference language is Mainstream American English (MAE).

Individualize this protocol on the CD and print it for your use.

AAE Language Characteristics		Score	
Omission of MAE Grammatical Features	Noun possessives (e.g., "it Kaneesha house" for *It's Kaneesha's house*)	☐ Yes	☐ No
	The plural morpheme (e.g., "she got five pencil" for *she has five pencils*)	☐ Yes	☐ No
	Third person singular (e.g., "he work downtown" for *he works downtown*)	☐ Yes	☐ No
	Forms of *to be* (*is, are*) (e.g., "he a nice man" or "They going on a vacation"	☐ Yes	☐ No
	The present tense form of auxiliary *have* (e.g., "I been here for two hours" for *I have been here for two hours*)	☐ Yes	☐ No
	The Past tense form of *have* (e.g., "he done it again" *for he has done it again*)	☐ Yes	☐ No
	The past tense morpheme (e.g., "he live in Africa" for *he lives in Africa*)	☐ Yes	☐ No
	The auxiliary *is* when the described action is temporary (e.g., "he working" "he be working;" see Chapter 4 for distinctions)	☐ Yes	☐ No
Replacement of certain MAE features with other features	Auxiliary *is* for auxiliary *are* (e.g., "they is doing fine!" for *they are doing fine*)	☐ Yes	☐ No
	Copula *is* for the copula *are* (e.g., "you is not bad!" for *you are not bad!*)	☐ Yes	☐ No
	Past tense *was* for its plural form (e.g., "they was doing well" for *they were doing well* or "you was nice to me" for *you were nice to me*)	☐ Yes	☐ No

African American English (AAE): Language Assessment Protocol (continued)

AAE Language Characteristics		Score	
Replacement of certain MAE features with other features *(continued)*	*None* for *any* (e.g., "he don't need none" for *he doesn't need any*)	☐ Yes	☐ No
	Them for *those* (e.g., "them houses, they be old" for *those houses are old* or "Where do you get them shoes?" for *where do you get those shoes?*)	☐ Yes	☐ No
	Gonna for future tense *is* and *are* auxiliary forms (e.g., "He gonna do it" for *he is going to do it* or "they gonna be fine" for *they are going to be fine*)	☐ Yes	☐ No
	Does for *do* (e.g., "he do cook well" for *he does cook well* or "It do make sense" for *it does make sense*)	☐ Yes	☐ No
Addition of Other Features	*at* at the end of *where* questions (e.g., "where is the cat *at*?" for *where is the cat?*)	☐ Yes	☐ No
	A second auxiliary (e.g., "I might could have done it" for *I could have done it*)	☐ Yes	☐ No
	A double negatives for emphasis (e.g., "I don't never want no cake" for *I don't want any cake* or "I have not seen no one" for *I have not seen anyone*)	☐ Yes	☐ No
	been to emphasize past events or actions (e.g., "I been had an accident when I was 20" for *I had an accident when I was 20* or "I been known that" for *I have known that*)	☐ Yes	☐ No
	done to a past tense construction (e.g., "he done painted the house" for *he painted the house*)	☐ Yes	☐ No
	An implied pronoun to restate the subject (e.g., "my mother, *she* cannot make it" for *my mother cannot make it*)	☐ Yes	☐ No

Diagnostic Criteria: These and other African American English language features observed in the child's speech are not a basis to diagnose a language disorder. Deviations must be observed in morphosyntactic structures that are *not typical of AAE* to justify the diagnosis.

Language Assessment Protocol 10
Asian American English: Language Assessment Protocol

Child's Name _____ DOB _____ Date _____ Clinician _____

Analyze the child's recorded speech-language sample. Check *Yes* if the Asian American English language is observed; give phonetically transcribed examples in your report. Take note of unique features not listed.

Individualize this protocol on the CD and print it for your use.

Asian American English Characteristics		Score	
Omission of grammatical features	Regular plural morphemes (e.g., "give me five book")	☐ Yes	☐ No
	Verbal auxiliaries (e.g., "he walking fast" or "they eating a lot")	☐ Yes	☐ No
	Verbal copula (e.g., "she very nice" or "they very big")	☐ Yes	☐ No
	Possessive morphemes (e.g., "that is Dad hat")	☐ Yes	☐ No
	Regular past tense morphemes (e.g., "he work hard last year")	☐ Yes	☐ No
	Articles (e.g., "give me book" or "cat is here")	☐ Yes	☐ No
	Conjunctions (e.g., "Paul [ ] Michelle are coming")	☐ Yes	☐ No
	Forms of have (e.g., "we [ ] been to the store")	☐ Yes	☐ No
Addition of grammatical elements	Past tense double marking (e.g., "he didn't went with his friends")	☐ Yes	☐ No
	Double negative (e.g., "they don't have No food to eat")	☐ Yes	☐ No
Misuse or incorrect use	Pronouns (e.g., "her wife is here")	☐ Yes	☐ No
	Prepositions (e.g., "she is in home")	☐ Yes	☐ No
	Comparatives (e.g., "this is gooder than that" or "this is nice than that")	☐ Yes	☐ No
	Lack of inflection on auxiliary *do* (e.g., "he do not have enough")	☐ Yes	☐ No
	Incorrect word order in interrogatives (e.g., "you are going Now?")	☐ Yes	☐ No

(continues)

Asian American English: Language Assessment Protocol (continued)

Diagnostic Criteria: These and other characteristics of English language productions influenced an Asian language are not a basis to diagnose a language disorder in bilingual Asian American children. To diagnose a language disorder in English, children should exhibit deviations other than what is typical of bilingual-Asian American children. Because of variations in Asian languages, each child's particular morphosyntactic characteristics need to be understood.

Language Assessment Protocol 11
Spanish-Influenced English: Language Assessment Protocol

Child's Name _____ DOB _____ Date _____ Clinician _____

Analyze the child's recorded speech-language sample. Check *Yes* if the Spanish-influenced English language feature is observed; give phonetically transcribed examples in your report. Take note of unique features not listed in the protocol.

Individualize this protocol on the CD and print it for your use.

Spanish-Influenced English Characteristics		Score	
Differences in word order	Nouns preceding adjectives (e.g., "The pencil red" for *The red pencil.*)	☐ Yes	☐ No
	Verbs preceding adverbs (e.g., "He drives very fast his motorcycle" for *He drives his motorcycle very fast.*)	☐ Yes	☐ No
Omission of grammatic morphemes	Regular plural allomorphs (e.g., "I see two book" for *I see two books.*)	☐ Yes	☐ No
	Regular possessive allomorphs (e.g., "The boy bicycle" for *The boy's bicycle.*)	☐ Yes	☐ No
	Regular past tense allomorphs (e.g., "They talk yesterday" for *They talked yesterday* or "We paint last month" for *We painted last month.*)	☐ Yes	☐ No
Varied grammatical expressions	Double negatives (e.g., "I don't want No more" for *I don't want any more.*)	☐ Yes	☐ No
	more instead of a comparative (e.g., "This house is more small" for *This house is smaller.*)	☐ Yes	☐ No
Varied prosodic features	Spanish stress patterns in English productions (e.g., "baking" with an emphasis on the final syllable)	☐ Yes	☐ No
	Reduced pitch range	☐ Yes	☐ No
	Lower pitch at the beginning of utterances that would normally be started at higher pitch in English	☐ Yes	☐ No

Diagnostic Criteria: These and other language characteristics are not a basis to diagnose a language disorder in children whose English is influenced by their Spanish. To diagnose such a disorder, the child's morphosyntactic features should deviate in other respects. Because a variety of Spanish dialects influence English, it is essential to understand the particular variety that affects English in a Spanish-English bilingual child.

PART IV
Assessment of Fluency

CHAPTER 10

Assessment of Fluency Disorders: Resources

- Descriptions of Fluency
- Measurement of Fluency
- Disorders of Fluency
- Stuttering
- Ethnocultural Variables and Stuttering
- Definition and Measurement of Stuttering
- Additional Features of Stuttering
- Cluttering
- Analysis and Integration of Assessment Results
- Differential Diagnosis of Fluency Disorders
- Postassessment Counseling

Fluency is an aspect of speech and language production. It is a somewhat neglected aspect of communication because impaired fluency, not normal fluency, has received much research and clinical attention. Historically, stuttering, a single disorder of fluency, was considered an entity unto itself; normal fluency, which is impaired in stuttered speech, did not receive the kind of attention that normal language or normal speech production received. There is no literature on the normal development of fluency in children that is comparable in scope to normal speech and language acquisition in children.

Because of an emphasis on impaired fluency, fluency itself is often defined negatively: it is speech that is relatively free from stuttering, cluttering, and such other disorders of fluency as neurogenic stuttering in adults. In measuring fluency, clinicians typically measure dysfluencies or stuttering, defined with varying degrees of specificity; if dysfluencies observed in the speech of a speaker are within a range that is socially acceptable, the speech is considered fluent. In more recent years, fluency has been described in some positive terms, however. Such descriptions are purely topographic: they inform how fluent speech feels and how the listeners may subjectively evaluate it.

Descriptions of Fluency

Generally, fluency is topographically described as speech that is relatively flowing, effortless, smooth, rhythmic, rapid, and continuous. Fluent speech flows without too many disruptions. It is produced without much muscular or ideational effort. Fluent speech has a rhythm to it because it has a pattern of rate and prosodic variations. To the contrary, speech that is relatively halting, effortful, rough, nonrhythmic, slow, and discontinuous is dysfluent (Guitar, 2006; Starkweather, 1987).

Fluency also can be described in terms of potential variables that may cause it. For instance, fluency is enhanced when a speaker has a good knowledge of the subject matter he or she is talking about; lack of knowledge may cause hesitations, impaired flow, and sparse and nonrhythmic speech with a high rate of dysfluencies (Hegde, 1987). Such other factors as an intact speech and language-related neuromuscular mechanism and command of language also may enhance fluency. An environment free from distracting variables that impinge on the speaker may promote fluency, provided other fluency-inducing variables are present.

Although several variables may normally lead to fluent speech production in all speakers, including those who stutter, it cannot be assumed that an absence of those variables causes stuttering. For instance, it is unlikely that stuttering is due to a lack of knowledge of the subject matter being spoken about; most people who stutter do so while talking on topics or subjects they know very well. They may frequently stutter on their own names and addresses, introducing themselves to others, asking for directions, ordering in restaurants, and so forth. Although certain neurological impairments in adults my cause a fluency problem, such impairments are not the typical causes of stuttering of early childhood onset (Hegde, 2008a). Nonetheless, some of the dysfluencies of children and adults who stutter may be due to the same variables that create disruptions in fluency in all speakers because people who stutter cannot be immune to them.

Measurement of Fluency

Although fluency is indirectly assessed by measuring dysfluencies or stuttering in speech, it may be essential to evaluate it more directly if treatment to be offered involves placing behavioral contingencies on fluent speech (as against stuttering). For instance, a clinician may want to positively reinforce fluency while ignoring stuttering. Before initiating such a treatment program, the clinician needs to evaluate fluency in a quantitative manner.

Two methods are available to quantitatively assess fluency. Both require a recorded sample of continuous speech. In the first method, fluency may be measured *topographically*. Topographic measurement of fluency specifies the number of fluent utterances heard in a speech sample. Fluent utterances are those that are free from dysfluencies and exhibit the previously described characteristics of fluent speech. The utterances may be further specified in terms of the number of words or syllables produced fluently. It is a response-unit based measurement of fluency.

The response-unit based measurement of fluency may specify the typical or modal utterance that a person speaks fluently (without dysfluencies). For example, a client may be typically fluent only on single words, two-word phrases, or sentences that do not exceed a certain number of words. Typicality is indexed by the statistical mode: the most frequently noted fluent utterance. Generally, the longer is the fluent utterance, the lower is the frequency of speech dysfluencies. Following such an assessment of fluency, the clinician may reinforce fluent utterances and measure their frequency to document improvement.

In the second method, fluency is measured in terms of *temporal durations*, instead of response units (Hegde & Brutten, 1977). In this method, the clinician measures the various time durations for which the client sustained fluency in continuous speech. Calculating the statistical mode for the observed durations, the clinician determines the most frequently observed fluent duration in speech. One client, for example, may be typically fluent for 10 seconds, whereas another may be fluent for 20 seconds. The longer is the durations of fluency, the lower is the frequency of dysfluencies. With this measure of fluency, the clinician may positively reinforce the typical durations of fluency and measure their frequency in all treatment sessions to find out if the frequency increases across sessions.

Disorders of Fluency

The concept of *fluency disorders* is relatively new; the term *stuttering* has a much longer history. In fact, the profession of speech-language pathology was established in the 1920s mainly because of a few individuals' research and clinical interest in stuttering. In the beginning, what is now known as speech-language pathology was mostly concerned with stuttering. Such pioneering speech pathologists as Wendell Johnson and Charles Van Riper were people who stuttered, and later on, became specialists in stuttering. It is only in subsequent decades that other speech disorders, including speech sound disorders, aphasia, language disorders in children, and swallowing disorders in adults became part of speech-language pathology.

Currently, several forms of fluency disorders are recognized although the bulk of research and clinical effort is concentrated on stuttering (Curlee, 1999; Hegde, 2008a)). Most clinicians working with children assess and treat children who stutter; their caseload may include a few children who clutter as well. But they are unlikely to work with neurogenic stuttering as it is found mostly in adults. This chapter is limited to the assessment of fluency disorders in children; clinicians should consult the companion volume, *Assessment of Communication Disorders in Adults* (Hegde & Freed, 2010), for resources and protocols to assess adult communication disorders.

Stuttering

In both children and adults, stuttering is the most commonly assessed and treated fluency disorder. It is characterized by a complex set of symptoms, but the most diagnostic of them is an increased rate of dysfluencies. Many other features also characterize the disorder, although a diagnosis of stuttering does not depend on their presence. We note the features that are mandatory for a diagnosis of stuttering as well as those that are found to varying extents in children (and adults) who stutter.

Stuttering is sometimes described as a *developmental fluency disorder*. The term may be somewhat misleading in that the disorder is not a stage of normal speech and language development. The term may only mean that it begins in early childhood, compared to neurogenic stuttering which has its onset in adulthood (see Duffy, 2005 and Hegde & Freed, 2011 for symptomatology and assessment of neurogenic stuttering in adults). We begin with an epidemiologic description of stuttering.

Epidemiology of Stuttering in Children

Stuttering begins in early childhood years. The onset may occur as early as age 18 months; onset in most children occurs before age 4. After age 6, onset of stuttering occurs in progressively fewer children. Onset of new cases is rare in the teenage and subsequent years. Adult onset of stuttering with no history of earlier difficulty is almost always suspected to have a neurologic basis (Bloodstein & Ratner, 2008; Hegde, 2008a).

A well-established fact of stuttering is that it is more common in males than in females. Although the sex ratio varies across studies, a general male:female ratio of 3:1 is often reported. In preschool years, the male:female ratio is closer than it is in older children or adults who stutter. Preschool male:female ratio is reportedly 1.4:1 or even 1:1. However, by the 11th grade, the sex ratio is 5.5 males to 1 female. It is generally thought that different sex ratios at different age levels is partly due to a greater number of girls than boys spontaneously recovering from stuttering (Bloodstein & Ratner, 1995). An additional reason may be the emergence of stuttering in more boys than girls.

Prevalence of stuttering, a measure of more persistent stuttering, is about 1% in the general population (Bloodstein & Ratner, 2008). The lifetime incidence of stuttering (i.e., persons who have ever stuttered during their lifetime) is between 5 and 10% of the population. The difference between the more persistent prevalence and the lifetime incidence is due to multiple variables, but recovery from stuttering due to treatment and other variables is a major variable. Both rates are also influenced by gender and family history of the disorder, suggesting the influence of genetic factors as well.

Stuttering tends to run in certain families, resulting in a higher familial prevalence of stuttering than in the general population (Bloodstein & Ratner, 1995; Guitar, 2006; Yairi & Ambrose, 2005). Some 40 to 50% of individuals who stutter are likely to have another member in the family, mostly fathers or siblings, who also stutter. Some studies suggest that familial prevalence may be as high as three times the prevalence in the general population. Up to 65% of those who stutter may have distant relatives who stutter. A father who stutters generally poses risk to sons; but a mother who stutters may pose risks to all her children, including daughters.

Another variable that suggests the importance of genetic factors is the *concordance rate* of stuttering in identical twins, which is higher than that in fraternal twins, and both of which are higher than that for ordinary siblings or other relatives (Yairi & Ambrose, 2005). The concordance rate in fraternal twins is lower than that for identical twins, but higher than that in ordinary siblings. The term *concordance* means that if one member of the twin pair stutters, the other member also does. The concordance *rate*, however is a measure of the *likelihood* that if one member of a twin pair stutters, the other also will stutter. Concordance is not perfect, which means that if one member of an identical twin pair stutters, the other one may not always stutter, but that there is an increased likelihood that he or she might. A slightly higher concordance rate for fraternal twins than for ordinary siblings suggests that environmental variables play a role in the prevalence of stuttering in all twin pairs (including perhaps identical twin pairs) because there is no genetic reason why fraternal twin pairs should experience higher concordance rates than ordinary siblings.

That a significant number of children who stutter recover from it without treatment is well established, but how many actually do so, and for what reason, are widely contested (Bloodstein & Ratner, 2008; Guitar, 2006; Yairi & Ambrose, 2005). Such recovery is typically described as *natural or spontaneous*, implying that no treatment was necessary for the recovery. Estimates of natural recovery vary between less than 30 to more than 75% (Ramig, 1993; Yairi & Ambrose, 2005. A more realistic estimate may be between 35 and 50%, however. Higher estimates may be evident if children are allowed to stutter up to 4 years or more (Yairi & Ambrose, 2005). It is possible that during this extended period of time, some kind of intervention, especially the informal, parent-induced kind, may have occurred. Whether, recovery is truly natural (no intervention of any kind, including informal parental measures) or assisted in some way is difficult to discern. Clinically more important is that it is difficult to predict who will and who will not recover spontaneously because the statistics apply to group data, not individual children (Gottwald & Starkweather, 1999; Millard, Nicholas, & Cook, 2008; Onslow, Packman, & Harrison, 2003; Zebrowski, 1997). Clinicians cannot give a valid answer to the parents' typical question whether *their child* will recover without treatment. Therefore, after making a diagnosis of stuttering, clinicians cannot counsel parents to avoid or postpone treatment for a specific child because of the uncertainty of natural recovery in that child.

Studies in which parents of children who stutter were compared with parents of children who speak normally fluently have not shown consistent and significant differences between them. Some parents of children who stutter may be anxious and overprotective of their children; such parental reactions may be due to the child's stuttering, however. There is no evidence that such parental reactions cause stuttering in their children.

Stuttering is found at all socioeconomic strata. Whether the incidence rates vary across socioeconomic strata is not clear. Similarly, stuttering is found in children and adults with any and all level of intelligence as measured through IQ tests. When people with diagnosed intellectual disabilities are excluded, IQs of people who stutter fall within the normal range. Among people who stutter, the range of IQ may vary from below normal to well above average. People who stutter may be found among highly accomplished artists, scientists, and professionals.

Although stuttering is found at all intellectual levels, its prevalence may be slightly higher in children and adults with diagnosed intellectual disabilities. For example, people with Down syndrome have a higher probability of stuttering (Bloodstein & Ratner, 2008). The prevalence rate reported varies from a low of 15% to a high of 53%; both much higher than that for the general population (about 1 to 1.5%).

Stuttering and phonological disorders may coexist in some children. Estimated number of children who have phonological disorders along with persistent stuttering varies from a low of 16% to a high of 70%. Some doubt whether stuttering and phonological disorders are inherently related (see Nippold, 1990 for a review of studies). Nonetheless, children who stutter do not have a unique pattern of phonological acquisition or disorders. Many children and adults who stutter have normal phonological skills.

One can expect stuttering to be correlated with language skills, but the evidence is currently contradictory. Nippold's (1990) and Watkins's (2005) reviews of research show that children who stutter may have normal, below normal, or above-normal language skills. Sampling variations may account for some of the discrepancy in the scientific literature on language skills of children who stutter. As noted, stuttering exists at all levels of intelligence. Because of a strong correlation between language skills and intelligence, stuttering may be associated with varied levels of language skills. Therefore, assessment for stuttering should include language (and speech) screening, and more complete assessment if the screening results warrant it.

Ethnocultural Variables and Stuttering

Stuttering has been reported in almost all cultures and societies (Bloodstein & Ratner, 2008; Hegde, 2008a); Robinson & Crowe, 2002; Van Riper, 1982). No society is completely immune to it, in spite of some early claims by anthropologists that it does not exist in certain societies (e.g., people of New Guinea or Polar Eskimos) and Johnson's claim (1944a, 1944b) that the disorder does not exit in American Indians. Johnson had hypothesized that stuttering is a matter of cultural practices in which a high premium is placed on fluency (Johnson, 1944a, 1944b; Johnson & Leuteneger, 1955). Children who speak normally have dysfluencies in speech and the parents who view this negatively may diagnose stuttering: a problem that did not exist but brought about by the diagnosis itself. This *diagnosogenic theory* of stuttering, based on Johnson's claimed evidence that the Native Americans did not stutter, has since been discredited by observations of Native Americans who do stutter (Zimmermann et al., 1983). Demographic evidence suggests that stuttering exists in North, Central, and South American, Native American, European, Asian, and African societies. Both rural and urban societies have people who stutter. Stuttering is reported in all continents (Bloodstein & Ratner, 2008; Robinson & Crowe, 2002; Van Riper, 1982).

Although stuttering is not absent in any society studied so far, its prevalence rates may be different across societies. It is difficult to judge the reliability and validity of reported prevalence data across different societies because of varied methods of studies, however. Possibly, stuttering is more common among African Americans than among whites, although the stuttering individuals in the two ethnocultural groups may exhibit similar types of dysfluencies. Some studies suggest a prevalence rate as high as 2.8% in African American children, compared to 1% for the general population. In the various countries in Africa, the prevalence is reported to be high: between 1.26 to 5.5.% of the populations. Similarly high prevalence rates are reported for the Caribbean population. However, stuttering in Hispanic and Asian populations seems to closely match the generally reported 1% for the U.S. population (see Robinson & Crowe, 2002 for a summary of studies).

There is speculation that cultural beliefs, attitudes, and myths about fluency and stuttering may influence the prevalence of stuttering. Whether cultural beliefs or myths about the causes of stuttering affect assessment or treatment is also an issue discussed in the literature (Robinson & Crow, 2002). Unfortunately, much of the discussion is based on clinical intuition and not research evidence. Nonetheless, it may be important for the clinician to understand the client's and the family members' views on the disorder, its etiology, and its effects on communication to evaluate their disposition toward, and motivation for, treatment. If the belief is that stuttering is not curable, for example, the progress in treatment may be harder to achieve for no other reason than poor attendance.

Potential cultural practice that may affect assessment and treatment of stuttering is the parent's reaction to stuttering in their child. It may be instructive to investigate how parents respond when the child has difficulty expressing himself or herself. Do they interrupt the child or do they patiently listen? Do they criticize the child or do they offer helpful suggestions? Did they seek help promptly or do they believe that stuttering will go away on its own? Answers to such questions obtained during assessment will have treatment implications. The clinician may have to modify the parental negative reactions that may exacerbate stuttering in the child.

Definition and Measurement of Stuttering

Stuttering has many definitions; some definitions are based on theories whereas others on listener evaluation studies. Studies on how people label or judge samples of dysfluent speech are known as *listener evaluation studies*. Definitions based on listener evaluations tend to be least theoretical. These studies are based on the assumption that there is nothing inherently wrong with repeating a word or a syllable; it is a disorder if listeners consistently evaluate it as such. Investigators have studied listener reactions to speech samples containing various kinds of "stutterings" or forms of dysfluencies (Hegde, 2008a).

Speech-language pathologists are fully aware that listener reaction alone, however, may be misleading in diagnosing a disorder of communication. Listeners may be mistaken about a characteristic of speech or the reaction may simply reflect a bias, prejudice, or a practice in one culture not shared by other cultures. Nonetheless, it is also clear that people in all cultures diagnose stuttering and react in certain ways to speech that is not fluent; such reactions seem to be free from ethnocultural biases. Therefore, studying how people react to samples of speech taken from speakers who stutter may give some clues as to what stuttering is according to social judgments. Although not studied in the typical listener evaluation studies, clinicians should recognize that unfavorable evaluations of speech or a characteristic of it are likely to generate negative emotions, avoidance behaviors, and other undesirable reactions in the speaker.

Some early listener evaluation studies had reported that speech samples would be called *stuttered speech* only if they contained part-word repetitions and speech sound prolongations (Sander, 1963; Williams & Kent, 1958). The investigators thus concluded that all other kinds of dysfluencies (e.g., word repetitions, interjections) were "normal" kinds of dysfluencies. This conclusion has led to the classic definition of stuttering: it is part-word repetitions, and speech sound prolongations. Unfortunately, in the early studies, the investigators often did not balance the frequency of different types of dysfluencies in the speech samples. The samples were biased in that they mostly contained part-word repetitions and speech sound prolongations. Later studies have demonstrated that if speech samples contain word repetitions or schwa interjections at frequencies that reached or exceeded 5% of words spoken, listeners would label them as *dysfluent* or *stuttered* speech (Hegde & Hartman, 1979a, 1979b). These findings have been replicated (e.g., Dejoy & Jordan, 1988; Hegde, Capelli, & De Cesari, 1984). Therefore, speech samples that contain 5% or more dysfluencies that were traditionally not considered forms of stuttering may still be judged stuttering. Accordingly, stuttering is defined as speech that contains at least a 5% dysfluency rate.

There is still reason to believe that people may have different thresholds of tolerance for different kinds of dysfluencies; some dysfluencies may be evaluated more negatively at lower frequency than other kinds of dysfluencies. Studies by Hegde and Dansby (1988) and Hegde and Stone (1991) have confirmed this. These studies have shown that part-word repetitions, speech sound prolongations, and broken words may be judged *stuttered speech* even at 3%, whereas other types of dysfluencies need to be 5% or more to be so judged. Therefore, definitions of stuttering may take into account the differential listener tolerance thresholds. Accordingly, stuttering may be defined either as: (a) a 3% dysfluency rate when only sound-syllable repetitions and speech sound prolongations are counted; or (b) a 5% dysfluency rate when all kinds of dysfluencies are counted. In essence, a less than 5% dysfluency rate is judged normal because, as Johnson had claimed, all speakers have dysfluencies in their speech. Although no speaker is completely free from speech dysfluencies, some are more dysfluent than most people. They are the ones who come to be regarded as people who stutter. Many clinicians use some quantitative criterion (e.g., a 3% or a 5% dysfluency rate) in assessing and diagnosing stuttering in children and adults. We take note in subsequent sections that stuttering is a complex disorder with many additional features. But most of those additional features seem to stem from an increase in dysfluency rates that exceed the normal range.

Among many other features of stuttered speech, the number of times a speech segment is repeated and the muscular tension and effort with which the dysfluencies are produced are especially important in diagnosing stuttering. A clinically significant frequency of dysfluencies (such as the proposed 5% for all types combined) may interact with these variables. It is possible that a dysfluency rate that exceeds the normal range will also contain multiple repetitions per unit of repetition (e.g., *t-t-t-t-time* as against *t-time*) as well as increased tension and effort. But this is not always the case. In the authors' experience with a large number of preschool children, it is possible to observe a child whose repetitions exceed 12 to 15 units per instance (e.g., "I want . . . " or "I do . . . " repeated up to 20 times on a single occasion). The child may or may not show excessive tension, effort, or undue overt emotional reaction. Therefore, frequency of dysfluencies is an overriding consideration in assessing and diagnosing stuttering, especially because at the time of onset or soon thereafter, tension, avoidance, and emotional reactions may not be as reliable an indication of a fluency problem as are the increased levels of dysfluencies.

Another potential and complicating variable that should be considered in diagnosing stuttering in children is the duration of dysfluencies, especially sound prolongations. A child or an adult may prolong each sound to such an abnormal extent that even if the frequency of dysfluencies remains less than 5% of words spoken, the clinician may be compelled to diagnose stuttering. Generally, clinicians categorize a sound prolongation as clinically significant if its duration approaches or exceeds 1 second (Van Riper, 1982). However, what if duration is very abnormal (say, 5 seconds or more), but the frequency is less than 3%? Most clinicians then may diagnose stuttering based on abnormal duration, ignoring frequency which may even be within the normal limits. In the authors' experience, though, it is unusual to find a child whose duration of dysfluencies is very long, but the frequency is very low. Long durations tend to be associated with high frequency. Therefore, once again, *frequency* of dysfluencies emerges as the solid criterion to diagnose stuttering.

There are other definitions of stuttering (Bloodstein & Ratner, 2008). Johnson had defined stuttering as an avoidance reaction; for him, dysfluency rates were not important. In Johnson's view, mostly because of parental punishment of normal dysfluencies, the child becomes apprehensive in speaking situations, becomes tense and anxious, and begins to avoid speech and speaking situations. For Johnson (Johnson & Associates, 1959), stuttering is what a person does to avoid stuttering. For Van Riper (1982), stuttering is excessive sound repetitions, sound prolongations, and word repetitions. Fo some clinicians, stuttering is a *moment* or an *event* in speech, so judged by an expert (Johnson & Knott, 1936; Martin & Haroldson, 1981). Problematically, such *moments* or *events* do not specify the behaviors that the experts call *stuttering,* and make it difficult to teach others how to objectively measure them. Definitions that define stuttering in terms of nonspeech behaviors (e.g., avoidance behaviors) do not make the necessary reference to a speech problem, which stuttering is.

In essence, stuttering is diagnosed when the rate of all types of dysfluencies combined reliably exceeds 5% of words spoken or read. Stuttering also may be diagnosed when the frequency of part-word repetitions and speech sound prolongations exceeds 3% of the words spoken or read aloud. The clinician, however, always keeps an eye for that unusual child or adult whose dysfluency rates do not meet the frequency criterion, but exhibits an excessively long duration of prolongations or multiple units of repetitions. Possibly, though unlikely, a clinician may encounter a client whose dysfluency rates are low, duration of prolongations are brief, the number of units of repetition is few, and yet exhibits excessive muscular tension and effort associated with those few dysfluencies. Stuttering may then be diagnosed on such people as well. In the authors' experience, excessive muscular tension and effort, unusually long duration of prolongations, and multiple units of repetitions are almost always found in people who exhibit a high frequency of dysfluencies. Hence, we place an emphasis on the frequency of dysfluencies in diagnosing stuttering. Dysfluency frequency that exceeds an accepted level (e.g., 5% of the words spoken) is our recommended diagnostic criterion. This means that to diagnose stuttering, the clinician should (a) have a clear knowledge of the different kinds of dysfluencies and (b) know how to measure them reliably (Hegde, 2008b).

Dysfluency Types and Their Measurement

As noted, it is the excessive production of dysfluencies that makes speech dysfluent or stuttered. A *dysfluency* is a speech behavior that disrupts fluency; it stops the flow of fluent speech; it interrupts the continuity of speech; it impairs the rhythm of speech; it may slow down the rate of speech, although not always. When the dysfluency frequency is low (e.g., below 5% of the words spoken), a clinical problem is not evident. Excessive amounts of dysfluency on the other hand, may pose a clinical problem not only because of the increased frequency, but also because their associated muscular effort and tension (especially in adults and older children), unfavorable negative emotions about self and others, and speech avoidance behaviors.

Dysfluency is a generic term; there are different categories of them. Assessment of stuttering in children requires a measurement of all of those categories (Table 10–1). Johnson and Associates (1959) originally described most of them. Johnson and his colleagues analyzed speech samples of adults and children to identify what they called normal *nonfluencies* because of the belief that what we now call dysfluencies are normal, no matter what frequency with which they are exhibited. Johnson and associates' categories, not necessarily their theoretical underpinnings, are still used in analyzing the different types of dysfluencies:

- Repetitions: A unit of speech, often meaningful and part of what is being said, is repeated; has at least three varieties:
  - Sound/syllable repetitions: A sound, often the initial sound of a word, is repeated; may be single unit repetition (e.g., *t-time*) or multiple units of repetitions (e.g., *t-t-t-time*).
  - Word repetitions: A word is repeated; may be a single-unit repetition (e.g., *What-what time is it?*) or multiple-unit repetitions (e.g., *What-what-what time is it?*)
  - Phrase repetitions: Two or more words are repeated (e.g., *"Can you, can you, can you do it for me?"*).
- Prolongations: Durations of speech or articulatory segments, often the sound or a syllable, that is longer than expected, abnormal, socially noticed, or unaccepted; has two main varieties:
  - Audible prolongations: Vocal speech segments that are more prolonged than the normal, usual, or acceptable; also called sound or syllable prolongations (e.g., *sssssoup*; *llllllong*); the length of prolongations may vary within and across individuals.

Table 10–1. Types and Examples of Dysfluencies Measured in Assessing Stuttering in Children

Dysfluency types	Examples

Repetitions
   Part-word repetitions
   Whole-word repetitions
   Phrase repetitions
	"What t-t-t-time is it?"
	"What-what-what are you doing?"
	"I want to-I want to-I want to do it"

Prolongations
   Sound/syllable prolongations
   Silent prolongations
	"Lllllet me do it"
	A struggling attempt to say a word when there is no sound.

Interjections
   Sound/syllable interjections
   Whole-word interjections
   Phrase interjections
	"um . . . um I had a problem this morning."
	"I had a well problem this morning."
	"I had a you know problem this morning."

Silent Pauses	A silent duration between words and sentences considered too long: "I was going to the (pause) store."
Broken Words (Intralexical Pauses)	A silent pause within words: "It was won—(pause)—derful."
Incomplete Phrases	A production that suggests an incomplete expression of an idea: "He wanted to—I think I will not say any more."
Revisions	A production that involves word change but expresses the same idea: "I will take a taxi, a cab."

- Silent prolongations: Sometimes described as tensed pauses, silent prolongations are extended articulatory positions or postures in the absence of voice; usually a sign of unusual effort and muscular tension (e.g., frozen lip and cheek posturing as in the production of a word starting with /b/ with no movement or voice).
- Broken words: A pause within a word; may be described as intralexical pauses; also accompanied by tension and articulatory posturing (e.g., go [pause] ing).
- Interjections: Intruded elements of speech that do not add to the meaning of what is being said; extraneous speech elements; has at least three varieties:
  - Sound/syllable interjections (e.g., interjections of uh and um)
  - Word interjections (e.g., well, Okay)
  - Phrase interjections (e.g., you know, I mean, let me see)

- Silent pauses: Inappropriate breaks in speech in which vocalization is ceased; brief pauses are normal at certain junctures of speech; inappropriate at other junctures, especially if they are too frequent or too long; may be associated with tension.

- Incomplete phrases: Speech productions that are grammatically and semantically incomplete; an idea being expressed is dropped (e.g., *I was going to say . . . well, what do you say?*)

- Revisions: Lexical modifications in speech with no significant change in the main idea being expressed; lexical (word) changes more significant than semantic changes (e.g., *Let us have some tea . . . coffee*); a brief pause (. . .) may precede the revision.

Reliable Measurement of Dysfluencies

Reliable measurement of dysfluencies is essential to diagnose stuttering and to show improvement during treatment or treatment research studies. *Reliability* is consistency of repeated measures (Hegde, 2003). Historically, reliable measurement of stuttering has been difficult and perhaps still is for the student clinician or a professional inexperienced in measuring stuttering. Clinicians who assess stuttering should demonstrate the two kinds of reliability: intraobserver and interobserver. With inexperienced clinicians, both forms of reliability generally may be low although intraobserver reliability may be slightly higher than interobserver reliability. Clinicians are more consistent with themselves than with others.

Intraobserver reliability is consistency of two or more measures obtained by the same individual on the same phenomenon. It is demonstrated by measuring the same phenomenon two or more times by the same clinician. If the multiple measures (at least two) are consistent, then the clinician who measured the phenomenon measured it reliably. Inconsistent measures are unreliable. Intraobserver reliability demonstrates that a clinician has learned to measure the phenomenon reliably. This is essential for both clinical and research work (Hegde, 2003).

Interobserver reliability is consistency of measures across two or more observers. This is demonstrated by having two or more clinicians measure the frequency of stuttering (or specific forms of dysfluencies) to assess consistency of measures across individuals. This type of reliability is essential to ensure that one clinician's measurement of stuttering agrees with another's (Hegde, 2003). Without interobserver reliability, a clinician's diagnosis of stuttering is questionable. See Chapter 3 for addition information on reliability and validity as they relate more to standardized tests.

Several factors affect reliability of stuttering measurement. Some of the more common factors include:

- **Definition of stuttering:** If the clinician is not clear about the behavior being measured, the measurement is unlikely to be reliable. This is especially the case with intraobserver reliability. To achieve consistency of measures, two or more clinicians should use the same definition of stuttering. If one clinician measures the frequency of specified dysfluencies and the other measures avoidance reactions, the two measures cannot agree.

- **Observer training:** Clinicians who are untrained in the measurement of stuttering are unlikely to demonstrate either intra- or interobserver reliability. Therefore, it is essential to use a specific definition *and* get training in reliable measurement from someone who measures stuttering reliably.

- **Observer experience:** Clinicians and researchers who have extensive experience in measuring stuttering are more reliable than beginning clinicians with little or no experience. The experience should be specific to measurement of stuttering, not just clinical experience with the disorder. Good training combined with experience in measuring stuttering usually results in reliable measures.

- **Severity of stuttering, especially the chained dysfluencies:** More severe stuttering is harder to measure than less severe stuttering. The clinician is likely to miss some dysfluencies if different forms of dysfluencies are produced rapidly and if a single instance of stuttering contains multiple dysfluencies (chained dysfluencies). A person who stutters, for example, may rapidly produce sound repetitions into which *uhs* and *ums* are interjected and a prolongation of a sound or two is added.

- **Certain types of dysfluencies:** Some forms of dysfluencies are more easily noticed than other forms. Beginning clinicians are usually tuned to notice part-word repetitions and speech sound prolongations. But they may miss pauses, word repetitions, word and phrase interjections, revisions, and so forth. As they gain experience, clinicians become adept at measuring the obvious as well as the subtle forms of dysfluencies.

Measurement Guidelines

Measurement of stuttering requires careful sampling of speech and oral reading, sometimes repeated sampling, repeated listening to recorded samples, and repeated measurement to make sure that all, or nearly all, dysfluencies have been counted. The process moves faster with training and experience; beginning clinicians will spend much time and effort to get their measurement skills refined. Without such an investment of time and effort, the clinician may never achieve reliable measurement.

Repeated observation and observation in multiple settings may be necessary in some cases. This is because dysfluency rates differ across time and situations. Variability in dysfluencies is found in people of all ages who stutter, but it is much more pronounced in preschoolers and younger children. Closer to its onset, the frequency of stuttering may vary widely. On the day of assessment, a young child may stutter more or less than what the parents will have observed at home. An older child's dysfluency rate in oral reading may be significantly different from the rate in conversational speech. Therefore, the following guidelines were developed to help control this variability across time and situations to achieve reliable measurement of stuttering (Hegde, 2008b).

Tape-record one or more conversational speech samples. To the extent possible, hold a naturalistic conversation with the child. Use such stimulus materials as toys and stimulus pictures sparingly and mostly with preschoolers; select stimuli that are familiar to the child. Most school-age children can carry on a conversation with the clinician. If conversational speech is difficult to evoke, give the child a topic (such as his or her birthday party, a visit to the zoo or a theme park) and ask the child to talk about it. With preschool children, use toys and picture stimuli to evoke continuous speech; select stimulus materials that are ethnoculturally appropriate. Tape-record the entire conversational exchange for later analysis. Use a high-quality tape recorder. Tape-record another sample of speech with the parent or other informant. Have them do this after they have observed how you recorded a sample. See Chapters 1 and 6 for additional information on recording productive speech and language samples.

Tape-record an oral reading sample. Record an oral reading sample from a child who is a reader. When you schedule an appointment for assessment, ask the parents to bring a couple of books that are the child's favorite. If none are brought by the parents, select books that are appropriate for the child's grade and ethnocultural background. Ask the parents or informants for suggestions. If it appears that the initial selection was difficult for the child's reading level, select a simpler book. Do take note of the kinds of reading errors and dysfluencies to understand the relationship between difficult words and dysfluency rates as well as the child's literacy skills. Take note of any errors of articulation as well.

Tape-record a monologue. Evoke a monologue with older children. A monologue gives a more flowing speech sample than conversational speech in which the child and the clinician take turns talking and listening. Ask the child to select a topic for monologue; if necessary, suggest several topics you think are appropriate for the child to select from. Inform the child that you will simply listen to what he or she has to say on the topic. Encourage the child to say as much as possible in the beginning and restrain from interrupting the child. If necessary, have the child select an additional topic for monologue.

Obtain a taped speech sample from home. This can be prearranged or can be obtained soon after the parents return home from assessment. At the time of scheduling the assessment, the clinician may ask the parents to tape-record a 5-minute sample of speech they think represents the amount of stuttering the child does at home. Ask them to repeat the sample if possible. Give them some general guidelines about recording a speech sample from the child. A parent who brings two or three brief speech samples, recorded across that many days or time periods, will assist the clinician to a great extent in understanding the dysfluency rates in the child's natural setting.

Listen to the samples once. To get familiarized with the taped samples of conversational speech, monologue, and the oral reading, listen to them first without counting dysfluencies. More experienced clinicians or those who are familiar with the child and his or her pattern of dysfluencies may skip this step. The clinician gets a general idea of the types and severity of dysfluencies, idiosyncratic expressions, speech and language production skills, and prosodic features of the child before beginning the serious job of counting the frequency of different types of dysfluencies. It is sometimes difficult to count all dysfluencies in an unfamiliar speech sample.

Count all types of dysfluencies on your second listening. Note that to establish the reliability of your own measures, you need to count a second time, preferably after one week. If you are a beginning clinician or a clinician with limited experience in measuring stuttering, you will definitely need to count them again, perhaps more than two times. The criterion is not how many times you measure them (beyond the essential two times), it is whether two or more measures are consistent. During all attempts at measurement, try to count as many dysfluencies as possible, using the following guidelines:

- Count **sound repetitions** as one instance, regardless of the number of units of repetitions in that instance (e.g., *t-time* or *t-t-t-time* are both counted as one instance of part-word repetition). The number of units of repetitions in instances of repetitions may be important in research studies or in gaining a deeper understanding of the severity of stuttering. In clinician practice, taking note of the typical number of units in most repetitions and commenting on them in the diagnostic report is adequate.

- Count **syllable repetitions** as either word repetitions or part-word repetitions (e.g., *I-I-I* or *my-my-my*) contains a word repetition whereas *t-t-t-time* contains a part-word or sound repetition).

- Count **prolongations** as one instance, regardless of their length (e.g., a relatively brief *mmmy* and a much longer *mmmmmy* are both counted as prolongations without distinction). This does not mean that the duration of prolongations is insignificant; it is, if one were to judge the severity. It is just practical to measure them that way in routine clinical practice. Like the number of units in a repetition, the duration of prolongation is an indication of severity of stuttering. Therefore, do take note of the average duration of most prolongations. Measurement of prolongations is more subjective than measurement of other kinds of dysfluencies, although one can measure them with specialized computer software or just a simple stop watch. A prolongation may be as brief as half a second, although even a quarter-second prolongation is noticeable to a trained ear. Comment on the duration of prolongations in the clinical report.

- Count the same type of dysfluency twice if it is separated by another dysfluency or a period of fluency (e.g., *um. . . wha, wha. . . um what time is it?* has two interjections separated by a part-word repetition).

- Be extra vigilant about pauses, which tend to be missed. Judge the appropriateness of pauses at their junctures. A pause in between sentences may be more acceptable than at other junctures. Count a pause if it strikes you as such; a one-second pause at wrong junctures is definitely a pause. As with prolongations, judgment of pause durations is subjective.

- Distinguish silent prolongations from audible prolongations. The former is a visual phenomenon with no sound; the latter is auditory, but may be visual as well.

- In a chain of mixed dysfluencies, count the different types of dysfluencies separately (e.g., *I-I-I um llllike to-to-to um d-d-do this this this mmmethod*).

This is chained dysfluency because one form of dysfluency is followed by another with no fluent productions in between. Dysfluencies in such chains are often produced rapidly, requiring close attention and sometimes repeated attempts to measure all of them.

Listen to the sample again and recount the dysfluencies. Unless you are an experienced clinician and you have previously established your reliability in measuring stuttering, you need to measure it a second, and possibly third, time. To practice the measurement skill, you can disregard the general rule of measuring a second time after a one-week interval, and measure the dysfluencies immediately after the first attempt. Later, you may measure samples with one week intervals to establish your own intraobserver reliability.

Count again if the first two dysfluency rates are inconsistent. There is no shortcut to reliable measurement of stuttering or any other behavior. By definition, reliability of a single measure is unknown. Two consistent measures are sufficient for clinical practice. Whether for clinical practice or research, two inconsistent measures require a third measure to establish a trend. If the second and the third measures are closer to each other, you know that the first measure was unreliable and the real dysfluency rate is closer to the second and the third measure.

Count the number of dysfluencies in oral reading. Use the same guidelines given for the speech sample. You may use the *Dysfluency Measurement Protocol* given in Chapter 11 to record the dysfluencies or use a double-spaced printed copy of the passage the child reads orally. If you used the latter, you may write abbreviations for different forms of dysfluencies on top of the word (e.g., *pwr* for part-word repetitions, *pro* for sound prolongations) or write abbreviations in between words (e.g., *si* for sound interjection, *pi* for phrase interjections).

Record the number of dysfluencies on a recording sheet. Using the *Dysfluency Measurement Protocol* given in Chapter 11, record the frequency of each dysfluency. Note that the protocol allows for measuring dysfluencies in one clinic speech sample, one clinic monologue, one clinic oral reading sample, and one speech sample from home. Print the protocol for your use from the CD. In the left-hand column of the protocol, all the different kinds of dysfluencies are listed for your convenience. In the corresponding empty right-hand column, place a tally mark to record each dysfluency heard in the sample. Not all forms of dysfluencies may be noted in given cases; some forms will be more frequent than others. In most children, part-word repetitions, word and phrase repetitions, speech sound prolongations, interjections of all kinds, and pauses are likely to be observed to a greater extent than broken words, revisions, and incomplete phrases. Each child will have a combination of dysfluencies.

Analysis of the Speech Sample

Because the diagnosis of stuttering depends on it, the main outcome to seek from the speech sample or samples is the *percent dysfluency rate*. This analysis is possible when the total number of dysfluencies and the total number of words spoken in a sample are calculated.

Calculate the total number of dysfluencies. On the *Dysfluency Measurement Protocol,* you find a place to enter the total number of dysfluencies for either a speech sample or an oral reading sample. First, add all the individual dysfluencies of a given kind (e.g., part-word repetitions or interjections) and enter the totals for each. Next, add all the totals for the different kinds to derive the grand total of dysfluencies observed in the speech sample.

Count the number of words spoken or read in a sample. In counting the number of words spoken, use the following guidelines:

- Exclude all interjected sounds, syllables, words, and phrases—they are counted as dysfluencies (e.g., do not add *ums* and *you know* to the word count; they are added to the dysfluency count)

- Count the single-syllable words as one word (e.g., the pronoun *I* is counted as a single word)

- Count the whole word as one word, disregarding the part that is repeated (e.g., *t-t-t-time* is counted as one word)

- Determine the total number of words for each speech sample and oral reading sample separately

Calculate the percent dysfluency rate. Calculate the rate separately for each speech and oral reading sample; that is the only way to find out if any two measures for either speech or oral reading are consistent. Use the following formula to calculate the percentage:

$$\frac{\text{The total number of dysfluencies in the sample}}{\text{The total number of words in the sample}} \times 100 = \text{\% dysfluency rate}$$

Obtain additional samples if the calculated percent dysfluency rates for two samples are inconsistent. It is likely that you will have at least one conversational speech sample, a monologue sample, and an oral reading sample. Dysfluency rates for the speech sample and the monologue should agree; if they do not, schedule another session in which a speech sample is recorded; also, get a home speech sample. The dysfluency rate for the oral reading sample may not and need not agree with that for conversational speech sample. Dysfluencies in oral reading are compared to those in conversational speech. Unless there is a particular clinical or research concern for reliably measuring dysfluency rates in oral reading, a single sample is sufficient for comparison. A child whose dysfluency rate is high in oral reading but low in conversational speech may be avoiding specific words on which stuttering is likely. A higher dysfluency rate is revealed when avoidance of specific words is prevented, as it happens in oral reading. Such a finding will have some therapeutic implications: treatment in final stages may have to target some persistent stuttering on certain words.

Additional Features of Stuttering

Although the core feature of stuttering is an increased dysfluency rate, assessment of additional features is important for a comprehensive understanding of this complex disorder in a child. Some of these features may be more prominent in adults than in children, but many features found in adults who stutter also may be found in children who stutter, albeit to varying degrees and different levels of severity.

Among these additional features, assessment of associated motor behaviors, mismanagement of airflow, emotional reactions, and avoidance behaviors is essential. Although a diagnosis of stuttering may be made without precisely measuring the frequency of these associated features, careful observation and description of such features is a part of good assessment.

Associated Motor Behaviors

Various motor (nonspeech) behaviors may accompany stuttering. Although their frequency and severity may be higher in adults, children, too, may exhibit a significant number of associated motor behaviors. Generally, they are less pronounced or fewer in preschool children. As the child gets older and stuttering persists, more pronounced and an increased number of associated behaviors may emerge.

By definition, these nonspeech motor behaviors are associated with stuttered speech, not fluent speech. It should be noted that associated motor behaviors do not show a linear increase in frequency and severity; some young children who stutter may exhibit more of them that are also more obvious than some adults who stutter. When they are severe or of high frequency, associated motor behaviors are more noticeable than the dysfluencies themselves. To varying extents, the clinician may find some or most of the following associated motor behaviors in children who stutter:

- Rapid and tense eye blink
- Tensed and prolonged shutting of the eyelids
- Rapid upward, downward, or lateral movement of the eyes
- Knitting of the eyebrows
- Nose wrinkling and flaring
- Pursing or quivering of the lips
- Tongue clicking
- Teeth clenching, grinding, and clicking
- Tension in facial muscles
- Wrinkling of the forehead
- Clenched jaw or jerky or slow or tensed movement of the jaws
- Jaw opening or closing unrelated to target speech production
- Tension in chest, shoulder, and neck muscles; including twitching and extraneous movements

- Head movements including turns, shakes, jerks, and lateral, upward, and downward movements

- Tensed and jerky hand movements including fist clenching and hand wringing

- Tensed and jerky arm movements including tapping on the thighs or pressing against the sides of the abdomen

- Tensed and jerky leg movements including kicking motions

- Tensed and jerky feet movements including grinding, pressing, rubbing, or circular movements on the floor

- Generally tense body postures.

During the interview and speech sampling, the clinician may take written notes on the particular kinds of associated motor behaviors a child exhibits. It is essential to observe the child closely, because a particular child may surprise the clinician with an unusual or never reported associated motor behavior. Parents usually are able to describe the major associated motor behaviors the child exhibits. However, a comprehensive Behavior Assessment Battery (Brutten & Vanryckeghem, 2007) that helps assess speech disruption and various associated, behavioral, emotional, and attitudinal aspects of stuttering in children also helps assess avoidance behaviors. This well-standardized test may be used. In the clinical report, the clinician should describe the most frequently noted associated motor behaviors, giving examples. The clinician may specify what kinds of behaviors are typically associated with what kinds of dysfluencies. Chapter 11 provides the *Associated Motor Behaviors Assessment Protocol* that clinicians may use.

Mismanagement of Airflow

Stuttered speech may be associated with what appear to be breathing abnormalities. However, children and adults who stutter typically do not have inherent respiratory problems that cause stuttering (Bloodstein & Ratner, 2008). Abnormalities that are seemingly respiratory are indeed a mismanagement of airflow in the process of speech production. Such a mismanagement is associated with dysfluencies, not fluency, and make the clinical picture more complex. In essence, it is a part of the stuttering problem, not its cause. In some children and adults who stutter, the mismanagement of airflow may be obvious; in others, it may be subtle. In some older children and adults, airflow mismanagement may be a dominant symptom, associated with marked dysfluencies. In some preschool children who stutter, airflow mismanagement may be barely noticeable.

Airflow management problems found in children and adults who stutter take several forms and not all may be noted in all children. Some of the more prominent airflow management problems noted in persons who stutter include:

- Attempts at speaking on limited or shallow inhalation

- Attempts at speaking during exhalation

- Running out of air at the end of phrases and sentences

- Apparent efforts to squeeze the air out of lungs to continue talking

- Inhalations and exhalations that interrupt each other

- Impounding of inhaled air with a sudden closure of the glottis and apparent attempts to speak while the air is impounded

- Sudden cessation of breathing during speech production

- Dysrhythmic respiration

- Audible inhalation, exhalation, or both

- Difficulty in maintaining an even airflow throughout an utterance.

Airflow mismanagement has been studied by clinical descriptions as well as through such instruments as a pneumotachograph (Bloodstein & Ratner, 2008). Clinical assessment of airflow mismanagement requires observation and description. A thorough description may be especially needed when treatment is recommended to address airflow mismanagement. Descriptive comments in the assessment report are sufficient for most clinical purposes.

Negative Emotions

Sooner or later, children who stutter begin to experience a variety of negative emotions about their speech problem, themselves as speakers, speaking situations, and people they interact with (Guitar, 2006; Yairi & Ambrose, 2005). Some of these negative emotions can be observed in preschool children as young as 3 years of age or even soon after the onset of stuttering around two years of age. Although the adults can talk about their negative emotions and describe them in detail, children, especially preschoolers, exhibit them in their nonverbal behaviors; sooner or later, they too, begin to verbalize them.

Generally, the more severe is the stuttering, the longer is its persistence; and more socially handicapping it is, the greater is the frequency and severity of emotional reactions. Not all speakers who stutter will exhibit all or even most of the following, but they need to be understood and kept in perspective during assessment:

- Anxiety or fear about speaking situations. Young children may not verbalize it, but clinicians can sense it or infer it from their behavior. Preschoolers may move away from speaking situations or silently seek comfort from caregivers when speech is demanded.

- Self-reported feelings of frustration in not being able to speak freely, spontaneously, and fluently. Older children may describe such feeling, but preschoolers may show it nonverbally, although the authors have observed some preschoolers as young as 2;6 say, "I don't want to talk."

- Self-reported negative statements about himself or herself, especially related to self as a competent speaker. These may be inferred in preschool children who may not make negative statements about themselves; but they may be heard in older children. The authors have noted a few preschoolers say, "I can't talk."

- A sense of helplessness when unable to move forward with fluent expressions, often described by older children and adults.

- Feelings of unpleasantness associated with speech and speaking situations. Preschool children may not verbalize them, although their facial expressions may reveal them. Older children might talk about those feelings when asked about them; adults freely verbalize them.

- Belief or impression that listeners are impatient, critical, or unsympathetic. These are verbalized mostly by older children and adults.

- Feelings of embarrassment in social situations. These are generally inferred from the behavior of young children. Some older children may admit to them when asked. Adults may freely express them.

- Belief that their stuttering may be due to some external, uncontrollable, and inexplicable force. This belief may be dominant in older children and adults.

- Self-reported lack of self-confidence in speaking situations. Such reports are mostly expressed by older students when specifically asked, and routinely by adults.

- Anxious or dreaded expectation of stuttering on certain words and in certain speaking situations (expectancy). Generally reported by older students to some extent and typically by adults.

The depth of assessment of negative emotions and feelings depends on the clinician's theoretical orientation. Some clinicians believe that negative emotions may be causally related to stuttering and, therefore, such emotions distinguish stuttering from other types of fluency disorders. Such clinicians consider an assessment of negative emotions and attitudes essential to a differential diagnosis of stuttering (Brutten & Vanryckeghem, 2007; Vanryckeghem, Hylebos, Brutten, & Pearlman, 2001). Clinicians who target negative feelings and emotions during treatment also assess them with the help of standardized or nonstandardized questionnaire-type of assessment tools (Brutten & Vanryckeghem, 2007; Cooper, 1999; Guitar, 2006). Such clinicians believe that unless the negative feelings and emotions are treated directly, fluency generated by any method will not last.

Often how the child feels about speech, speaking situations, and how he or she reacts to both the speaking situations and conversational partners may be assessed by asking the child carefully worded questions. Parents may be asked about the child's feelings about stuttering and how the child reacts in social situations. Whether the child expresses frustration, fear, anxiety, and describes himself or herself in negative terms (e.g., "I can't talk good," "I don't feel like talking") may be evaluated during the interview of parents. Many children, even preschoolers, may begin to avoid certain words or speaking situation, as noted in a subsequent section.

There are published tools available to assess negative emotions and feelings of children who stutter (Hegde, 2008b). For instance, the previously mentioned comprehensive Behavior Assessment Battery (BAB) for children (Brutten & Vanryckeghem, 2007) has three checklists: the *Speech Situation Checklist,* the *Behavior Checklist,* and the *Communication Attitude Checklist.* The assessment battery helps assess the children's negative emotional reactions to speaking situations, the kinds of speech disruptions that follow negative emotional experiences, the coping strategies the children who stutter use, and the speech-associated attitudes the children who stutter exhibit. The BAB may be administered to children between the ages of 6 and 16. A similar assessment tool, called the KiddyCat: the Communication Attitude Test for Preschool and Kindergarten Children, is also available (Vanryckeghem & Brutten 2007) and may be administered to preschool children.

Depending on the age of the child, clinicians may use both of these well-researched assessment tools.

Some clinicians believe that negative emotions and attitudes are a consequence of stuttering and, therefore, it is not essential to target emotions and feelings during treatment. They believe that when stuttering is directly reduced and fluency is increased, there will be no reason for children or adults to harbor negative feelings and emotions about their speech and speaking situations. Such clinicians may not formally assess negative emotions and attitudes in great detail. Nonetheless, they will take note of them during interview (of the client, the parent, or both) and describe in their clinical reports the negative feelings and emotions the child with stuttering experiences. Clinicians who take this approach also wish to see that the child's negative emotions and attitudes toward speech and speaking situations are eliminated or diminished; they believe, however, that to achieve this goal, one needs to improve fluency.

Persistent negative emotions in certain speaking situations may be related to still persistent stuttering in those situations. Therefore, treatment needs to monitor fluency in various situations. When fluency is generalized to most speaking situations, the child's negative emotions in those situations may be reduced. Generally, negative emotions and feelings associated with stuttering coexist with avoidance behaviors.

Avoidance Behaviors

A significant feature of stuttering is avoidance of speaking situations, certain kinds of conversational partners, and specific words. These avoidance behaviors are largely due to the negative experiences and unpleasant emotional reactions associated with stuttering. Stuttering may generate its own negative emotions of tension, anxiety in speaking situations, and a sense of frustration. Unfavorable reactions from the listeners, even if they are mild or only occasional, may exacerbate such emotional reactions in persons who stutter. Even a parental suggestion to "slow down" or "think before you speak" may carry its own negative emotional consequence for the child. Avoidance behaviors are a typical consequence of unpleasant situations and unfavorable conversational partners. By avoiding unpleasant speech tasks and speaking situations, persons who stutter free themselves from the negative consequences of those tasks and situations. Such avoidance behaviors are reinforced negatively: the relief the avoidance behaviors provide from negative emotions and feelings is the reinforcement for those behaviors.

People who stutter exhibit a wide range of avoidance behaviors. The number and frequency of such behaviors vary across individuals, but they tend to be stronger and persistent in people who have a consistent tendency to stutter on certain words and in certain speaking situations. Some of the more frequently reported or observed avoidance reactions include:

- *Avoidance of certain speaking situations.* People who stutter are especially prone to avoid speaking on the telephone, ordering in restaurants, buying something at a counter, speaking to a group, introducing self, verbally giving personal phone numbers or addresses, saying one's own name, responding to roll calls, and asking for directions when lost. Experienced clinicians will know that individual clients will surprise them with unusual avoidance reactions. A tendency to depend on others for their communication needs may be a part of the coping strategy, necessitated by avoidance. For example, persons who stutter may ask others to order for them in restaurants, gesture someone to answer telephone calls for them, and take a friend along to shop.

- *Avoidance of certain conversation partners.* Persons who stutter tend to avoid strangers, authority figures, supervisors or bosses, and persons of the opposite sex; but individual children and adults may avoid specific situations depending on their unique past experiences.

- *Avoidance of certain words.* This is common among children and adults who stutter. Most adults can list sounds or words that give them particular difficulty. They become adept at word substitutions and circumlocutions that help them avoid difficult sounds or words.

- *Avoidance of talking on certain topics.* Such topics may include their stuttering. And emotional experiences associated with it. It may be that such talk is unpleasant or that they would stutter more if they do.

- *Avoidance of eye contact.* This behavior may be reinforced because it helps minimize social embarrassment due to stuttering.

- *Avoidance of talking as much as possible.* Some but not all who stutter may reduce their overall verbal output, a behavior reinforced by reduced negative consequences of stuttering.

Generally, the longer is the history of stuttering and more severe is the stuttering, the greater is the number of avoidance behaviors. Thus, an adult with severe stuttering is likely to have more avoidance reactions than a preschool child who just began to stutter. It cannot be assumed, however, that a preschool child who stutters will not have developed any avoidance reaction. Because the avoidance reactions of very young children are not well documented in the literature, we present specific examples observed in some of the 40 or more preschool children (2.5 years to below 6) we have treated for their stuttering:

- Whispering to avoid stuttering; the mother of a 3-year-old who stuttered reported that her daughter began to whisper at home, and the behavior was documented in the clinic (stuttering is greatly reduced when whispered).

- Saying, "I don't want to talk" following a severe stutter; one 4-year-old boy said so to his mother at home and repeated it during treatment.

- Talking in an impersonated tone, with an exaggerated articulation or loudness increase; one 3;6-year old boy talked like a cartoon character to avoid stuttering (an unusual mode of talking may reduce stuttering).

- Talking with an unusual physical posture; during treatment sessions involving conversational speech, a 5-year-old boy would suddenly leave the chair, stand up, and begin talking with a bulging chest, tucked-in stomach, and raised shoulders. He would shout his words (this avoidance strategy worked well for the child).

- Pretending ignorance of a word on which stuttering is likely; one 2.6 year-old-girl shrugged her shoulders and made a hand gesture that meant, "I don't know" when asked, "What is this?" while showing the picture of a doll. Earlier, she had produced the word *doll* in conversational speech and had multiple repetitions of the initial /d/.

- Pretending to be thinking of an answer when a question was asked; one 3-year-old boy pressed his left index finger to his cheek and fixed his gaze on the ceiling for a few seconds before giving simple and obvious answers to such questions as, "What is your Mom's name?" Or, "What is your baby sister's name?"

- Pretending not to hear a question; a 5-year-old girl often began to get abruptly busier with something when the clinician began to ask questions. After a while, she would ask, "Did you say something?"

- Pointing, instead of speaking; a common strategy with very young children, with or without a communication disorder; however, if the required verbal response is observed at other times and was stuttered, then the clinician may infer avoidance.

- Refusing to say a particular word; a 4 year-old boy said, "I don't want to say that word" when shown the picture of a monkey; asked, "Why?" he replied, "It's a *em* word." He tended to prolong the /m./

- Sudden reduction in vocal intensity following a severe stuttering; a 3-year old girl's voice would become unusually soft following a stutter (sometimes a softer or a louder voice than the typical may reduce stuttering).

- Moving away from the speaking situation; when a 3-year-old girl began to repeat the phrase "I do" more than a dozen times, a 5-year-old boy listening to her blurted out, "Hey! Just say it." Immediately, the girl briskly moved away from the speaking situation, came to where the supervisor was sitting in the same large room, and climbed on to his lap.

Avoidance behaviors are motivated by negative emotional reactions; when a difficult speaking situation is avoided, children and adults who stutter in them feel a reduction in their negative feelings, including perhaps a fear of that speaking situation. This reduction in negative feelings is the negative reinforcement for the avoidance behaviors. Therefore, a good measure of avoidance reactions is also a good measure of negative emotional reactions that prompt those overt actions.

Therapeutically, too, avoidance behaviors have significant implications. It is likely that words and situations a child persistently avoided in the past may still be avoided in the final stages of treatment when the child is mostly fluent. Still avoided words and situations need to be built into treatment work to reduce avoidance. For instance, a child may need to practice "smooth speech" while saying words on which stuttering persists. An older boy who still avoids telephones or stutters while talking on the phone may be given practice talking on phones. In the authors' clinical experience, generalized fluency is the key to reducing both avoidance reactions and the motivating negative feelings.

Because of all the treatment implications, it is important to assess avoidance behaviors in children and adults who stutter. Most adults and older children will describe their avoidance behaviors during interview. Many clients may answer questions about such behaviors on the case history form. To make a more formal assessment, the clinician may use the Behavior Assessment Battery (Brutten & Vanryckeghem, 2007), described earlier, which helps assess avoidance behaviors along with emotional reactions and speech disruptions. In addition, a clinician may design a client-specific avoidance behavior checklists and use it during assessment. The *Avoidance Behaviors Assessment Protocol* provided in Chapter 11 offers such a checklist for a quick completion of this task.

Cluttering

Cluttering is a disorder of fluency predominantly affecting speech rate but also may involve (controversially) language and thought processes. Cluttering may coexist with stuttering; however, stuttering does not coexist with cluttering. In other words, cluttering is associated with stuttering; but stuttering is not associated with cluttering; a person who stutters is unlikely to clutter as well; but a person who clutters is likely to stutter as well (Hegde, 2008a, 2008b).

Also known as tachyphemia, cluttering is characterized by rapid and irregular speech rate and indistinct articulation. A hurried speech even under normal circumstances is its main characteristic. The prevalence rate of cluttering in the United States is not well established, and it is probably underdiagnosed. The classic literature on cluttering is in German. In recent years, there have been significant increases in English publications on cluttering (see review of literature by Daly, 1986; Daly & Burnett, 1999; Myers & St. Louis, 1992).

Etiology of cluttering is mostly unknown. Although no genetic basis has been identified for cluttering, many investigators believe that genetic factors are important in its etiology. Some evidence suggests that cluttering may have a familial tendency (Myers & St. Louis, 1992). Some neurophysiologic abnormalities are suggested by deviant electroencephalographic (EEG) findings in about 50% of people who clutter.

A complex set of speech and language features characterize cluttering in children and adults, and include (Daly, 1986; Daly & Burnett, 1999; Myers & St. Louis, 1992):

- **Excessively fast rate of speech.** The rate may progressively accelerate, a tendency called *festinating.* Rate may increase within and between words and there may be periodic rushes of highly compressed or telescoped speech. More than the rapid rate, it is the articulatory breakdown that is associated with such rate that distinguishes cluttering; there are speakers who speak very rapidly and yet clearly.

- **Errors of articulation.** These errors are not always an indication of an independent speech sound disorder; they are possibly due to hurried speech. Errors include omission of sounds, syllables, and even words; reduction of consonant clusters to singletons; sound transpositions within words; inversion of the order of sounds; and reduced speech intelligibility due to such errors. The /r/ and /l/ seem to be especially difficult for people who clutter.

- **Various kinds of dysfluencies.** Typical forms of dysfluencies include repetition of longer words and phrases, revisions and interjections; silent pauses at inappropriate junctures, but lack of normal pauses between words or sentences. Unless the person who clutters also stutters, repetition of sounds and short words and sound prolongations may be less frequent, although there are individual differences. Unlike people who stutter, those who clutter are less likely to exhibit struggle during dysfluent speech productions, significant associated motor behaviors, word substitutions and circumlocutions, or anxiety about speech and speaking situations.

- **Worsening of dysfluencies when relaxed.** Reading a well-known text also may increase dysfluencies. To the contrary, there may be improved fluency under stressful or demanding conditions (tendencies that are opposite to what are observed in people who stutter). Fluency also may improve when attention is drawn to dysfluencies, while giving short answers, talking in foreign language, and speaking after interruption.

- **Language difficulties.** Possibly significant in several individuals who clutter, but may not be significant in all individuals. Language problems may include poor syntactic structures, run-on sentences, and incorrect use of prepositions and pronouns; such poor narrative skills as improper sequencing of ideas or events, inappropriate interjections of topics, poor topic maintenance, and word-finding problems; generally inadequate language formulation; poor listening skills, which may be due to short attention span; a general verbosity; tangential expressions; and poor eye contact.

- **Prosodic problems.** The speech rhythm may be impaired. These problems may be a function of irregular and festinating rate of speech.

- **Voice problems.** Voice may be loud to begin with, but fade toward the end of sentences. Monotonous voice may be an additional feature.

- **Disorganized thought processes.** These problems are inferred from poor language expressions of people who clutter. Short attention span, lack of self-monitoring, and an inability to take into account the perspective of the listener and the listener's difficulty understanding one's own speech are all features of this general problem.

- **Motor incoordination.** Symptoms include hasty and uncoordinated movements; clumsy movements and impaired sequencing of complex actions; and difficulty imitating simple rhythmic patterns. Some of the writing problems associated with cluttering may be a function of poor motor control.

- **Reading difficulty.** Some may begin to read a passage normally, but soon may make numerous mistakes in what they read.

- **Writing problems.** Poor spelling, sentence fragments, run-on sentences, omission and transposition of letters; omission of words; and generally disintegrated writing characterize writing problems.

- **Academic problems and learning disabilities.** These may be possibly due to thought and language problems associated with cluttering.

- **Unconcerned about the speech problem.** Persons who clutter may be described as being unaware of their difficulty, but this is unlikely. They are just less concerned about it and its effects on the listeners. These features of people who clutter contrast with those who stutter. People who clutter may believe that somehow listeners have a problem understanding them. Because of their lack of concern, people who clutter are less willing to seek treatment than those who stutter.

- **Some exceptional skills.** Excellent mathematical or scientific achievement may be noted in some cases, in spite of their language and speech problems.

Assessment of cluttering needs a comprehensive effort to understand the various verbal and nonverbal features of the disorder. Differential diagnosis may be challenging in that the clinician needs to distinguish cluttering form stuttering, an articulation disorder, and a language disorder. Assessment of reading, writing, and fine and gross motor skills may be necessary as well. Please see Chapter 11 for a *Cluttering Assessment Protocol.*

Analysis and Integration of Assessment Results

The clinician will tailor the analysis of assessment results to the particular type of fluency disorder the child exhibits. It may be stuttering or cluttering. Regardless of the type of fluency problem, however, the clinician will integrate the results of common assessment procedures with those of fluency assessment. For instance, the clinician will summarize the case history and interview information and the results of the orofacial examination and hearing screening. Information obtained from other professionals also is considered in the analysis.

If the assessment results suggest stuttering, the clinician will make an analysis of the dysfluency types and their frequency in conversational speech and oral reading (if relevant), observed associated motor behaviors and such other problems as airflow mismanagement, negative emotional reactions and speech-related attitudes, and avoidance reactions. Parental reactions to stuttering, their efforts to control it, and their disposition toward the fluency problem and its treatment will be analyzed. In addition, previous assessment and treatment information also will be a part of the analysis. The clinician will then integrate all the assessment results to construct a coherent picture of the child's stuttering and the family concerns and reactions.

If the assessment results suggest cluttering, the clinician will concentrate on the speech rate variations and all the associated speech-language problems listed previously.

Differential Diagnosis of Fluency Disorders

Fluency disorders are not commonly confused with a typical articulation or language disorder. In most cases, the parents will already have made a diagnosis of stuttering in their child; such a parental diagnosis is usually correct. On occasion, a parent may misdiagnose cluttering as stuttering. Therefore, in our clinical experience, stuttering is rarely misdiagnosed by parents, but cluttering may be. To the contrary, there may be children whose stuttering is not diagnosed in its earliest stages because the parents have not paid attention to the child's speech. In essence, then, there may be far fewer false positive parental diagnoses of stuttering than the false negatives.

Based on the assessment results, **diagnose stuttering** if:

- The child's overall dysfluency rate exceeds 5% of the words spoken, when all kinds of dysfluencies are counted.
- The child's part-word repetitions, speech sound prolongations, and broken words are at least 3% of the words spoken.
- The child exhibits extremely long silent or audible prolongations, even though their frequency is below accepted criterion (such as 3 or 5%).

Note that a diagnosis of stuttering is further supported by the presence of associated motor behaviors, negative emotions and feelings, mismanagement of airflow during speech production, and avoidance behaviors (Hegde, 2008a, 2008b). Nonetheless, these additional features are neither essential to diagnose stuttering nor require a diagnosis of stuttering when they are present but the dysfluency rates or durations of dysfluencies do not warrant a diagnosis. People may avoid certain words, speaking situations, or listeners for a variety of reasons, including unpleasant experiences unrelated to stuttering. People may experience unpleasant feelings about speech for reasons other than stuttering (e.g., a person may "hate talking to groups" because of past failures, not necessarily fluency failures). Airflow mismanagement during speech production may be observed in people who have dysarthria. By definition, abnormal motor behaviors in people who stutter are associated with their dysfluent speech; therefore, they are unlikely to be observed when speech is normally fluent. Uncontrolled facial and limb movements may be seen in some people during speech, but in such cases, a neuromotor disorder based on neuropathology may be documented.

Based on the assessment results, **diagnose cluttering** if:

- The child's overall rate of speech is judged to be too fast.
- The unusually fast rate is associated with articulatory breakdowns, causing reduced speech intelligibility. The child exhibits sound, syllable, or even word omissions, transposition of sounds within words, and telescoping or compression of speech.
- The articulatory proficiency and speech intelligibility improve when the speech rate is slowed down, but it is difficult for the child to maintain a slower rate unless constantly monitored.
- The child exhibits a higher than the normal level of dysfluencies that tend to get worse when relaxed or when reading a well-known text but improve under stressful or demanding conditions.
- The child exhibits syntactic problems along with prosodic variations (possible additional features).
- The child exhibits voice problems (possible additional features).
- The child exhibits reading and writing problems, likely features.
- The child appears to be relatively unconcerned about his or her speech problem, a most likely feature.
- The child demonstrates notable mathematical or scientific skills (a possible additional feature).

Note that a child may clutter and stutter as well. If this seems possible, then evaluate the child's assessment data in light of both stuttering and cluttering diagnostic criteria.

Postassessment Counseling

Conclude your assessment session with the postassessment counseling. On completion of assessment, counsel the client, the family members, or both about the results of assessment. Although you will not have analyzed the results of the assessment, you will have gained valid enough clinical impressions to summarize the results, make a tentative diagnosis, offer recommendations, describe treatment options, suggest prognosis, and answer the parents' questions.

Make a Tentative Diagnosis

Summarize your observations and describe your main impressions that are based on your observations. You can say whether in your judgment, the child has a fluency disorder, and if the child does, what kind of a disorder. In a majority of cases, the disorder will be stuttering. Describe the main features of the child's disorder. To justify your diagnosis, you might point out the child's dysfluencies; associated motor behaviors; airflow mismanagement; avoidance of words and speaking situations; and any evidence of negative feelings about self, listeners, and speaking situations.

If the child's fluency disorder is diagnosed as cluttering, differentiate it from stuttering to help parents understand the difference. Compare the two disorders and emphasize the unique features of each.

Make Recommendations

In the case of preschool children, some clinicians wait until the child is 6 or 7 years old before starting treatment. Others believe that the treatment should be started when a diagnosis is made. In our experience with preschool children who stutter and their parents, it is better to start treatment as soon as a diagnosis is made. Treatment may be postponed only if the diagnosis is uncertain or the dysfluency rates fluctuate so much that there are many days of normal fluency. In such cases, additional assessment sessions or home speech sampling may be necessary to diagnose or rule out stuttering.

Generally, if the dysfluency rates vary but the parents are still concerned about the overall rate, there is no justification for postponing treatment. Possibility of spontaneous recovery does not reassure many parents when it is not possible to predict it with certainty in their children. Also, in our experience, the parents who know there is effective treatment available for preschool children who stutter, request, or even demand, treatment for their child.

Suggest Prognosis

Prognosis for improved fluency, even normal fluency that is sustained, is good if children are treated. Generally, the younger the age at which a child is treated, the better the prognosis for normal-sounding, unmonitored, and well-maintained fluency. Fluency in older children and adults, too, significantly improves with effective and competently administered treatment. It is possible that adults who are treated may need to monitor their fluency on a more or less regular basis; this need may be more acute when the treatment procedure used is prolonged speech as against pause-and-talk (time-out).

Poor prognosis is often a result of several factors, including ineffective, inefficient, or improperly administered treatment; lack of follow-up and booster treatment; or failure to complete an effective treatment program. The clinician should point out that the prognosis is good if the client and the family complete the recommended treatment program, implement the maintenance program at home, keep in touch with the clinician so follow-ups may be conducted, and receive booster treatment when stuttering tends to increase. The clinician also may point out that a family history of stuttering or a severe stuttering does not necessarily mean poor prognosis for improvement.

Answer Frequently Asked Questions

Most parents of children who stutter typically ask several questions about stuttering and its treatment. Family members may have reviewed various Web sites on stuttering, its potential causes, and treatment options. Student clinicians often ask the clinical supervisors how best to answer such questions. It is important to give honest and scientific answers to the family members' questions. The answers given should reflect the state of the knowledge and should be formulated in objective and probabilistic terms. The clinician should mention research when necessary to convince the clients and their family members of the validity of answers offered. Some commonly encountered questions and their answers follow; you may need to modify the terms you use to suit the age, education, and the judged sophistication of families in formulating your answers. To suggest specific treatment procedures depending on the age of the child, see Hegde (2007).

What Causes Stuttering or Cluttering?

Although we know about several potential causes of stuttering, it is difficult to say what caused it in individual cases. Scientific knowledge we have about causation of stuttering (or cluttering) is based on groups of persons, not specific individuals. As a group, some genetic factors may be involved in about 45 to 50% of people who stutter or clutter. This means that nearly half the number of individuals who stutter or clutter may have a blood relative who also may have a similar problem. However, no specific gene has been identified. Even in those cases where a family history is positive, environmental factors may be important as well. Negative reaction to stressful speaking situations, a tendency to experience anxiety associated with speech, traumatic emotional experiences, and reactions to negative criticism may all play a role, although research is not definitive about such environmental factors.

We know more about how stuttering gets exacerbated or diminished than we do about its origin. For example, stuttering typically increases while talking to strangers, speaking under stressful situations, talking to authority figures, talking in a hurry, ordering in restaurants, talking over telephones, and so forth. Stuttering typically decreases when talking to close friends or family members, especially to infants and small children. Singing and talking while assuming the role of someone else may also increase fluency. Fortunately, most fluency problems can be effectively treated regardless of their original causes.

How Long Does It Take to Treat Stuttering Effectively?

It depends on several factors. Generally, it takes less time to treat a younger child than it does to treat an older child or an adult who has been stuttering for longer durations. Progress will be faster if family members follow up on suggestions to hold informal treatment sessions at home, support and help sustain fluency, and informally monitor fluency and stuttering in naturalistic speaking situations. Generally, about 6 to 12 months of treatment, offered twice a week, may be needed to experience substantial improvement in most cases.

How Effective Are Some of the Gadgets Promoted on the Internet?

Some of the gadgets, especially those that delay auditory feedback of speech, feed mechanical noise to the ears, or provide rhythmic metronome-like auditory stimuli tend to decrease stuttering. There also are many variations of these devices, but some of them are not experimentally tested. We should avoid devices whose effects have not been established through scientific research. Good news is that stuttering can be effectively treated without mechanical devices, more so in children. Therefore, investment in costly instruments is often unnecessary, may even be inappropriate for children. Unfortunately, many kinds of devices in the past have not succeeded in the market place. Because of bankruptcy of manufacturers, expensive instruments, once bought, may be unserviceable; if they run on a computer, it may be impossible to upgrade the software, rendering the unit useless.

What About Maintenance of Fluency Following Treatment?

This too, depends on the individual. Generally, young children who receive effective treatment maintain fluency better than adults who do. Stuttering that returns is not an indication of failed treatment; it only means that another round of treatment is necessary to make fluency last. A schedule of regular follow-up and prompt treatment when stuttering increases will eventually help wean a person away from treatment. To get booster treatment—which is treatment offered sometime after the initial dismissal from treatment—it is important for you to contact me or another clinician when there is an increase in stuttering. Booster treatment can be just a few sessions. In some cases, an extended telephone conversation may be all that is needed. A few simple things you can do at home—based on what we will have demonstrated to you in the clinic—may help restore fluency in your child.

What Are Some of the Treatment Options?

There are various well-researched treatment options for children who stutter. Slow speech almost always induces more fluent speech, although it may not sound very natural; it may also be difficult for the child to maintain a consistently slow speech. We generally do not recommend slow speech for preschoolers, although some older children may be good candidates.

In recent years, there have been alternatives to slower speech that have proven effective. These alternatives avoid the undesirable effects of slow speech, mostly the unnatural sounding speech. In one such procedure, we consistently and strongly reinforce or reward the child for speaking without stuttering. We do not teach the child to speak slowly or do anything to avoid stuttering. We just strengthen the fluency that does exist in the child's speech. We can also use a token system in which we give a token to the child when the speech is fluent and take a token back when the speech is stuttered. This system is effective with preschoolers and younger school-age children. We usually select a technique that is best for the child.

When Do We Start Treatment?

We recommend that we start treatment sooner rather than later for better and lasting outcome. We can set up a date now or you can call me or the clinic office later to begin treatment. [*Depending on the service setting, the clinician offers additional information on when and how to begin a treatment program for the child.*]

CHAPTER 11

Assessment of Fluency Disorders: Protocols

- Note on Common Protocols
- Note on Specific Protocols
- Interview Protocol
- Dysfluency Measurement Protocol
- Associated Motor Behaviors Assessment Protocol
- Avoidance Behaviors Assessment Protocol
- Cluttering Assessment Protocol

Note on Common Protocols

In completing a fluency assessment, the clinician may use the common protocols given in Chapter 2, also available on the CD. To make a comprehensive assessment of fluency disorders in children, the clinician may modify as needed and print for use the following common protocols from the CD:

The Child Case History Form

Orofacial Examination and Hearing Screening Protocol

Use this protocol along with the *Instructions for Conducting the Orofacial Examination: Observations and Implications.* If the preliminary findings of the orofacial examination suggests the possibility of velopharyngeal inadequacy or incompetence, use the *Resonance and Velopharyngeal Function Assessment* protocol in Chapter 13.

Assessment Report Outline

Expand the fluency section in the outline to include all relevant information gathered through the case history, interview, assessment, and reports from other professionals.

Note on Specific Protocols

This chapter contains a collection of protocols that can be used individually or combined in a variety of ways to facilitate the evaluation of a child's fluency problems. Each of these protocols is also available on the CD.

The protocols on the CD may be individualized and printed out as a group and used for a complete fluency assessment. Also, one or more protocols may be selectively printed out and used as needed. In assessing children with multiple disorders of communication, the clinician may combine these protocols with protocols from other chapters. For example, the clinician may combine these fluency assessment protocols with speech assessment protocols (Chapter 7), language assessment protocols (Chapter 9), or voice assessment protocols (Chapter 13).

Fluency Assessment Protocol 1
Interview Protocol

Child's Name _____ DOB _____ Date _____ Clinician _____

Note that your interview of the parents or caregivers and the child (if appropriate) is mainly concerned with getting additional information on the child's fluency problem, any associated clinical conditions or communication disorders, and academic concerns including literacy problems.

Individualize this protocol on the CD and print it for your use.

Preparation

☐ Review the "interview guidelines" presented in Chapter 1.

☐ Make sure the setting is comfortable with adequate seating and lighting.

☐ Record the interview whenever possible.

☐ Find out if the parent is comfortable having the child in the same room during the interview. If so, have something for the child to do (toys, books, etc.). If not, make arrangements for someone else to supervise the child in a different room during the interview.

☐ Review the case history ahead of time, noting areas you want to review or obtain more information about.

Introduction

☐ Introduce yourself. Briefly review your assessment plan for the day and give an estimate of the duration of assessment.

    Example: "Hello Mr. /Mrs. [*the parent's name*]. My name is [*your name*] and I am the speech-language pathologist who will be assessing _____ [*the child's name*] today. I would like to start by reviewing the case history and asking you a few questions. Once we are finished talking, I will work with _____ [*the child's name*]. Today's assessment should take about _____ [*estimate the amount of time you plan to spend*]."

Interview Questions

Ask the following kinds of questions to get clarifications or additional information. Skip or rephrase questions as found appropriate. Some parents need to be questioned in greater detail about the kinds of dysfluencies the child exhibits because they only describe the problem in general terms; others give more specific descriptions. Note that many answers the parents give to the initial question may require additional follow-up questions not specified in the outline. During the interview, replace the term "he" or the phrases "your child," and "your son" with the child's name. Although

(continues)

Interview Protocol (continued)

the outline shows the questions that need to be asked and answered, avoid relentless questioning. Frequently, paraphrase what the informants say by way of answers to your questions. Ask about the informants' views, thoughts, or feelings. If appropriate, express approval of what they say. Note that it is not just the clinician who asks questions; parents or other informants, too, will have questions that the clinician needs to answer. If they have questions about the typical features of stuttering, causes of the problem, treatment options, and so forth, answer briefly and promise more detailed information later.

☐ What is your primary concern regarding your son's [or daughter's] speech?

☐ Can you describe the problem?

☐ So you think your son stutters. What exactly does he do when you say he stutters?

☐ Does he repeat sounds? For example, have you heard him repeat the first sound in a word like "t-t-time" or "p-p-pen"?

☐ Does he repeat the first syllables in words? For example, have you heard him repeat like "Sa-Sa-Saturday" or "Lai-lai-like it"?

☐ Does your son prolong the sounds of speech? For example, have you heard him say "Llllike it" or "Mmmmmommy"?

☐ Have you heard your son repeat words and phrases? Can you give some examples?

☐ Have you heard him start a sentence and not finish it? Can you give some examples?

☐ Have you heard him revise something he begins to say? For example, does he say things like "I want juice, milk, Mom"? We all revise, but do you hear them very frequently?

☐ What about such interjections as "um" and "you know" and "OK" and "I mean?" Once again, all speakers say them, but do you hear them too frequently?

☐ Does he sometime pause too much when you don't expect him to pause? For example when a stranger asks "What's your name?" does he take a bit too much time to say his name?

☐ I think what you have described is typical of most children who stutter. They repeat sounds and words, prolong sounds, interject extraneous materials, say incomplete sentences, and drop an idea and revise repeatedly. Any other behavior that concerns you? For instance, does he show any facial expressions that draw attention to his speech difficulty? Can you describe some of them?

☐ Does he make any hand or feet movement when he stutters?

☐ What other kinds of extraneous movements does he make when he stutters?

☐ Let us now talk a little bit about how it all started. When was the problem first noticed? Who noticed it?

☐ What were the very first signs or symptoms that made you think there might be a problem?

☐ I would like you to think back and recall anything special that may have been associated with the beginning of stuttering in your child. Did anything unusual happen at the time you first noticed stuttering in your son?

☐ How did you react to your son when you heard him stutter? How did any one else [*your husband, your wife, the child's brother, or sister*] react to it?

☐ Did you give some suggestions for the child to avoid the problems? What kind of suggestions?

☐ Did you ask the child to speak slowly or think before saying something?

☐ Did you give any other suggestions? What were they?

☐ How did he react to your suggestions?

☐ Did your suggestions help the child? Did he do what you told him to do? In what ways did the suggestions help? [*Ask follow-up questions about the strategies suggested to the child, their effects, the child's reaction, and the additional steps the family members took to help the child speak more fluently.*]

☐ How did your child's stuttering change over the course of time? Did it get worse, improve, or stabilize?

☐ Does your son's stuttering vary over time and situations?

☐ How does it vary? When or under what conditions is he more fluent?

☐ When or under what conditions does he stutter more?

☐ If it has, when did his stuttering become more stable across situations and time?

☐ Once again, what you have told me is typical of stuttering. Stuttering tends to vary across time and situations. Now I want to discuss some associated problems that may be a reaction to stuttering. For instance, does your son avoid saying some words? Can you think of words he avoids?

☐ What does he do when he doesn't want to say certain words? Does he use similar words, beat around the bush, use vague words, or describe instead of naming something?

☐ Does he avoid speaking to certain individuals? Is he ever reluctant to talk? Whom does he typically avoid speaking to?

☐ Does he freely speak to some individuals? In other words, whom does he not avoid?

☐ Does he appear frustrated when he can't get the words out?

☐ How does he express his frustration?

☐ Has your child told you anything about how he feels about his speech problem?

☐ Has your son told you anything about how other children or adults have reacted to his speech? [*Ask follow-up questions about the child's emotional reactions and feelings associated with stuttering and other avoidance reactions.*]

☐ Do you feel that your son's stuttering is affecting his social interactions?

☐ Do you feel that your son's stuttering is affecting his school performance?

☐ Do you think your child's reading and writing skills are fine? [*ask this question when appropriate to the child's age; ask follow-up questions on literacy skills*]

☐ What kind of concerns have you heard from your son's teachers? [*Ask follow-up questions about the effects stuttering had on the child's social, academic, and personal life.*]

(continues)

Interview Protocol (continued)

☐ Does your child have any language problems that you are concerned with?

☐ Do you think his language skills—I mean his vocabulary, grammar, and general language skills—are OK for his age?

☐ Considering his age, have you noticed any problems in producing the speech sounds correctly? What English speech sounds does he still mispronounce or not pronounce at all?

☐ Is there any difficulty understanding what he says because he does not say English sounds correctly?

☐ What do you think of his voice? Does his voice sound normal to you? [*Ask follow-up questions about other communication disorders the child may have.*]

☐ What is your first language? What is your [husband's, wife's] first language?

☐ Is English your son's first language? If not, what other language or languages does he speak? Also, what language is routinely spoken at home?

☐ Does he speak the two languages equally well? If not, which language is stronger?

☐ If English is not the primary language, do you feel your son stutters to the same extent in both the languages? If not, in what language does a stutter less?

☐ Who reads stories to your son, talks more, and spends more play time with him? You or your [husband, wife]? Maybe both of you do to the same extent. [*Ask follow-up questions about the family's ethnocultural background, bilingual status, and family communication patterns.*]

☐ Did you or your [husband, wife] ever stutter?

☐ Did your son's sister [sisters] or brother [brothers] ever stutter? If they ever did, do they still do? Did he [she] ever receive treatment?

☐ Is there a family member who you know stutters? Maybe on your side of the family or your [husband's, wife's] side. Because some, but not all children who stutter, may have a family history of stuttering, I want to know if there is any blood relative that you know stutters, whether the person had treatment, and whether he or she still stutters. [*Ask follow-up questions about the family history of stuttering, treatment received by other members of the family, and the current status of their stuttering.*]

☐ Why do you think your son stutters? Do you have any thoughts about the causes of stuttering in your son?

☐ Do you know of any treatments for stuttering? How did you learn about them? [*Discuss the caregivers beliefs about stuttering and its treatment; answer any questions they may have about the causes and remedies for stuttering briefly, and tell them that you will offer more information later.*]

☐ Do you think your son hears normally?

☐ Did your son have ear infections in the past? Does he have any ear infections now?

☐ Has your child ever had a hearing test? If yes, when and where? What were the results?

☐ Has your child seen any other specialists for his stuttering? If so, who and when? What were their recommendations? How have you followed up on this?

☐ Has your child received therapy for stuttering? When and where?

☐ What did they work on in therapy? Can you describe the types of activities that were used? How did your child respond? Do you feel the therapy was helpful? Why or why not?

☐ Did your child receive any other kind of speech therapy? [*Ask follow-up questions about previous treatment for stuttering or any other communication disorder and the nature and effects of such treatment.*]

☐ Are there any other kinds of concerns you have about your child that you wish to let me know? [*Ask follow-up questions about any other problem the informants may mention; may include behavior problems, autism, intellectual disabilities, neuromotor problems, academic difficulties, vision problems, and so forth.*]

Before concluding the interview, review the case history and follow up with any additional questions you need to ask. Fill in any "blanks" in the medical, developmental, social and educational histories.

Close the Interview

Before you close the initial interview, summarize the major points you have learned from the interview, allowing the parent or the caregiver an opportunity to interrupt or correct information. Close the interview with the following:

☐ You have given me sufficient information to begin my assessment. I know that your child repeats sounds, syllables, and words; prolongs sounds; interjects syllables and words; and does other things as you have described to me. Now, do you have any questions for me at this point?

☐ Thank you very much for you input. The information has been very helpful.

☐ Now, I will work with [the child's name]. When we are finished, we will discuss the findings. I will also answer your questions about stuttering and its treatment.

Fluency Assessment Protocol 2
Dysfluency Measurement Protocol

Child's Name _____ DOB _____ Date _____ Clinician _____

Individualize this protocol on the CD and print it for your use.

	Frequency			
Dysfluency Types	Speech	Monologue	Oral reading	Home speech
Repetitions Part-word Whole-word Phrase				
Prolongations Sound/syllable Silent				
Interjections Sound/syllable Whole-word Phrase				
Silent Pauses				
Broken Words (intralexical pauses)				
Incomplete Phrases				
Revisions				
Total of dysfluencies/ Number of words				
Percent dysfluency rate				

Comments:

Fluency Assessment Protocol 3
Associated Motor Behaviors Assessment Protocol

Child's Name _____ DOB _____ Date _____ Clinician _____

Individualize this protocol on the CD and print it for your use.

Rate each behavior: 0 = Not observed   1 = Infrequent   2 = Frequent

Associated Motor Behaviors Checklist	Rating *(0, 1, or 2)*
Rapid and tense eye blink	
Tensed and prolonged shutting of the eyelids	
Rapid upward, downward, or lateral movement of the eyes	
Knitting of the eyebrows	
Nose wrinkling and flaring	
Pursing or quivering of the lips	
Tongue clicking	
Teeth clenching, grinding, and clicking	
Tension in facial muscles	
Wrinkling of the forehead	
Clenched jaw or jerky or slow or tensed movement of the jaws	
Jaw opening or closing unrelated to target speech production	
Tension in chest, shoulder, and neck muscles (e.g., twitching and extraneous movements)	
Head movements (e.g., turns, shakes, jerks, and lateral, upward, and downward movements)	
Tensed and jerky hand movements (e.g., fist clenching and hand wringing)	
Tensed and jerky arm movements (e.g., tapping on the thighs or pressing against the sides of the abdomen)	
Tensed and jerky leg movements (e.g., kicking motions)	
Tensed and jerky feet movements (e.g., grinding, pressing, rubbing, or circular movements on the floor)	
Generally tense body postures	
Other behaviors observed or reported:	

Comments:

Fluency Assessment Protocol 4
Avoidance Behaviors Assessment Protocol

Child's Name _____ DOB _____ Date _____ Clinician _____

Individualize this protocol on the CD and print it for your use.

To complete this assessment, observe the child, and interview the child and the parents. Place a check mark against the behavior the child typically exhibits.

Avoidance of Speaking Situations; typically, the child avoids:	Scoring
Saying one's own name	☐
Responding to roll calls	☐
Speaking situations (moves away from the speaking situation)	☐
Ordering in restaurants	☐
Speaking on the telephone	☐
Introducing self	☐
Giving personal phone numbers or addresses	☐
Speaking in front of the class or a social group	☐
Reading aloud in front of a class	☐
Answering questions in the classroom	☐
Saying the names of family members [specify]:	☐
Asking for directions when lost	☐
Asking for help when something is difficult (e.g., solving a math problem or putting together a puzzle)	☐
Avoidance of other speaking situations observed or reported:	
Strategies to Avoid Stuttering; typically, the child:	
Depends on others for communication needs	☐
Gestures instead of speaking	☐
Has a family member ask for something in a store	☐
Pretends not to hear a question	☐
Pretends to be thinking when questions are asked	☐
Pretends not to know an answer	☐

Pretends ignorance of a word on which stuttering is likely	☐
Lets others finish a word or complete a sentence	☐
Coughs or clears throat before saying a difficult word	☐
Whispers	☐
Talks in a soft voice (sudden reduction in vocal intensity on certain words)	☐
Talks in a loud voice (sudden increase in vocal intensity on certain words)	☐
Talks in an impersonated tone (e.g., a cartoon character)	☐
Talks with an unusual physical posture	☐
Talks with an exaggerated articulation	☐
Other strategies to avoid stuttering, observed or reported:	
Avoidance of Conversational Partners; typically, the child avoids talking to:	
Adult strangers	☐
New kids in school	☐
Teachers and other authority figures	☐
Persons of the opposite sex	☐
The mother	☐
The father	☐
Other members of the family [specify]:	☐
Peers in the neighborhood	☐
Avoidance of other conversational partners, observed or reported:	
Avoidance of Certain Words; typically, the child:	
Substitutes one word for another	☐
"Beats around the bush" instead of saying something directly	☐
Pretends not to know a word	☐
Refuses to say a particular word (e.g., "I don't want to say that word")	☐
Says *this thing* and *that thing* frequently	☐
Stutters on the following sounds [list them]:	☐

(continues)

Avoidance Behaviors Assessment Protocol (continued)

Stutters on the following words [list them]:	☐
Other word-avoidance strategies, observed or reported:	
Avoidance of Talking About Stuttering; typically the child:	
Switches topic when stuttering is mentioned	☐
Leaves the room when conversation is initiated on stuttering as a topic	☐
Gets upset when asked about his [her] stuttering	☐
Refuses to talk about the classmates' reactions to one's stuttering	☐
Refuses tot talk about teachers' reaction to one's stuttering	☐
Does not talk about his [her] stuttering and emotional experiences associated with it	☐
Other strategies to avoid talking about stuttering, observed or reported:	
Avoidance of Talking in General; typically, the child:	
Says "I don't want to talk" following a severe stutter	☐
Keeps quiet when a question is asked	☐
Plays by himself or herself when other children are present	☐
Does not take part in social conversations	☐
Avoids eye contact during conversation	☐
Has reduced the amount of talking in general	☐
Other strategies of avoiding talking in general, observed or reported:	

Fluency Assessment Protocol 5
Cluttering Assessment Protocol

Child's Name _____ DOB _____ Date _____ Clinician _____

Individualize this protocol on the CD and print it for your use.

Observed positive and negative signs are checked and examples are given.

Positive Signs	Negative Signs
☐ Speech rate abnormalities:	☐ Difficulty controlling the rate, even with contingent feedback
☐ Errors of articulation:	☐ Can produce the sounds under slower speech rate
☐ Dysfluencies:	☐ Repetition of sounds and sound prolongations ☐ Few or no associated motor behaviors, word substitutions and circumlocutions, minimal or no struggle during dysfluent speech
☐ Worsening of dysfluencies when relaxed, and while reading familiar texts ☐ Improved fluency under stress, while giving short answers, and speaking after interruption	☐ Absence of anxiety about speech and speaking situations ☐ Unconcerned about the speech problem and its effects on listeners ☐ Unwilling to seek or continue treatment
☐ Language difficulties:	
☐ Prosodic problems:	
☐ Voice problems:	
☐ Disorganized thought processes:	
☐ Motor incoordination:	
☐ Reading difficulty:	
☐ Writing problems:	
☐ Academic problems:	

PART V
Assessment of Voice

CHAPTER 12

Assessment of Voice: Resources

- Prevalence of Voice Disorders in Children
- Children's Voice Disorders
- Etiologic Factors Associated with Voice Disorders
- The Need for Medical Evaluation
- Assessment of Voice Production
- Instrumental Evaluation
- Laryngeal Imaging
- Clinical Assessment of Voice
- Stimulability of Voice Production
- Assessment of Voice in Ethnoculturally Diverse Children
- Analysis and Integration of Assessment Results
- Differential Diagnosis of Voice Disorders
- Postassessment Counseling

Voice assessment and treatment procedures have been changing in response to recent research and the technologic advances that now allow the clinicians to objectively measure vocal behaviors that were once subjectively described. These advances, along with speech-language pathologists' long-standing clinical skills and procedures, create an opportunity to work in collaboration with the medical community to achieve the most accurate and comprehensive voice diagnosis possible. This, in turn, provides an opportunity for speech-language pathologists (SLPs) to collaboratively develop efficient and effective medical and behavioral treatment protocols to best serve children and adults with voice disorders.

The assessment and treatment of voice problems in young children has been some-what controversial in recent history. It has been suggested that hoarseness, the most common reason for childhood voice referrals, is maturational. Hoarseness is rarely the result of a life-threatening condition in children, and many will develop normal voices as adults (Mori, 1999). In addition, children, particularly those under the age of 5, are often unaware of their voice differences (e.g., hoarseness), and are therefore unlikely to be motivated to make the behavioral changes needed to correct them.

On the other hand, voice abnormalities might be a sign of a more serious medical condition such as papilloma, web, laryngopharyngeal reflux (LPR), or chronic nodules. The timely and accurate diagnosis of these problems may lead to medical and behavioral treatments that successfully manage or remediate them. Although many children achieve improved vocal quality as they get older, Powell, Filter, and Williams (1989) showed that 38% of these children will continue to have voice problems for 5 years or more after their initial screening. Even though young children may be unaware of their voice problem or the way it affects their everyday functioning, deviant voice may have a negative effect on social communication. Voicing problems might be the cause or result of such difficulties in socialization as screaming to get attention. Leeper (1992) and Ruddy, McCrea, Fichera, and Lehman (2008) found that voice disorders affect a child's performance in the class-room. Moreover, children with voice disorders are often perceived as more negative, more aggressive, or as having more behavioral problems than their peers with normal voice qualities (Lass, Ruscello, Stout, & Hoffmann, 1991; Ruscello, Lass, & Podbeseki, 1988). Ruddy et al. (2008) found that children with voice disorders had fewer peer interactions. It has also been reported that children and adolescents feel their voice disorders resulted in negative attention and limited their participation in some activities (Connor et al., 2008).

Studies have supported the use of direct therapy and behavior modification (including the promotion of healthy vocal behaviors) to reduce or eliminate vocal misuses or abuses that could be potentially damaging to the vocal folds. For example, in a study of 31 school-age children with vocal nodules, Deal, McClain, and Sudderth (1976) demonstrated that after 2 months of treatment, 68% had reduced nodule size and 23% had normal larynges. Four months later, 65% had normal larynges. Data such as these support the value of voice assessment and treatment, even in very young children (Allen, Bernstein, & Chait, 1991; Allen, Pettit, & Sherblom, 1991; Baker & Blackwell, 2004; Hooper, 2004; Johnson & Parrish, 1971; Kahane & Mayo, 1989; Moran & Pentz, 1987; Mori, 1999; Ramig & Verdo-lini, 1998, Sandage & Zelazny, 2004).

Prevalence of Voice Disorders in Children

Incidence and prevalence estimates of voice disorders in children vary widely. Most authors agree, however, voice disorders may be found in 6 to 9% of school-age children (Andrews,

1986; 2002; Johnson & Child, 1988; McNamera & Perry, 1994; Moore, 1982; Senturia & Wilson, 1968; Warr-Leeper, McShea, & Leeper, 1979). Lecoq and Drape (1996) conducted a study in which they screened the voices of 259 primary school children. They found that 10% had dysphonia associated with either a laryngeal problem or resonance problem. Still, others have estimated that voice disorders may be found in 1.2 to 23.9% of children (Deal, McClain, & Sudderth, 1976; Gillespie & Cooper, 1973; Powell, Filter, & Williams, 1989; Silverman & Zimmer, 1975). In a survey, SLPs in the schools reported that 2 to 4% of children in their caseload had voice disorders (Davis & Harris, 1992). Several studies have demonstrated that, in the school-aged population, the prevalence of voice disorders related to abuse or misuse is higher for boys than it is for girls (Akif Kilic, Okur, Yildirim, & Guzelsoy, 2004; Carding, Roulstone, Northstone, & Team, 2006).

Most childhood voice disorders are associated with laryngeal hyperfunction, which is caused by vocal abuse or misuse (Glaze, 1996; Hooper, 2004; Johnson & Child, 1988; McNamera & Perry, 1994). It has been estimated that 45 to 80% of childhood dysphonia cases are the result of vocal nodules secondary to vocal abuse (Baynes, 1966; Herrington-Hall, Lee, Stemple, Nieme, & McHone, 1988). More recently, gastroesophageal reflux disease (GERD) and laryngopharyngeal reflux (LPR) have been identified as major contributors to vocal hoarseness, which is the most common presenting complaint of children with voice disorders (Cezard, 2004; Kaufman, Sataloff, & Touhill, 1996; Theis, 2011). According to Faust (2003), the reported occurrence of hoarseness in school-aged children ranged from 6% to 23%.

Although laryngeal hyperfunction and vocal nodules are the most common diagnoses among school-aged children with voice disorders, very young children are more likely to present with diagnoses of laryngomalacia, subglottic stenosis, or vocal fold paralysis (Saniga, & Carlin, 1993). These conditions may occur in medically complex children who, due to advances in neonatal care, have undergone sometimes numerous invasive medical procedures at a very young age. Children with congenital abnormalities of the larynx and those that have undergone surgery to the airway have a higher incidence of voice disorders (Gherson & Wilson Arboleda, 2010; Woodnorth, 2004). In addition, children who have experienced tracheostomies or prolonged periods of intubation are at high risk for speech and language delays secondary to prolonged periods of aphonia (Kelchner, de Alarcon, Weinrich, & Brehm, 2009; Smith, Marsh, Cotton, & Myer, 1993). It has also been shown that articulation and language disorders, mild hearing problems, upper respiratory infections, allergies, and asthma often coexist with voice disorders (Greene & Mathieson, 2001; St. Louis, Hansen, Buch, & Oliver, 1992). Therefore, when assessing voice disorders in children, the possibility of concurrent medical problems, as well as speech, language, or developmental delays, needs to be considered.

Children's Voice Disorders

Voice disorders are variously classified (Andrews, 2006; Boone, McFarlane, & Von Berg, 2005; Sataloff, 2005). In some classifications, medical pathology is confused with a voice disorder. For instance, it is not uncommon to describe *laryngeal cancer* as an *organic voice disorder* or *vocal nodules* as a functional voice disorder. Cancer and vocal nodules may be the causes of the associated voice disorders, but they are not voice disorders.

Another difficulty with the traditional classification is the distinction between the *organic* and *functional* voice disorders. Except for pure functional aphonia, a high-pitched voice in a male, and selective mutism that may exist without any organic changes in the laryngeal or neural mechanisms, almost all other voice disorders are organic (Hegde, 2008b). Traditionally, hoarseness due to vocal nodules is classified as functional, but it is the nodules (organic changes) that cause the vocal deviation. That the nodules are due to faulty vocal behaviors does not make the voice disorder *functional*.

Voice disorders should be classified strictly according to the vocal parameters. Underlying medical pathology should not be confused with voice disorders. Causes of voice disorders may be *organic* or *behavioral* (functional). Within this conceptual framework, voice disorders may be classified broadly as *dysphonias* and *aphonia*. *Dysphonias* refer to a variety of vocal characteristics that are deviant in some or several dimensions; most voice disorders fall under this category. Dysphonias may be further classified as *disorders of pitch (frequency)*, *disorders of loudness (intensity)*, *disorders of quality*, and *disorders of resonance*. Technically, *aphonia* is absence of voice, although a constant and total absence of voice is rare in children or adults. Among a few special conditions, *elective* or *selective mutism* may be noteworthy in some children (Hegde, 2008b).

Disorders of Pitch (Frequency)

Frequency is a measure of the physical property of a sound. In voice production, the frequency of vocal fold vibration is measured in terms of hertz (Hz) or cycles per second. The average frequency of vocal fold vibrations in an individual is called the *fundamental frequency*. Progressively higher frequencies of vocal fold vibrations in a speaker evoke comparably higher sensations of pitch in the listener (Hegde & Freed, 2011). The unit of pitch measurement is called a *mel*. The pitch of a 1000 Hz tone is arbitrarily fixed at 1000 mels to serve as a reference pitch. If a listener judges a tone as half as high in pitch as that of the 1000 Hz tone, then the pitch of that tone is 500 mels. The pitch of a tone judged twice as high would be 2000 mels (Raphael, Borden, & Harris, 2007).

It is normal for pitch patterns to vary within a speaker and across speakers. Stathopoulos, Huber, and Sussman (2011) found greater fundamental frequency variability in children and older adults than in younger adults. However, when pitch patterns deviate significantly from the practices of peers within the verbal community, a disorder of pitch may occur. A speaker's age, size, and gender provide reference points to judge whether the pitch is deviant or within normal limits. Two measures that are commonly used in the assessment of vocal pitch are *habitual pitch* and *pitch range*. The habitual pitch of a speaker is defined as the average pitch heard in a sample of continuous speech (Boone, McFarlane, Von Berg, & Zraich, 2010; Case, 2002). The pitch range is determined by measuring the lowest possible pitch (basal) and the highest possible pitch (ceiling). Instrumentation, such as those described later in this chapter, may be helpful in measuring these aspects of vocal pitch.

Disorders of pitch arise due to inappropriate frequency with which the vocal folds vibrate, breaks in the cycles of vocal fold vibrations, lack of normal variations in the frequency of vibrations, and asynchronous vibrations of the two folds. Pitch disorders may be caused by both behavioral and organic deviations.

Inappropriate Pitch. In this disorder, the vocal pitch is described as inappropriate in relation to the child's size, age, and gender. The voices of young boys and girls usually have a similar pitch level, but as they get older, the pitch levels are differentiated. The age at which the fundamental frequencies of boys' and girls' voices begin to differ from each other is believed to be between 7 and 12 years (Shrivastav, 2002). At age 7, boys and girls have roughly the same pitch, with a range of 220 to 310 Hz and an average habitual pitch of 260 Hz. At the age of 18, male voices average 125 Hz, nearly a 70% reduction when compared to 400 Hz prevalent at age 1. In contrast, at age 18, female voices average 205 Hz, only a 50% reduction when compared to the same 400 Hz prevalent at age 1 (Wilson, 1987). Voices that do not change with maturity might result in *mutational falsetto* or *puberphonia* which is characterized by the use of a very high pitch in postpubescent males and females. In most cases, this is a behavioral or functional voice disorder associated with faulty learning. An excessively low pitch in children is unusual, but could occur as a result of severe reflux, significant vocal fold edema, or faulty learning.

Pitch Breaks. Unexpected breaks in vocal pitch are a deviation in the smooth rates with which vocal folds normally vibrate. Pitch breaks generally occur for one of three reasons. First, they may occur as a normal part of maturational voice changes (mutation) in boys. In this case, the pitch breaks generally become evident toward the end of puberty and should not last longer than 6 months. This would not be considered a clinically significant problem requiring treatment. The second cause of pitch breaks is a habitually produced inappropriate pitch. If the child's habitual pitch is inappropriately high, then the voice is likely to break toward a lower pitch, and if it is inappropriately low, the voice is likely to break to a higher pitch. Therefore, close analysis of the pitch breaks when they occur might provide direction for therapy. Third, pitch breaks may occur due to vocal fatigue associated with vocal hyperfunction. According to Boone et al. (2010), speaking with excessive muscular effort can lead to both pitch breaks and phonation breaks.

Monopitch. When a child's voice lacks the normal pitch variations, it is described as monopitch. This may be characteristic of a neurologic disorder. Monopitch is often associated with dysarthria, especially ataxic and hypokinetic dysarthrias. In children, dysarthria is frequently associated with *cerebral palsy*, which is addressed in Chapter 6. In the absence of a history and evidence of neurologic damage, monopitch is classified as a functional voice disorder associated with faulty learning.

Diplophonia. The term *diplophonia* means that two distinct frequencies are being produced simultaneously. Diplophonia occurs when the two vocal folds vibrate at different rates because of a lesion, swelling, scarring, or vocal fold paralysis, or when there is another vibrating source in addition to the vocal folds. Other laryngeal structures that can be set into motion to produce vocal sound are the ventricular folds, the aryepiglottic folds, or a laryngeal web.

Disorders of Loudness (Intensity)

Intensity is a measure of the physical properties of a sound stimulus whereas loudness is a judgment listeners make based on their auditory sensation (Raphael et al., 2007).

Intensity may be measured by a sound level meter or similar instrumentation; however, *loudness* is measured as a response listeners give to a sound stimulus. Raphael et al. (2007) describe a scaling procedure in which the measured unit of loudness is called a *sone*. In this measuring procedure, 1 sone equals the loudness of a 1000 Hz tone at 40 dB. Using this as a reference point, listeners may be asked to judge whether two sound intensities are equal in loudness, half as loud, twice as loud, and so forth. More commonly, measurements of loudness are based on nonverbal or verbal reactions to sound stimuli such as moving away from a sound source or declaring, "That's too loud." For this reason, loudness is sometimes described as a subjective judgment based on the intensity of the sound stimulus (Hegde & Freed, 2011).

Vocal, loudness refers to the amplitude (magnitude) of vocal fold vibrations. The greater the amplitude of vibrations, the higher the judged loudness of the voice will be. The vibratory amplitude and resulting vocal intensity is largely a function of subglottic air pressure. Greater subglottic air pressure during phonation will result in a higher amplitude of vocal fold vibration and a correspondingly louder voice. The typical loudness of conversational speech is around 60 dB SPL at 1 meter. The softest phonation (not whispered) voice is about 40 dB and the highest intensity the larynx is capable of is 100 to 110 dB (Kent, 1994).

Loudness of speech varies depending on several factors, including the speech situation, the listener characteristics, and the speaking environment (Hunter, Halpern, & Spielman, 2012). Loudness of speech is also a matter of individual differences with some individuals who habitually speak louder or softer than others. In addition, vocal loudness may partly be a cultural phenomenon in that some cultures promote relatively soft conversational voice when compared to other cultures. Yet, any extreme in the range of normal vocal intensity variation is a disorder of loudness and may need clinical attention. In assessing loudness deviations, the clinician generally considers the social appropriateness of the vocal intensity, as well as, any negative impact it might have on communication. For example, an excessively loud voice may be judged as more or less aversive and an excessively soft voice may be handicapping because of its failure to meet the social and educational needs of the child.

> ***Excessively Loud Voice.*** Voice that is too loud in most everyday speaking situations is socially inappropriate and calls attention to itself. This may be associated with a hearing loss, but is usually a functional disorder associated with faulty learning. Excessive loudness is not only socially inappropriate, but it can lead to more serious problems, including the development of nodules, polyps, or laryngeal hyperfunction.

> ***Excessively Soft Voice.*** This means that the child's voice is so soft that it interferes with communication and fails to meet social demands of interaction. A barely audible voice may require increased listener effort in order to hear the speaker. This may reduce communication effectiveness in a classroom environment or during social interactions with other children. An excessively soft voice may be caused by neurologic damage or laryngeal pathologies such as nodules or polyps. Excessively soft voice in most children, however, is a functional disorder associated with faulty learning. As noted, soft voice partly may be due to the child's cultural background.

Disorders of Quality

The term *voice quality* refers to several variables related to the manner in which phonation is produced and the various ways in which listeners evaluate the phonated sound. Phonation produced with audible air leakage or excessive tension, aperiodicity of vocal fold vibrations, and pitch variations may all contribute to vocal quality disorders.

Breathiness. Breathiness as judged by a listener is closely linked to increased glottal opening and noise in the voice signal (Linville, 2002). A voice is described as *breathy* when excessive audible air leakage is associated with phonation. Inadequate approximation of the vocal folds causes audible air leakage. Failure to adequately approximate the vocal folds may be associated with neurologic damage, but in most children, it is usually the result of vocal fold edema, nodules, or polyps. McAllister, Sederholm, Sundberg, and Gramming (1994) found a high incidence of glottal opening and breathiness or hoarseness in 60 10-year-old children with reduced voice range profiles (sound pressure levels and fundamental frequencies). Stroboscopic examinations revealed that 10% of the children had vocal nodules and 23% had glottal openings. Breathiness can also occur as the result of faulty learning.

Harshness. Vocal harshness is characterized by an unpleasant, strident, or rough voice because of aperiodicity of vocal fold vibration. Harshness may be associated with excessive vocal effort, hard glottal attacks, abrupt initiation of voice, and constriction of the vocal tract. Possible etiologic factors include neurologic disorders, laryngeal structural problems, vocal abuse, or faulty learning.

Hoarseness. Vocal hoarseness is a combination of harshness and breathiness. In addition, it is characterized by a grating or husky voice that includes phonation breaks, diplophonia, and low pitch. A hoarse voice may sound dry or wet. A wet voice is generally caused by excessive mucus in the larynx. Hoarseness may be associated with various organic etiologies such as edema, nodules, polyps, cysts, papilloma, reflux, laryngitis, allergies, asthma, or other upper respiratory infections (Greene & Mathieson, 2001; Koufman, Sataloff, & Touhill, 1996). Hoarseness may also be the result of vocal abuse and misuse, or faulty learning. It is frequently associated with laryngeal hyperfunction. St Louis et al. (1992) found that the majority of students in grades 1 through 12 with either severe or moderate voice disorders exhibited vocal hoarseness.

Tense voice. A tense voice is the result of phonation produced with excessive adduction and medial compression of the folds. The voice sounds tight, strained, and effortful. A tense voice is often associated with various organic conditions that promote compensation resulting in hyperadduction of the folds. Hyperadduction of the folds may exacerbate the organic condition or contribute to laryngeal hyperfunction even further. A tense voice can also be associated with faulty learning.

Disorders of Resonance

Modification of the laryngeal tone by the cavities of the throat, mouth, and nose that lie above the vocal folds is called *resonance*. Resonance changes the vocal tone. If, for mostly organic reasons, the various cavities do not contribute to this resonance or contribute excessively, the voice of a speaker does not sound normal. Resonance disorders include hypernasality, hyponasality, cul-de-sac resonance, and assimilation nasality.

Hypernasality. Hypernasality is excessive nasal resonance on non-nasal speech sounds. Etiologic factors associated with hypernasality include craniofacial anomalies such as a short palate or velum, clefts of the hard or soft palate, submucous clefts, and velopharyngeal insufficiency (VPI). In addition, it is associated with deafness, faulty learning, and cerebral palsy in some children. Hypernasality in children may also occur as a consequence of tonsillectomy or adenoidectomy because of reduced tissue mass that is now insufficient to achieve a more adequate closure of the velopharyngeal valve.

Hyponasality. Hyponasality is inadequate nasal resonance. A hyponasal voice is characterized by too little nasal resonance so the child sounds "stuffed up." Hyponasality affects the production of the nasal phonemes /m/, /n/, and /ŋ/. Hyponasality may occur as the result of an obstructed nasal passage or nasopharynx, excessive or thick secretions secondary to chronic upper respiratory infections or allergies, structural deviations of the nasal septum or sinus cavities, enlarged adenoids, significant hearing loss, or faulty learning. Other organic factors associated with hyponasality include pharyngitis, tonsillitis, diseases of the nasal cavity, nasal polyps, papilloma, foreign bodies in the nasal cavity, and nasal neoplasm (tumor).

Cul-de-sac Resonance. *Cul-de-sac* voice refers to "bottom of the sac" resonance that is usually produced because of posterior retraction of the tongue deep into the oral cavity and hypopharynx. In children, it is generally associated with oral apraxia, cerebral palsy (athetoid dysarthria), deafness, or faulty learning.

Assimilation nasality. Assimilation nasality occurs when the oral sounds surrounding nasal sounds become nasalized. This is usually associated with velopharyngeal insufficiency (VPI) or faulty timing in the opening and closing of the velopharyngeal port. The velopharyngeal port that was open during the nasal sound production remains open during the adjacent oral sound production, thus inducing unwanted nasal resonance on the oral sounds. This problem is often associated with such neurologic disorders as cerebral palsy, resulting in spastic dysarthria. It is thought that faulty learning also may be responsible for assimilation nasality in some cases.

Nasal emission. Nasal emission is the audible escape of unvoiced air through the nares during the production of speech. Nasal emission is associated with the production of such pressure consonants as stops, fricatives, and affricates and usually indicates velopharyngeal incompetency or insufficiency. Nasal emission may co-occur with hypernasality, but the two are separate problems.

Functional Aphonia

Functional aphonia refers to the loss of voice or the inability to produce phonation for speech, although there is no organic pathology. Children with functional aphonia will produce phonation during such nonspeech acts as coughing, throat clearing, or laughing.

Functional aphonia can be constant or intermittent, but persistent total loss of voice is rare. Some children may communicate using whispers and gestures whereas others may be mute. Other children may communicate with an extremely faint voice with breathiness. Still other children may produce a weak and shrill voice.

Functional aphonia has a relatively sudden onset. This is a behavioral or psychological disorder that is sometimes described as a *hysterical reaction* or conversion reaction in psychoanalytic terms. In Freudian theory, a conversion reaction is an observable problem (such as lack of voice or sudden paralysis of the arms with no organic pathology) that is not the real problem. The real problem may be some socially unacceptable, unconscious, and unobservable desire or impulse that has been transformed (converted) into the observable problem. There is no convincing evidence supporting such a theory of behavior disorders. In behavioral analysis, functional aphonia is a positively reinforced behavior; the child may derive some benefit (positive reinforcement) from his or her inability to talk. The child, for instance, may be excused from oral presentations to the class. Therefore, in diagnosing functional aphonia, evidence of positive reinforcement is more easily detected than some unconscious impulse or conflict.

Functional aphonia may develop secondary to a physical condition such as the flu, an upper respiratory infection, or laryngeal surgery that resulted in temporary voice problems. The child may have been advised not to talk during the period of recovery. However, the child may continue to be aphonic even after the organic condition resolves and there is no longer a reason for aphonia. Such a voice problem may be diagnosed as *functional aphonia*.

Elective or Selective Mutism

Elective or selective mutism is the partial or complete withholding of vocal communication. The child is fully capable of producing phonation (and speech) but apparently refuses to speak. Possibly, an aphonic child believes that he or she cannot produce phonation but a child who is electively mute knows that speech is possible, produces speech in certain situations, but in certain other situations, *elects* to be mute. Elective mutism is typically described as a behavioral or psychiatric disorder (American Psychiatric Association, 2000; Cline & Baldwin, 1994; McInnes & Manassis, 2005; Wintgens, 2005).

To diagnose elective mutism, it should: (a) be limited to specific situations, (b) not be due to social embarrassment, ethnocultural differences, gender variations, or a lack of knowledge on a topic of discussion, and (c) last at least one month and should persist after the first month in school (American Psychiatric Association, 2000). Like those with functional aphonia, children who are selectively mute may communicate with gestures, facial expressions, and limited verbalizations produced in a monotonous and altered voice.

Etiologic Factors Associated with Voice Disorders

Voice disorders in children or adults have a variety of potential etiologic factors. Most voice disorders, whether classified as organic or functional, have laryngeal tissue changes associated with them (e.g., hoarseness and breathiness associated with nodules or polyps). As noted earlier, only a few voice disorders exist without any laryngeal tissue changes (e.g., functional aphonia, selective mutism, a high-pitched voice in a male). Many laryngeal pathologies are the result of certain vocally abusive behavior patterns (e.g., nodules or polyps associated with yelling, screaming, or cheering). What follows is a review of etiologic factors associated with voice disorders in children.

Vocally Abusive Behaviors and Vocal Misuse

The term *vocal abuse* refers to injurious vocal habits or misuse of voice. Vocal abuse includes yelling, screaming, cheering, making noises while playing, grunting, excessive crying, and chronic throat clearing or coughing. *Vocal misuse* refers to abnormal pitch and loudness characteristics (American Speech-Language-Hearing Association, 2004b). Vocally abusive behaviors and vocal misuse frequently contribute to the development of a voice disorder. A survey conducted by McNamara and Perry (1994) found that 44% of respondents stated that "most" of their caseload in the schools was associated with vocal abuse and misuse. Another 34% stated that "some" of their caseload was associated with vocal abuse and misuse. Therefore, the identification of these behaviors is an important part of assessment, and the elimination of these behaviors is the goal of voice therapy.

A list of specific vocally abusive behaviors and vocal misuses commonly found in children is presented later in this chapter. In addition, a detailed *Vocal Abuse and Misuse Inventory* is available in Chapter 13. These behaviors are also addressed in the *Child Voice Evaluation* Protocol in Chapter 13.

Laryngeal Hyperfunction

The term *laryngeal hyperfunction* refers to a pervasive pattern of excessive effort and tension in producing voice that negatively affects the muscles and structures of the larynx. As stated earlier, most childhood voice disorders are the result of hyperfunction associated with vocal abuse or misuse. Laryngeal hyperfunction may also develop in an effort to compensate for such structural deviations or vocal fold lesions as congenital malformations, webs, papilloma, paralysis, nodules, polyps, granuloma, or edema. These conditions often interfere with proper vocal fold adductions. In response, the child attempts to squeeze the larynx closed. This effort to produce a louder voice or more clear tone by squeezing the vocal folds together may result in supraglottic compression, edema, and an overall laryngeal muscle imbalance.

Laryngeal hyperfunction also may develop in response to such acute or chronic medical conditions as bacterial or viral infections, allergies, or medication effects. These conditions may create excess mucus, dryness, or swelling. These conditions may stimulate such vocally abusive behaviors as coughing, throat clearing, and effortful phonation. Laryngeal hyperfunction may be habitual or temporary. Habitual patterns are more likely to have a significant negative effect on the voice. Several authors have identified hyperfunction as the most likely disorder associated with voice problems in children; therefore the identification of hyperfunction is an important part of any pediatric voice assessment (Andrews, 1995; Glaze, 1996).

Vocal Nodules

Vocal nodules are an inflammatory degeneration of the superficial layer of the lamina propria with associated edema and fibrosis (Stemple, Glaze, & Klaben, 2000). They are associated with swelling in the mid-membranous portions of the true vocal folds that interferes with vocal fold vibration and glottal closure (Heman-Ackah, Kelleher, & Sataloff, 2002). This often results in vocal hoarseness. They represent the most common benign vocal fold lesion seen in children, accounting for approximately 38 to 78% of those presenting with hoarseness (Andrews, 2006; Gray, Smith, & Schneider, 1996). Dobres, Lee, Stemple, Kummer, and Kretchmer (1990) found that nodules were present in 17.5% of the children seeking evaluation and treatment at a children's hospital otolaryngology clinic. Vocal nodules occur in boys more often than in girls. According to the American Speech, Language and Hearing Association (2004b), boys are diagnosed with nodules 2 to 3 times more often than girls. Highest risk school-age populations include cheerleaders and boys described as *aggressive* or *attention seeking*.

Nodules are usually bilateral, but can be unilateral, particularly in the early stages. They are generally located on the medial edge of the vocal folds, at the junction of the anterior and middle thirds of the vocal folds. Nodules may be acute or chronic. Acute nodules are often caused by trauma or hyperfunctional voice use. If they are not long-standing, they may be somewhat soft or gelatinous in appearance. Chronic nodules appear harder and more fibrotic because of thickening of the epithelium over time. They usually are the result of chronic vocal abuse or misuse. Nodules can also occur secondary to vocal irritation related to long-term exposure to airborne irritants, excessive mucus, or dryness. The effects of nodules on the voice are variable depending on their location, size, and extent of the lesion. Mild-to-moderate dysphonia, with associated edema and hyperfunction, are commonly associated with nodules.

Polyps

Polyps are rare in children, but may occur as the result of an acute vocal trauma or voice abuse. Polyps are a fluid-filled lesion of the superficial lamina propria. Polyps are usually unilateral, but can be bilateral. They generally develop on the middle third of the vocal folds and can be sessile (blister like) or pedunculated (attached to a stalk).

Polyps may result in a mild-to-severe dysphonia depending on the size, extent, location, and type. The voice associated with polyps may sound hoarse and breathy. These voice problems are largely due to the asynchronous vibration of the vocal folds because of their mass differences and inadequate glottal approximations.

Papilloma

Papilloma are nonmalignant, wartlike lesions that develop in the epithelium and invade deeper into the lamina propria and vocalis muscle. They are persistent tumors that tend to grow in clusters. Because of their propensity to recur after surgical removal, the disorder is often referred to as recurrent respiratory papillomatosis (RRP), and in children it is further classified as juvenile onset RRP (JORRP). JORRP is typically identified in infancy or between the ages of 2 to 4 years. It usually presents as hoarseness or stridor (noisy respiration) and is characterized by extensive involvement of the larynx with frequent recurrences. Papilloma are caused by infection with the human papilloma virus (HPV). They occur equally in boys and girls, and may be life threatening because they can obstruct the airway. They often decrease with age and disappear during puberty. Papilloma however, can, persist into adulthood. The overall prevalence is 4.5 per 100,000 children and 2 per 100,000 adults (UC Davis Health System, 2012).

Papilloma spread rapidly throughout the larynx, pharynx, trachea, and bronchi. Therefore, a primary concern is airway maintenance. Often this requires aggressive medical treatments such as CO_2 laser excision, interferon, cidofovir injection, and even tracheotomy. The lesions also have a strong tendency to multiply and recur rapidly after excision, so treatments are usually ongoing. Papilloma affects the mass and stiffness of the vocal folds, often resulting in a severe dysphonia. Breath support for phonation may be reduced secondary to airway obstruction. In addition, the need for repeated medical treatments could result in vocal fold scarring and associated voice problems that tend to persist.

Recently, it has been noted that individuals with RRP tend to have a high prevalence of laryngopharyngeal reflux (LPR), described later in this chapter. It is uncertain whether the presence of papilloma predisposes one to reflux or whether irritation caused by refluxed stomach contents contributes to the development of papilloma. In addition, individuals with LPR undergoing treatment for papilloma are at greater risk of surgical complications, most notably, the development of a laryngeal web (UC Davis Health System, 2012).

Paradoxic Vocal Fold Dysfunction

Paradoxic vocal fold dysfunction (PVCD) is a respiratory pattern in which the vocal folds adduct during inspiration, resulting in dyspnea (difficulty breathing) and stridor (noisy breathing). Other symptoms include laryngitis, hoarseness, or choking. It is most often found in women, ages 40 to 60, but can occur in children (Sandage & Zelazny, 2004; Trudeau, 1998). Hartnick and Boseley, (2010) describe it as one of the most common causes of central airway obstruction in children. PVCD generally occurs in discrete episodes that vary in duration and frequency of occurrence. Typical triggers of PVCD include exercise, shouting, singing, stress, and anxiety.

Potential causes of PVCD include behavioral ("psychogenic") reactions, hyperfunction, chronic laryngopharyngeal reflux (LPR), and laryngeal dystonia secondary to neurologic conditions. Without a known etiology, it often masquerades as asthma, reflux, or vocal fold paralysis, although it can also present comorbidly with these conditions (Hartnick & Boseley, 2010). Chronic or frequent episodes of PVCD may result in laryngeal hyperfunction or vocal fold trauma with subsequent effects on voice in the form of a mild-to-moderate dysphonia.

Laryngeal Trauma

Traumatized laryngeal structures cannot produce normal voice. Laryngeal trauma may result from a variety of causes or forces. The resulting voice disorder, if there is one, will vary depending on the location and severity of the injury and the type of medical intervention provided.

Causes of laryngeal trauma are varied, but include three main categories. The first category includes injury caused by external force applied to the laryngeal area. Automobile accidents, assault and gunshot wounds, and accidental penetration of the laryngeal area by sharp objects are among the common causes of laryngeal injury. The second category includes the burning of the laryngeal area due to smoke or gas inhalation. The third category of potential causes of laryngeal injury includes surgical sequelae. Intubation injuries are discussed further under *Subglottic Stenosis and Intubation Injuries*.

Gastroesophageal Reflux and Laryngopharyngeal Reflux

Gastroesophageal reflux disease (GERD) and laryngopharyngeal reflux (LPR) have been identified as common pediatric disorders (Bach, McGurit, & Postma, 2002; Halstead, 1999; Scott, 1998; Silva & Hotaling, 1994). Over the past few years LPR has gained increased recognition as a contributor to voice problems in children (Block & Brodsky, 2007; Carr, Nagy, Pizzuto, Poje, & Brodsky, 2001; Shah, Harvey, Woodnorth, Glynn, & Nuss, 2005). GERD is the backward flow of stomach contents into the esophagus. It is due to inadequate functioning of the lower esophageal sphincter. The backward flow of strong acids and enzymes the stomach produces to help with the digestion can burn and irritate the linings of the esophagus. Symptoms may include heartburn, indigestion, emesis, swallowing difficulties, or gagging (Halstead, 1999).

In some patients reflux passes through the esophagus and affects the larynx and pharynx. This problem is diagnosed as LPR (Gupta & Sataloff, 2009; Koufman, 2002a). Patients with LPR may not experience heartburn or indigestion because small amounts of reflux move through the esophagus very quickly and settle in the larynx or pharynx. For this reason, it has also been called *atypical reflux* (Koufman, 2002a). According to Kaufman (1991, 2002b) and Karkos, Leong, Apostolidou, and Apostolidis (2006), symptoms of LPR may include *globus pharyngeus* (feeling like there is a lump in the throat), vocal hoarseness, excess mucus, chronic cough, chronic throat clearing, and laryngospasm. In addition, GERD patients are predominantly supine (night-time) refluxers, whereas LPR patients are predominantly upright (daytime) refluxers.

The prevalence of reflux in general, presumably including GERD and LPR is estimated at 20 to 40% in infants and 7 to 20% in children (Cezard, 2004; Vandenplas & Sacre-Smits, 1987). GERD in general, and LPR in particular, have been associated with voice disorders (Cohen, Bach, Postma, & Koufman, 2002; Grontved & West, 2000; Hanson & Jiang, 2000; Kuhn, Toohill, & Uluaip, 1998). Koufman, Wiener, Wu, and Castell (1988) estimated that approximately 10% of patients with laryngeal and voice disorders had LPR. A study conducted by Little et al., (1997) looked at 222 children between the ages of 1 and 16 years who had been diagnosed with laryngeal disorders, pulmonary disorders, recurrent emesis, nonrespiratory disorders, or were post-Nissen fundoplication (a surgical procedure designed to decrease reflux). In addition, they included randomly selected patients from a pediatric intensive care unit. Little and his associates found that 95% of the children had abnormal pH readings on the esophageal probe (GERD), 49% had reflux indicators on both the esophageal and the pharyngeal probe (GERD and LPR), and 46% had pharyngeal reflux in the absence of abnormal esophageal ratings (LPR). In 2000, Koufman, Amin, and Panetti found that out of 113 patients with documented laryngeal and voice disorders who participated in their study, 50% had pH-documented reflux.

Diagnosis and treatment of GERD and LPR in children is important. It may be associated with several life-threatening and respiratory conditions such as apnea, laryngomalacia, subglottic stenosis, recurrent upper respiratory tract infections, asthma, recurrent bronchitis, laryngeal papilloma, paradoxic vocal fold motion, stridor, chronic cough, chronic nasal pain, and aspiration pneumonia (Heatley & Swift, 1996; Ulualp &

Brodsky, 2005; Wilson, Theis, & Wilson, 2009; Yellon, 1997; Zalesska-Krecicka, Krecicki, Iwanczak, Blitek, & Horobiowska, 2002). In addition, these conditions hold particular interest for speech-language pathologists because of their association with voice disorders and such laryngeal pathologies as vocal hoarseness, nodules, granuloma, ulcers, and functional voice disorders (Andrews, 2006; Bach, McGuirt, & Postma, 2002).

Acute or Chronic Laryngitis

In general, the term *laryngitis* refers to an inflammation of the vocal fold mucosa causing dysphonia. It is usually characterized by breathiness, a low pitch, and intermittent phonation breaks. In severe cases, aphonia may develop.

The cause of acute laryngitis is unknown, but it is often associated with a viral or bacterial upper respiratory infection. In young children laryngitis can be associated with a diagnosis of *croup* or *laryngotracheobronchitis.* These terms refer to a group of conditions involving inflammation of the larynx and upper airway in children between the ages of 3 months and 5 years. Croup in most cases is caused by viruses; however, it can also be caused by bacteria or an allergic reaction. It is characterized by narrowing of the subglottic airway, a loud "barking" cough, hoarseness, and inhalatory stridor (Medline Plus, 2006; Stemple, Glaze, & Klaben, 2000).

Chronic laryngitis results from long-standing inflammation of the mucosa and epithelial layer that is not associated with an infection. Causes include repeated episodes of acute laryngitis, vocal misuse and abuse, asthma, allergies, GERD or LPR, repeated vomiting associated with bulimia, and poor hydration. Roland, Bhalla, and Earis (2004) stated that asthma may be an important underlying etiology of children's voice disorders. Frequent coughing and throat clearing associated with asthma traumatizes the vocal folds and may contribute to the development of laryngitis, nodules, and polyps. In addition, inhaled bronchodilators and steroids may dehydrate the vocal folds further contributing to vocal symptoms. Environmental allergy responses can also lead to vocal fold edema, increased upper airway secretions, sneezing, coughing, and throat clearing which can all contribute to chronic laryngitis (Sicherer & Eggleston, 2007). Chronic laryngitis is characterized by laryngeal fatigue and a mild-to-severe dysphonia.

Craniofacial Disorders

Craniofacial malformations take many forms, including clefts, velopharyngeal insufficiency (VPI), or nasal obstructions. Such malformations will have a significant effect on the resonance of the voice, often resulting in hypernasality, assimilation nasality, or hyponasality. Depending on the location and extent of a malformation, laryngeal behavior might also be influenced. It is not unusual for congenital anomalies of the larynx to be associated with other craniofacial abnormalities.

Laryngeal anomalies are often the result of unilateral or bilateral underdevelopment of the laryngeal structures. For example, in Opitz syndrome, the larynx is often small with short, thick vocal folds. Another anatomic problem is laryngomalacia which may result in laryngeal stridor, webbing, subglottic stenosis, and laryngotracheal cleft. These types of structural anomalies of the larynx generally cause problems with vocal quality and pitch.

Hearing Impairment

Hearing impairment is a general term that includes the hard of hearing and the deaf. Children who are hard of hearing can learn oral language, often with the help of amplification. Those who are deaf do not have sufficient auditory acuity to normally learn the oral language. The effects of hearing loss on voice depends, among other factors, on the age of onset of the loss, the degree of loss, the quality and timing of initiation of an aural rehabilitation program, and the parental involvement and support. Hearing loss affects not only voice, but all aspects of oral communication. Generally, most significant negative effects on speech, voice, and language are experienced by children who have more severe loss with an early onset. Prelingually deaf children experience the most severe consequences. Deaf individuals who acquire oral speech with special assistance also exhibit many vocal deviations.

Hearing loss, especially deafness, is commonly associated with voice problems. Individuals with significant hearing loss often present with variations in vocal quality, resonance, pitch, and loudness control. A high-pitched voice, harshness, hoarseness, breathiness, and hypernasality as well as hyponasality may all characterize the voice of children with significant hearing loss. Possibly, the lack of sensory feedback disrupts the typical acquisition of voicing and may also increase susceptibility to vocal abuse and misuse as the child tries to compensate for inadequate or absent auditory feedback of voice production (Andrews, 2006).

Neuromuscular Impairment

Voice problems may be associated with neuromuscular impairments resulting from central nervous system (CNS) or peripheral nervous system (PNS) damage. Voice disorders due to neurologic problems are seen more often in the older persons than in children. However, congenital or acquired neurologic diseases may affect voice in children.

Head injury may be a significant factor in affecting vocal control and thus causing voice problems in children. Other factors that can affect the neural control of the vocal folds or velopharyngeal mechanism include cerebral palsy, brain tumors, strokes, infections, and anoxia. Any kind of neurologic involvement is likely to affect not only voice, but also speech production. Therefore, voice problems in neurologically involved children often co-occur with dysarthria, which includes problems with respiration, phonation, articulation, resonation, and prosody. In addition, dystonia may be noted.

Laryngeal Hypofunction and Vocal Fold Paralysis

Laryngeal hypofunction is a general term used to describe inadequate tone in the laryngeal musculature and associated structures. Inadequate laryngeal tone results in poor vocal fold adduction, allowing excessive air to escape. The vocal characteristics of laryngeal hypofunction include breathiness due to inadequate vocal fold adduction, a weak voice, reduced vocal endurance due to air wastage, reduced loudness, and reduced speech intelligibility. In severe cases, aphonia may develop (Hutchinson & Hanson, 1979; Morris & Spriestersbach, 1978).

Laryngeal hypofunction may be associated with brain injury, neurologic disorders, or diseases that result in flaccid dysarthria, vocal fold paresis, or vocal fold paralysis. Vocal fold paralysis implies complete immobility, whereas vocal fold paresis includes folds that are partially mobile with reduced abduction or reduced adduction. Faulty innervation of the "paralyzed" fold, rather than complete denervation, is likely the reason for the various descriptions regarding impaired laryngeal movement with vocal fold paralysis or paresis (Maronian, Robinson, Waugh, & Hillel, 2004). Bilateral vocal fold paralysis (BVFP) is more commonly seen in neonates, whereas unilateral vocal fold paralysis (UVFP) in more frequent in older children (Smith & Sauder, 2009). Vocal fold paresis or paralysis can occur as the result of recurrent laryngeal nerve damage, laryngeal trauma, or intubation injuries. In studies where UVFP was more frequently reported than BVFP, it coincided with a high volume of congenital cardiac surgery (Zbar & Smith, 1996). The left recurrent laryngeal nerve is vulnerable to damage during the surgeries required to correct congenital cardiac anomalies, thus these surgeries are a frequent cause of vocal fold paralysis in infants, particularly those under 30 weeks gestational age (Smith et al., 2009).

The most likely cause of laryngeal hypofunction in children is prolonged hyperfunction. With prolonged hyperfunction, the muscles can become exhausted until they are unable to produce normal tonus. Weakness follows, reducing vocal fold adduction. This "hyperfunctional-hypofunctional" cycle has been considered an important component in the diagnosis of voice disorders associated with vocal nodules (Hall, 1995; Hillman, Holmberg, Perkell, Walsh, & Vaughan, 1989).

Congenital and Acquired Laryngeal Webs

A laryngeal web is a bridge of tissue that forms between the two vocal folds. It usually begins at the anterior commissure and extends to various lengths along the vocal folds. A congenital web (noticed at the time of birth) is due to a failure, on the part of the vocal folds, to separate during the tenth week of embryonic development. This may result in a compromised airway at birth, requiring immediate medical intervention to establish an adequate airway.

Acquired webs may develop in the anterior commissure following vocal fold surgery or vocal trauma. Depending on the extent of the web, characteristics may include dyspnea and stridor, and vocal characteristics ranging from normal to severe dysphonia. The treatment for a laryngeal web is surgery to separate the folds. Following surgery, voice therapy may be needed.

Subglottic Stenosis and Intubation Injuries

Subglottic stenosis refers to narrowing of the area below the vocal folds, often due to prolonged intubations or the use of a large endotracheal tube in children. Dobres, Lee, Stemple, Kummer, and Kretchmer (1990) collected data on 731 patients seeking evaluation and treatment at a children's hospital otolaryngology clinic. They found subglottic stenosis in 31% of the children, and that it was the most frequently occurring laryngeal pathology in the 0 to 3-year-old-group.

Laryngeal tissues may be traumatized by tracheostomy and endotracheal intubation (Burns, Dayal, Scott, Van Nostrand, & Bryce, 1979; Whited, 1979, 1984). These factors may lead to laryngeal irritation, edema, webbing, and granulomas of the vocal processes of the arytenoids cartilages. Other intubation injuries may include interarytenoid fixation, arytenoid dislocation, vocal fold paresis or paralysis, perforation of the pyraform sinus or esophagus, ulcers, and laryngeal or tracheal stenosis. The subsequent effect on airway maintenance and voice production will be dependent on the location and extent of the injury or lesion. According to Burns et al. (1979), the most common signs of laryngeal intubation trauma are hoarseness, dysphagia, dyspnea, and aspiration.

Endocrine Abnormalities

Abnormalities of the endocrine system may have a negative effect on the still growing larynges in children, leading to voice disorders. Glandular abnormalities that affect physical growth, including the growth of the larynx, are associated with voice problems.

Disorders of the pituitary gland affect general growth and that of the larynx. Consequently, an underdeveloped larynx may prevent the normal voice change in pubescent children. The effect is more noticeable in the male children whose voice will sound abnormally high pitched. Hypofunction of the adrenal gland also may be associated with high-pitched voice in boys.

The Need for Medical Evaluation

Prior to treating any child or adult with a voice quality or resonance disorder, a referral should be made to a laryngologist. According to McMurray (2003), any type of voice change associated with airway symptoms or swallowing difficulties may be indicative of a life threatening condition and should be medically evaluated and treated immediately. The laryngologist evaluates the larynx with indirect mirror examination or a fiberoptic endoscopic examination. The laryngologist will try to identify any organic or neurologic conditions associated with the voice disorder. Such structural changes as edema, nodules, polyps, ulcers, and tumors can be identified and such physical conditions as LPR or papilloma can be diagnosed and medically treated.

Based on the findings, the laryngologist may recommend additional testing (e.g., CT scans, biopsy, blood tests), surgical intervention, medical management, and voice therapy. Unfortunately, speech-language pathologists working in the public schools often have difficulty obtaining a laryngeal examination for children with voice disorders. Reasons given for this included lack of parental follow-up, lack of physician follow-up with referral to a specialist (otolaryngologist), and difficulty obtaining the results of a laryngeal examination that are relevant to voice production. As a result, children may indefinitely remain on a waiting list for service, or treatment may be based on an inaccurate or incomplete diagnosis of the child's voice disorder (Leeper, 1992).

To improve voice services to school children, Leeper (1992) developed a program involving several low-cost voice clinics in conjunction with New Mexico State University. Overall, 61% of the students who attended the clinic subsequently were enrolled in voice therapy and 17% had modifications made to ongoing treatment activities because of new assessment information provided to the clinicians. Creative assessment models, such as the one used in this study, may facilitate more accurate and timely identification and subsequent treatment of children with voice disorders in the school population.

In summary, it is important that the speech-language pathologist and laryngologist cultivate a good working relationship to offer effective services to children with voice disorders. As noted earlier, voice treatment designed to alter vocal quality or resonance should not begin until a laryngologic examination is completed. A comprehensive treatment plan, based on input from both the speech-language pathologist and the laryngologist may include medical management as well as voice treatment. In addition, periodic follow-up examinations by the laryngologist may help document the positive effects of voice treatment on the laryngeal pathology (e.g., reduction in the size of the vocal nodules).

Assessment of Voice Production

A thorough voice evaluation will include several components. In general, a voice evaluation will consist of all or some combination of, the following activities:

- A written case history
- Parent or caregiver interview
- Hearing screening
- Orofacial examination and diadochokinetic tasks with added emphasis on assessing breathing and breath support, laryngeal tension, and velopharyngeal function, as needed
- Spontaneous speech-language sample and reading sample (when appropriate) to assess vocal pitch, loudness, quality, and resonance as well as to assess speech and language production, as needed
- A variety of clinical assessment tasks used to assess vocal pitch, loudness, quality, and resonance
- Instrumental evaluation (if available) of pitch, loudness, quality, resonance, aerodynamic parameters of voice, phonatory efficiency, and glottal closure
- Perceptual evaluation of vocal quality using a rating scale protocol
- Assessment of voice stimulability
- Differential diagnosis
- Recommendations
- Postassessment counseling

Written case history, clinical interview, hearing screening, diadochokinetic tasks, and the orofacial examination are described in Chapter 1. Detailed protocols for each of these are available in Chapter 2. In addition, specific protocols for the assessment of voice in children are provided in Chapter 13 and on the accompanying compact disk (CD). These protocols were designed specifically for assessing voice in children. They can be printed out individually or compiled for a complete, ready-to-use, voice evaluation. What follows is a discussion of the remaining components.

Instrumental Evaluation

A speech-language pathologist skilled and experienced in assessing and treating voice disorders can conduct a competent voice evaluation with or without instrumentation. Instrumentation however, may, improve documentation and quantification, and may offer data on reliability of judgments or measurements made. Technologic developments offer a variety of opportunities to objectively analyze and document voice parameters (Behrman, 2007). Laryngeal function studies or phonatory function tests are objective measurements of the phonatory system that may be conducted if instrumentation is available. An overview of several types of instrumental assessment procedures follows.

Acoustic Analysis

In the context of voice and its disorders, an acoustic analysis is the determination of various physical properties or parameters of sound produced by the vocal folds. The analysis includes an assessment of several vocal parameters. Acoustic measures may involve quantification of fundamental frequency, to include the average, minimal, and maximal fundamental frequency of voice along with the frequency range. Measures of vocal intensity might include the average, minimal, and maximal intensity or loudness of voice along with the loudness range. Additional properties measured include maximum phonation time, average percent jitter (frequency perturbation), average percent shimmer (amplitude perturbation), and harmonics-to-noise ratio (HNR).

Instrumentation can also be used to measure the degree of nasality in an individual's speech. The Nasometer II, Model 6450 by KayPENTAX is the latest version of this instrumentation. The Nasometer II uses separate microphones to pick up the oral and nasal components of an individual's speech. The signal from each microphone is then filtered, digitized, and processed by a computer. The resultant measure is a ratio of nasal to nasal-plus-oral acoustic energy that is multiplied by 100 and expressed as a *nasalance score*. The nasalance score represents the degree of nasality in a person's speech and may be a reflection of his or her velopharyngeal control. Information gathered using the Nasometer II may prove valuable during the assessment of voice disorders associated with craniofacial anomalies and VPI (Dalston, 1989; Dalston, Warren, & Dalston, 1991).

Reliable quantitative recordings and voice analyses can contribute to a thorough evaluation of children's voices and facilitate the documentation of measurable treatment outcomes following behavioral therapy or medical intervention (Theis, 2010). Campisi et al. (2002) established a database of pediatric normative values based on 100 control subjects (50 boys and 50 girls) aged 4 to 18 years. They utilized the Multi-Dimensional Voice Program (MDVP) to extract up to 33 acoustic variables from each voice analysis. Computer-assisted voice analysis options such as the MDVP, and others listed below, are an important diagnostic advancement because they are tolerated well by children and provide objective, reproducible, and noninvasive acoustic measurements (Campisi et al., 2000). Heylen et al. (1998) describe a Voice Range Profile Index for Children (VRPIc) that can be used to screen children for voice disorders or quantitatively assess the effectiveness of voice treatment. The VRPIc uses a specific combination of the child's age, the highest vocal fundamental frequency, the lowest intensity, and the slope of the upper VRP contour.

Instruments that might be used to assess one or more of the acoustic parameters described above include the following:

- Sound level meter
- Fundamental frequency analyzer/indicator
- Visi-Pitch III® (Kay Elemetrics Corp.)
- KayPENTAX Real-Time Pitch®
- KayPENTAX Computerized Speech Lab CSL®
- KayPENTAX Multi-Dimensional Voice Program (MDVP)®
- KayPENTAX Nasometer II, Model 6450®
- C-Speech®
- Dr. Speech (Tiger Electronics)®
- Speech Studio® (Laryngograph Ltd.)

Electroglottography (EGG)

Electroglottography (EGG) measures changes in the impedance (resistance) to low-voltage electric current that is allowed to pass through the vocal folds through electrodes attached to the surface of the neck. Vocal fold actions, including vibration and approximation, result in systematic changes in resistance to the current flow (which is not felt by the individual). Open vocal folds offer more resistance to the flow of electricity than closed ones. The electroglottograph generates a waveform that corresponds to the relative contact of the two folds during phonation. Thus, the instrument helps assess the area of vocal fold contact during the vibratory cycle.

Commercially available electroglottographs include:

- KayPentax Electroglottograph®
- Electroglottograph EG2-PC® (Glottal Enterprises)
- Digital Laryngograph® (Laryngograph Ltd.)

Electromyography (EMG)

Electromyography helps assess the functioning of the laryngeal musculature and may be helpful in the diagnosis of vocal fold paralysis. It is not widely used by speech-language pathologists in the United States, except in major research centers with medical affiliations. Hirano (1981) describes the necessary equipment and electrode placement.

Several authors have used EMG to assess muscle activity in specific laryngeal muscles. Electromyography can be completed using surface electrodes attached to the skin of the anterior neck or over the laryngeal, infralaryngeal, or supralaryngeal areas (Sapor, Baker, Larson, & Ramig, 2000; Yiu, Verdolini, & Chow, 2005). Fujita, Ludlow, Woodson, and Naunton (1989) and Gallena, Smith, Zeffiro, and Ludlow (2001) measured posterior cricoarytenoid muscle activity using a transnasal surface hypopharyngeal electrode. Electromyography can also be done by placing wire electrodes directly into the laryngeal muscles using a hypodermic needle. This technique has typically been used to measure muscle activity in the thyroarytenoid muscle, the posterior cricoarytenoid muscle, and the cricothyroid muscle. Insertions are typically more reliable in the thyroarytenoid and posterior cricoarytenoid muscle (Gallena, Smith, Zeffiro, & Ludlow, 2001; Smith, Denny, Shaffer, Kelly, & Hirano, 1996).

Aerodynamic Measures

Aerodynamic measures for voice assessment are important because phonation is an aerodynamic phenomenon (Behrman, 2007). Airflow through the glottis and air pressure regulation below and above the glottis is essential in phonation and speech articulation. Various airflow measures help identify potential laryngeal pathologies and include such measures as pulmonary function testing, airflow rates, transglottic airflow, subglottic air pressure, supraglottic pressure, glottal impedance, glottal resistance, and vital capacity.

Instruments designed to assess the aerodynamic parameters of voice include the following:

- Spirometer (measures volume of air inspired and expired by the lungs)
- KayPENTAX Aerophone II® (calculates 22 speech and voice aerodynamic parameters)
- Nagashima Phonatory Function Analyzer® (measures multiple aerodynamic and voice parameters)

Laryngeal Imaging

Laryngoscopy is the viewing of the larynx and surrounding structures. This can be done using a laryngeal mirror, a rigid fiberoptic endoscope, or a flexible fiberoptic endoscope. A laryngeal mirror is a small round mirror mounted at an angle on a long, thin handle. Indirect mirror laryngoscopy involves placing the laryngeal mirror back into the oropharynx with the mirror angled downward to view the vocal folds and surrounding structures. The examiner will be looking at the reflection or "mirror image" of the structures in view.

The *rigid endoscope* is a rigid tube that is inserted into the oral cavity and oropharynx. It lies just above the tongue and projects a high-intensity light down at an angle to view the larynx and surrounding structures. Because it is placed in the oral cavity, articulation is difficult during the examination. Therefore, during the examination, the client's activities may be limited to breathing, coughing, laughing, and phonation of vowel sounds.

The *flexible endoscope* is a flexible tube that is inserted into the nasal passage. It can be placed above the velum in the *nasopharynx* to assess velopharyngeal structures and function. The scope can also be passed into the oropharynx or below to observe the larynx and surrounding structures. Images obtained with the flexible nasoendoscope are somewhat smaller and darker than those obtained with a rigid endoscope. Because the scope is passed transnasally (not intraorally), the velopharyngeal mechanism and the larynx may be viewed with the scope in place during the production of consonant sounds or even continuous speech. The flexible scope is now widely used for the assessment of VPI in children. The information gained from such an assessment can assist physicians as they plan surgical or nonsurgical management options.

Stroboscopy refers to the use of a strobe light in conjunction with a flexible or rigid endoscope. The intermittent illumination of the strobe light is slower than the rate of vocal fold vibration, thus allowing the human eye to perceive movement patterns of the folds in slow motion. The use of digital stroboscopy, such as the KayPentax Digital Video-stroboscopy System®, has become standard in many voice clinics and hospitals.

It is the official position of the American Speech-Language-Hearing Association (ASHA) that endoscopy is an imaging procedure included within the scope of practice for speech-language pathologists (American Speech-language-Hearing Association, 2008). The identification and diagnosis of laryngeal pathology is outside the scope of practice of speech-language pathologists and remains the responsibility of laryngologists. However, speech-language pathologists with specialized training in flexible/nasal endoscopy, rigid/oral endoscopy, and/or stroboscopy may employ these techniques for the evaluation and treatment of speech, voice, resonance, and swallowing disorders.

Clinical Assessment of Voice

A variety of clinical tasks help assess voice in children. The types of tasks used depend to some extent on the specific kind of voice problem the child exhibits. In general, clinicians design specific tasks that help: (a) identify vocally abusive behaviors, (b) assess breathing and breath support for voice production, (c) measure pitch, (d) measure loudness, (e) assess vocal quality, and (f) evaluate laryngeal tension.

Procedures to obtain the specific measures include direct observation of the child during various speech and nonspeech tasks, behavioral check lists, and instrumental measurements. A brief description of the main tasks and their procedures follows.

The Identification of Vocally Abusive Behaviors and Vocal Misuse in Children

As mentioned earlier, a significant number of childhood voice disorders are associated with laryngeal hyperfunction due to vocal abuse or misuse. Therefore, the identification of these behaviors is an important part of any voice assessment. If it is determined that a vocal behavior is contributing to the development or maintenance of a disordered voice and hyperfunctional larynx, then reduction or elimination of that behavior should be targeted in therapy. As described previously, *hyperfunction* refers to a pattern of excessive effort and tension in the larynx and surrounding structures and muscles. A hyperfunctional larynx may be characterized by muscle dystonia, edema, supraglottic constriction, paradoxic vocal cord motion (PVCM), or lesions such as nodules or polyps.

In general, vocal misuse that needs to be assessed would include habitual use of one or more of the following:

- Inappropriate pitch
- Inappropriate loudness

- Poor respiratory patterns
- Hyperfunctional phonation patterns
- Inappropriate rate of speech.

Vocal abuse occurs when the vocal folds are forced to adduct too vigorously. Vocally abusive behaviors commonly found in children that need to be assessed include:

- Shouting, yelling, and screaming
- Loud talking
- Incessant talking
- Vocal noises during play
- Frequent and chronic coughing
- Frequent and chronic throat clearing
- Faulty respiratory habits
- Hard glottal attacks
- Participation in such vocally strenuous activities as singing or performing on stage.

Vocal abuse and misuse are assessed through an inventory (behavioral checklist). A detailed *Vocal Abuse and Misuse Inventory* is available in Chapter 13 and is also included in the *Child Voice Evaluation* Protocol in the same chapter.

Clinical Assessment of Breathing and Breath Support for Phonation

Respiration provides the essential power source for phonation: airflow through the vocal folds. Therefore, an inefficient or faulty breathing pattern may reduce phonation times, limit loudness, or contribute to hyperfunctional behaviors. Normally, most people use one of three general breathing patterns:

1. *Thoracic breathing* is characterized by slight expansion of the chest during breathing. Most people breathe in this manner.

2. *Clavicular breathing* is characterized by shoulder elevation, strain in the neck muscles, and thoracic tension in the area of the clavicle. This is an inefficient and effortful type of breathing. Excessive tension and muscle activity involved in this type of breathing may contribute to a hyperfunctional voice disorder.

3. *Diaphragmatic or abdominal breathing* involves contraction of the diaphragm and expansion of the abdomen during inhalation. This in an efficient and healthy way to breathe, taking some of the focus away from the upper thorax, shoulders, and larynx. Diaphragmatic breathing is often evident in singers or professional speakers who are trying to adopt an efficient breathing pattern while maintaining laryngeal relaxation.

In addition to instrumental assessment of breath support and airflow for phonation described previously, the following clinical tasks may also be useful in assessment:

1. Assessment of the child's general breathing pattern through observation during speech and quiet breathing. The clinician also may note effortful or noisy inhalation, stridor, airflow obstruction, or "mouth breathing."

2. Assessments of nasal patency by having the child breathe with his or her mouth closed. The clinician also may take note of any nasal flutter and whether the nasal breathing is noisy or effortful.

3. Measurement of *maximum phonation time,* which is a reflection of vital capacity, respiratory control, and glottal efficiency. The child is asked to take a deep breath and sustain the vowel /a/ for as long as possible at a comfort level. The pitch may be low or high. Most children (6 to 10 years of age) should be able to sustain /a/ for at least 10 seconds.

4. Measurement of *words per breath.* If respiratory support is inadequate or if air wastage is occurring due to glottal inefficiency, then a child may produce fewer words per breath. The child may also have to breathe more often. This could result in speech that sounds "choppy" or dysfluent. Normative data for words per breath are lacking, although clinical observations suggest that normal speakers typically produce 12 or more words per breath (Haynes & Pindzola, 2004). More important than the actual measurement is to observe whether the breathing pattern interferes with speech production or draws attention to itself. The clinician should note any noisy inhalation or stridor as these may reflect vocal fold approximation during inhalation (PVCD) or airway obstruction.

5. Measurement of the *s/z ratio,* which is a quick screening task designed to assess the differential contributions respiratory and phonatory inefficiency (laryngeal problems) make to a person's voice problem. Although this procedure might be helpful for clinicians who do not have the benefits of instrumentation, it should be cautioned that this is a crude representation of respiratory and laryngeal function. Findings from the s/z ratio cannot stand alone and should be supported by other clinical assessment procedures (Boone, McFarlane, & Von Berg, 2005; Fendler & Shearer, 1988). Typically, the s/z ratio is assessed as follows (adapted from Deem & Miller, 2000):

    *   The child is instructed to sustain /s/ for as long as he or she can on three trials. The clinician records the longest /s/ production in seconds.
    *   The child is then instructed to sustain /z/ for as long as he or she can, also on three trials. The clinician records the longest /z/ production in seconds.
    *   To create a fraction, the clinician takes the longest /s/ time and places it over the longest /z/ time.
    *   The clinician then divides the longest /s/ by the longest /z/ to calculate the *s/z ratio:* _____ (longest /s/) ÷ _____ (longest /z/) = _____ (s/z ratio).

    Possible results of the s/z ratio include (adapted from Eckel & Boone, 1981 and Prater & Swift, 1984):

a. If the longest /s/ duration is 10 seconds or more *and* the s/z ratio is 1.2 or less, then the findings are normal and do not suggest a respiratory problem or a laryngeal problem.

b. If the longest /s/ duration is 10 seconds or more *and* the s/z ratio is greater than 1.2, then the findings indicate laryngeal pathology (Eckel & Boone, 1981).

c. If the longest /s/ duration is less than 10 seconds *and* the s/z ratio is 1.2 or lower, then the findings indicate a respiratory problem.

d. If the longest /s/ duration is less than 10 seconds *and* the s/z ratio is greater than 1.2, then the findings suggest both a respiratory problem and a laryngeal pathology.

The *Child Voice Evaluation Protocol* in Chapter 13 provides a space for recording the s/z ratio.

Clinical Assessment of Pitch

Habitual pitch is the average pitch of a child's speech. It is measured in cycles per second or hertz (Hz), and refers to the rate of vocal fold vibration. Normative data for the fundamental frequencies of children in the age range of 1 through 9 years are found in Table 12–1 and normal fundamental frequency ranges for females and males, ages 10 through 16 years are found in Table 12–2. The fundamental frequencies for children under the age of 10 are almost identical for males and females. At the age of 10 years, the separation between the fundamental frequency averages for males and females increases, with the

Table 12–1. Normal Fundamental Frequency Ranges for Children, Ages 1 Through 9 Years

Age (years)	Acceptable Range for Fundamental Frequency
1–2	340–470 Hz
3	255–360 Hz
4	240–340 Hz
5	225–325 Hz
6	220–315 Hz
7	220–310 Hz
8	210–300 Hz
9	200–290 Hz

Source: Adapted from D. K. Wilson, *Voice Problems of Children* (3rd ed.), p. 119. Baltimore, MD: Williams and Wilkins, 1987.

Table 12–2. Normal Fundamental Frequency Ranges for Females and Males, Ages 10 Through 16 Years

Age (years)	Acceptable Range for Fundamental Frequency	
	Female	Male
10	205–290 Hz	195–280 Hz
11	200–285 Hz	195–275 Hz
12	200–280 Hz	195–275 Hz
13	195–280 Hz	140–275 Hz
14	190–270 Hz	140–215 Hz
15	185–260 Hz	135–205 Hz
16	180–225 Hz	125–180 Hz

Source: Adapted from D. K. Wilson, *Voice Problems of Children* (3rd ed.), p. 119. Baltimore, MD: Williams and Wilkins, 1987.

male voice about 10 Hz lower than the female voice. At the age of 13 years, the fundamental frequency of the male voice drops significantly, as seen in Table 12–2.

To calculate habitual pitch, the clinician may have the child count from 1 to 10 and sustain a production of /a/. In addition, a spontaneous speech sample and a reading sample (if the child can read) may be recorded. A pitch pipe, piano, frequency analyzer, Computerized Speech Lab, or other such instrumentation can be used to determine the child's pitch at several points during the production of one or more of these clinical tasks.

In addition to habitual pitch, clinicians need to explore the child's *pitch range*. A pitch pipe, piano, frequency analyzer, Computerized Speech Lab, or other such instrumentation can be used to identify the highest pitch, the lowest pitch, and the overall pitch range of the child's voice during the following clinical tasks:

- produce the lowest pitch possible and produce glottal fry
- produce the highest pitch possible—usually a falsetto while producing /i/
- "step" up and "step" down the musical scale
- "glide" down from the highest pitch to the lowest or "glide" up from the lowest pitch to the highest.

While the child is performing these tasks, the clinician may listen for any changes in the quality of the voice that occur as a consequence of pitch changes.

Clinical Assessment of Loudness

A sound level meter, Computerized Speech Lab (CSL) or other instrumentation (discussed earlier) can be used to measure the child's vocal loudness during the following tasks:

- Counting, starting with a whisper for the first number (#1), and gradually getting louder with each number until the child gets to his or her loudest. This task can help identify the child's loudest voice, the softest voice, and the loudness range.

- A spontaneous speech sample is recorded to identify the mean loudness of the child's voice. With the help of the chosen instrument, the clinician measures the child's vocal intensity at several points during the sample to calculate the average decibel level.

Clinical Assessment of Vocal Quality

The assessment of vocal quality is an important part of any clinical voice evaluation. Poor vocal quality may be a reflection of laryngeal hyperfunction, inappropriate glottal closure, or reduced phonatory efficiency, among other things. As discussed previously, some aspects of vocal quality (e.g., jitter, shimmer, HNR) can be measured instrumentally. Yet, despite many years of research, it still is not clear how to measure overall perceived vocal quality in a reliable and valid way (Kreiman & Gerratt, 2010).

Over the years, a number of rating scale protocols have been proposed. Kreiman and Gerratt (2010), questioned the validity of such measures stating that "Rating scale protocols for quality assessment never have been based on a model of voice quality, and because the construct being measured is not well defined, it is not possible to determine that a given set of scales or acoustic measurements is the "correct" one for measuring it." (p. 63). These authors identify the need for a comprehensive theory that would establish causal links between laryngeal pathology, voice acoustics, and vocal quality before attempting to design a valid and reliable tool for measuring vocal quality. In the mean time, however, these types of measures continue to be widely used in an attempt to standardize procedures for the evaluation and documentation of vocal quality.

Hartnick and Boseley (2010) stated that a traditional GRBAS scale or CAPE-V (description of both follows) may be used for rating vocal quality in children; however, the need for children to take more breaths and have greater rib cage movement during speech acts must be accounted for. A study conducted by Zraick et al. (2011) found that both CAPE-V and GRBAS reliability coefficients varied across raters and parameters, yet slightly improved rater reliability was established when the CAPE-V was used to make perceptual judgments of voice quality as compared to the GRBAS scale. Clinical tasks that can help assess laryngeal functioning and overall vocal quality include:

1. *Conversational speech.* The clinician may listen to the child's voice during connected speech production to describe the overall quality in terms of breathiness, hoarseness, harshness, strained, whispered aphonia, intermittent aphonia or phonation breaks, and hard glottal attacks. The GRBAS scale may be helpful in documenting vocal characteristics during the conversational speech sample.

    The GRBAS Scale was developed by the Committee for Phonatory Function Tests of the Japan Society of Logopedics and Phoniatrics (Hirano, 1981). It is used to evaluate five characteristics of voice production: grade (G), rough (R), breathy (B), aesthenic (A), and strained (S). *Grade* (G) refers to the overall degree of hoarseness in the voice. *Rough* (R) refers to the listener impression of the irregularity of vocal fold vibrations and corresponds to irregular fluctuations in fundamental frequency, amplitude of vibration, or both. *Breathy* (B) refers to the impression of air leakage through the glottis. *Aesthenic* (A) refers to the degree of weakness or lack of power in the voice. *Strained* (S) refers to the impression of vocal hyperfunction. Each of these characteristics is rated using a 4-point scale where "0" is normal, "1" is slight, "2" is moderate, and "3" is extreme (Stemple, Glaze, & Klaben, 2010; Zraick et al., 2011). The GRBAS does not include a specific protocol or guidelines regarding administration and analysis, which may negatively influence the reliability of voice quality assessments done using this instrument (Kempster et al., 2009; Zraick et al., 2011).

2. *The Consensus Auditory-Perceptual Evaluation of Voice (CAPE-V).* The CAPE-V protocol was created as a direct outcome of the 2002 Consensus Conference on Auditory-Perceptual Evaluation of Voice sponsored by the American Speech, Language, and Hearing Association's (ASHA) Special Interest Division 3 for Voice and Voice Disorders (Kempster, Gerratt, Verdolini Abbott, Barkmeier-Kraemer, & Hillman, 2009). The CAPE-V was designed for use with adults and requires the individual being assessed to perform three vocal tasks: (a) sustain the vowels /a/ and /i/ three times each, (b) read six specific sentences with different phonetic contexts, and (c) converse naturally in response to the standard question, "Tell me about your voice problem."

   Masaki (2009) developed a pediatric version of CAPE-V that included age-appropriate sentence tasks designed to elicit similar vocal behaviors when compared to the adult form sentences, and a spontaneous speech sample as a substitute for the third task. These three samples are rated based on overall severity of the voice disorder, as well as, the consistent or intermittent presence of the following attributes: roughness, breathiness, strain, pitch, and loudness. Areas for describing additional features such as tremor, falsetto, fry, diplophonia, aphonia, wetness, and other relevant characteristics are also included. Several studies have been conducted to establish reliability and validity of this measure (Berg & Eden, 2003; Karnell et al., 2007; Zraick et al., 2011). For a detailed description of the development of the CAPE-V, procedural instructions, and a copy of the protocol, readers are referred to Kempster et al. (2009) or the ASHA Web site (http://www.asha.org).

3. *The s/z ratio.* Described previously, this ratio will help to identify the possible presence of poor respiratory support or a laryngeal pathology that may be negatively affecting vocal quality. Any vocal pathology that interferes with glottal closure will result in increased breathiness. Attempts to compensate for poor glottal closure may result in laryngeal tension or hyperfunction. This may result in a tense or strained voice. In addition, laryngeal pathologies that affect the pattern of vocal fold vibration may create jitter or shimmer. Poor respiratory support can also contribute to hyperfunctional behaviors and negatively affect vocal quality, as described earlier.

4. *Vocal endurance.* Testing for vocal endurance involves having the patient count vigorously from 1 to 100. Any loss of voice or worsening of the vocal quality during this task is a sign of vocal fatigue. Vocal fatigue is often the result of chronic laryngeal hyperfunction or neurologic involvement; however, the latter is less likely in children.

5. *Coughing and throat clearing.* These tasks require adequate glottal closure. Poor glottal closure will result in increased breathiness and air wastage. Attempts

to compensate for poor glottal closure may result in laryngeal tension or hyperfunction. Vocal fold lesion, paresis, or paralysis may be suspected if the cough and throat clear are weak.

6. *Hard glottal attacks.* These can be tested by having the client count from 80 to 89, stopping briefly between each number. The repeated production of "8" at the start of each number will make any hard glottal attacks more obvious. The use of hard glottal attacks during speech production may contribute to vocal hyperfunction or laryngeal pathology with a subsequent effect on vocal quality.

Clinical Assessment of Laryngeal Tension

To clinically assess tension in the laryngeal muscles that may be affecting the voice, the clinician should gently palpate the external laryngeal musculature and thyroid cartilage. The clinician may gently shift the position of the larynx. Musculoskeletal tension is evident if these maneuvers are painful for the child or if the larynx is held rigidly in place so the clinician cannot move it.

Laryngeal imaging through laryngoscopy may reveal the following signs of laryngeal hyperfunction: anterior-to-posterior constriction (shortening) of the vocal folds during phonation, supraglottic compression, or laryngeal edema. As noted previously, any muscle tension also may be instrumentally measured with the help of electromyography. Most clinicians, however, assess muscle tension clinically, as described.

Clinical Assessment of Resonance

Many voice disorders are not characterized by significant resonance problems. Therefore, a brief assessment conducted as part of the orofacial examination and speech sample analysis is often adequate to rule out a resonance disorder. If, however, a resonance disorder is suspected, then a more detailed evaluation will be required to determine the type of resonance problem that may be present and its possible etiologic factors. As discussed earlier, oral and nasal airflow parameters and nasilance can be measured instrumentally. In addition, a variety of clinical tasks are available for this purpose.

A detailed description of these tasks is available in the *Resonance and Velopharyngeal Function Assessment Protocol* in Chapter 13. As described previously, resonance disorders in children include hypernasality, hyponasality, assimilation nasality, and cul-de-sac resonance. The clinical tasks described in this protocol may be conducted to confirm or rule out the presence of hypernasality, hyponasality, nasal emission, or assimilation nasality. Furthermore, observations made during these clinical tasks will assist in determining whether the resonance problem is the result of an organic condition, such as VPI, or the result of faulty learning.

Stimulability of Voice Production

There are several clinical tasks that can be used to assess stimulability of voice. These tasks are generally used for one of two purposes: to evoke phonation in an aphonic child, or to facilitate an improved vocal quality in a dysphonic child. Although somewhat controversial, the child's response to these stimulability activities can provide prognostic information and direction for therapy. A brief description of each activity follows. Detailed, procedural directions for these tasks are described in the *Voice Stimulability Assessment Protocol* in Chapter 13.

1. *Coughing, throat clearing, and laughing:* These nonspeech acts are sometimes useful in helping children with functional aphonia "find" their voice. If phonation is produced during these activities, the clinician may assume that the aphonia is functional. Phonation can then be shaped into a hum or vowel production as a precursor to producing words, phrases, and conversational speech.

2. *Inhalation phonation:* This type of phonation requires vibration of the true vocal folds. Therefore, it may be helpful in evoking phonation in a child who demonstrates aphonia or in a child who produces ventricular phonation.

3. *Glottal fry:* Glottal fry requires that the vocal folds vibrate in a relaxed manner. Therefore, this is a useful stimulation technique for patients who have a hyperfunctional voice disorder. Glottal fry is produced at a low pitch with very little airflow or subglottic air pressure. A child who produces glottal fry may achieve a more relaxed phonatory pattern under treatment than the one who cannot produce it. On the other hand, a child who cannot produce glottal fry may have significant laryngeal hyperfunction.

4. *Yawn-sigh:* The yawn-sigh is an excellent technique for minimizing laryngeal tension. Therefore, it is a useful stimulability technique with children who have a hyperfunctional voice disorder. Any improvement in vocal quality observed during the "sigh" is a good prognostic indicator. In therapy, the "sigh" can be shaped into "h-words" or open mouth vowels, which can be shaped into words, phrases, and conversational speech.

5. *Tone focus:* This technique may be a useful stimulability procedure for children who have vocal hyperfunction or who have a voice that sounds as if it is being produced too low, deep down in the throat. It may help the child to resonate a little higher up in the facial mask, thus taking the focus off the laryngeal area. Any improvement observed in the child's vocal quality while using tone focus is a good prognostic indicator for the use of tone focus or Resonant Voice Therapy in treatment.

6. *Exploring the child's pitch range:* A common vocal misuse in children is speaking at an inappropriate pitch. Therefore, the clinician might explore the child's pitch range to find out if a slight elevation or lowering of pitch results in improved vocal quality. If it does, then this is a good prognostic indicator that therapy for pitch adjustment will be successful in improving vocal quality and possibly reducing hyperfunction.

Assessment of Voice in Ethnoculturally Diverse Children

Research on voice disorders in children from diverse backgrounds is limited. For the most part, published research has compared vocal characteristics across different ethnocultural groups, and investigated the incidence of voice disorders in different ethnocultural groups.

Awan and Mueller (1996) compared the fundamental frequencies (F_0), pitch sigma, and speaking pitch ranges of White, African American, and Hispanic kindergarten-age children. They found significant differences between racial groups on measures of F_0 and speaking pitch range. Specifically, the Hispanic children demonstrated increased mean fundamental frequencies in comparison with the African American children, and reduced speaking ranges when compared to both the African American children and the White children.

Wheat and Hudson (1988) investigated the vocal frequency characteristics of 50 male and 50 female African American 6-year-olds. They concluded that there were no significant differences in mean or range values as a function of the child's gender. Furthermore, in a comparison to the fundamental frequencies of White children, these investigators concluded that the fundamental frequencies of the African American children were consistently lower than those of White children reported by Gilbert and Campbell (1980).

The incidence of children's voice disorders in various ethnocultural groups has not been well documented. Most of the research pertains to adults, and more specifically to laryngeal, pharyngeal, oral, and esophageal cancers. Available research on voice disorders in children does not provide empirically derived incidence or prevalence data on racial and ethnic differences. Nonetheless, several authors have suggested that the incidence and severity of certain voice conditions might differ across cultural and racial groups (Agin, 2000; Baker, 1984; Duff, Proctor, & Yairi, 2004; Haller & Thompson, 1975). In contrast, a more recent investigation of preschool-age children (2 to 6 years) found no significant difference in the prevalence of voice disorders based or ethnicity, age, or gender (Duff, Proctor, & Yairi, 2004).

Although empirically based evidence on vocal characteristic differences and voice disorders in children from diverse backgrounds is both limited and conflicting, the clinician should consider the possibility that F_0 differences may be culturally influenced. There may be other differences that have not been researched. Parental dispositions toward voice disorders and their treatment may be variable across ethnocultural groups. Therefore, the clinician should follow the guidelines offered in Chapter 4 while assessing voice in ethnoculturally diverse children.

Analysis and Integration of Assessment Results

To determine whether a voice disorder exists, the clinician should analyze the assessment information gathered using the various strategies described and integrated it with information from other sources, particularly the ENT examination results and any information from the child's school setting. The analysis may not be completed before conducting the postassessment interview; however, most experienced clinicians will have sufficient information to suggest a tentative diagnosis and prognosis, and to make appropriate recommendations.

1. Develop a profile of the child and the family. Consider information provided in the case history and interview when formulating a profile of the child's and the family's communication patterns; describe the onset and development of the voice disorder, associated medical or clinical conditions, family's reaction to the child's voice problem, and ethnocultural factors affecting the child's voice; describe the child's interests, hobbies, and any special talents or favorite activities.

2. Summarize information provided by other professionals, particularly the ear-nose-throat specialist; describe the academic and vocal demands the child faces in school; describe any previous assessment and treatment results.

3. Establish an inventory of the child's vocal abuse and misuse behaviors. Consider the child's vocal behaviors within the home, school, and other environments. Use the *Vocal Abuse and Misuse Inventory* in Chapter 13.

4. Diagnose a voice disorder based on the following criteria (Hegde, 2008a) and use the *Child Voice Evaluation* in Chapter 13:
   • Abnormal loudness
   • Abnormal pitch, pitch breaks, or pitch deviations
   • Deviant vocal quality including breathiness, hoarseness, or harshness
   • Deviant resonance including hypernasality, hyponasality, assimilation nasality or cul-de-sac resonance; use the *Resonance and Velopharyngeal Function Assessment Protocol* in Chapter 13.
   • Abnormal vocal characteristics including muscle tension, hard glottal attacks, and abnormal aerodynamic measures
   • Evidence of vocal abuse or misuse
   • Evidence of organic pathology from medical examinations in conjunction with listed deviations in voice.

5. Support your diagnosis with information from the case history, interview, orofacial examination, instrumental analysis, laryngeal imaging, and other observations; identify any contributing etiologic factors and velopharyngeal deficits; and suggest a medical examination to rule out or confirm a laryngeal pathology.

6. Determine the effect of the child's voice problem on overall communication, academic achievement, and socialization. Information from the case history, academic records, other professionals who have seen the child, and the interview can be integrated with the results of the evaluation to make this determination.

7. Summarize the results of stimulability testing; use the *Voice Stimulability Assessment Protocol* in Chapter 13.

8. Determine the prognosis for improved voice with intervention. Several prognostic indicators should be considered when formulating the prognostic statement. These indicators include the type of voice disorder, the severity of the voice disorder, the need for medical management, the motivation of the client and parents, and stimulability or response to trial therapy.

9. Make recommendations based on the results of your assessment.

Differential Diagnosis of Voice Disorders

Initially, it is determined that a voice disorder exists based on the observation of abnormal loudness; abnormal pitch, pitch breaks or pitch deviations; deviant vocal quality; deviant resonance including hypernasality, hyponasality, assimilation nasality, or cul-de-sac resonance; and abnormal vocal characteristics including muscle tension or hard glottal attacks. These vocal parameters are considered abnormal or deviant if they are so outside the norm that they call attention to themselves, have the potential to cause pathologic changes in the larynx, or interfere with the child's ability to communicate. In addition, a voice disorder may be diagnosed on the basis of abnormal aerodynamic measures; evidence of vocal abuse or misuse; or evidence of organic pathology from medical examinations. Beyond an initial diagnosis of a voice disorder, differential diagnosis is needed to distinguish between various voice disorders and etiologies.

Diagnose **dysphonia** if:

- The child is diagnosed with a voice disorder of pitch, loudness, quality, or resonance.
- The child demonstrates vocal misuse or vocally abusive behaviors that are related to the diagnosed voice problem.
- The child is diagnosed by a physician as having a laryngeal pathology associated with vocal misuse or vocally abusive behaviors.

Diagnose **functional aphonia** if:

- The child demonstrates a complete loss of voice or the inability to produce phonation for speech; a physician or a laryngologist has ruled out organic pathology or etiology.
- There is case history evidence of some gain from the problem (positive reinforcement of aphonia); there is possible evidence of stressful conditions associated with the onset.
- Alternatively, there is evidence of an upper respiratory or similar illness requiring complete vocal rest that preceded aphonia.
- The child produces phonation on such nonspeech acts as coughing, throat clearing, or laughing.

Diagnose **selective mutism** if:

- The problem is limited to specific social situations
- It is not due to such extraneous factors as shyness, social embarrassment, or ethnocultural differences
- Lasts at least one month after the beginning of school
- The child successfully communicates with gestures and facial expressions.

Diagnose an **organic** or **neurologic voice disorder** if:

- The child demonstrates a voice disorder of pitch, loudness, quality, or resonance
- The voice disorder is associated with a medically diagnosed organic or neurologic condition (e.g., such medical conditions as LPR, upper respiratory infections, structural changes secondary to laryngeal trauma, craniofacial disorders such as cleft palate, conductive hearing loss, laryngeal papilloma, laryngeal web, and

such neurologic conditions as vocal fold paralysis, sensorineural hearing loss, neuromuscular diseases, or cerebral palsy).

Diagnose **velopharyngeal incompetence (VPI)** if:

- The child, on clinical tasks, demonstrates hypernasality or assimilation nasality, in the absence of any unrepaired palatal clefting.
- Velopharyngeal incompetence is confirmed through a medical examination.

Diagnose a **hyperfunctional voice disorder** if:

- The child demonstrates a voice disorder of pitch, loudness, quality, or resonance that is associated with a pervasive pattern of excessive effort and tension that affects the muscles and structures of the larynx.
- The presence of laryngeal hyperfunction is confirmed by direct or indirect examination of the larynx completed by an otorhinolaryngologist.
- Laryngeal hyperfunction is associated with vocal abuse or misuse.
- Laryngeal hyperfunction is associated with an effort to compensate for such structural deviations as congenital malformations, webs, papilloma, paralysis, nodules, polyps, granuloma or edema, as confirmed through a medical examination of the larynx.

Postassessment Counseling

Conclude your assessment session with postassessment counseling. This is an opportunity to share information with the child's parents or other caregiver(s) who have accompanied the child. Although you will not have fully analyzed the results of the assessment, you will have gained clinical impressions that are valid enough to summarize the results, make a tentative voice diagnosis, offer recommendations, describe treatment options, suggest a prognosis, and answer the most frequently asked questions. If a laryngeal examination has already been completed by an ENT specialist, then those findings will influence your diagnosis, prognosis, and recommendations. Knowing the physical and neurologic status of the larynx will allow you to provide information and answer frequently asked questions with greater confidence. If the child has not been examined by a laryngologist, then this referral should be made so that potential laryngeal pathologies can be ruled out or confirmed.

Make a Tentative Diagnosis

Summarize your observations and the clinical impressions gained from those observations. To the extent the observations justify, make as clear a voice diagnosis as possible. Describe the pitch, loudness, quality, and resonance features of the child's voice that justify your diagnosis of a voice disorder. You might point out any vocal misuse or vocally abusive behaviors that may be contributing to the voice problem, and the fact that these behaviors can lead to such physical changes inside the larynx as swelling, nodules, or polyps. It is often helpful at this point, to provide some basic education regarding vocal production and healthy vocal behaviors so that the parent or caregiver begins to develop an understanding of how the child's behaviors may be influencing his or her voice.

If it appears that the child's voice disorder might be associated with some type of laryngeal pathology, point out typical associations, but assure the parent or caregiver that a physical condition can only be confirmed or ruled out by a medical examination of the larynx, and that this needs to be done by an ENT specialist as soon as possible. The diagnosis of laryngeal pathologies cannot be done simply by listening to the voice and is outside the scope of practice for speech-language pathologists. If a laryngeal examination has been completed and pathology has been identified, the clinician may describe the pathology and its relationship to the voice disorder, as well as to any observed vocal misuses or vocally abusive behaviors. It is important to facilitate an understanding of any relationship that exists between identified vocal pathology, the child's behaviors, and the diagnosed voice disorder.

Make Recommendations

Treatment should be postponed until after the child's larynx has been examined by an otorhinolaryngologist to rule out or confirm any potential laryngeal pathology. Any recommendations made prior to that examination should be considered tentative, and will be finalized once the medical report is available. Research data and expert clinical experience support the use of voice therapy in the management of patients with acute and chronic voice disorders. Voice therapy contributes to increased effectiveness and efficiency in the production of voice and social communication. Voice therapy can result in a decrease in severity or resolution of some vocal pathologies; this in turn helps avoid surgery. When surgery is necessary, voice therapy can improve surgical outcomes, prevent additional injury, and limit treatment costs. Studies support the success of direct therapy and behavior modification to reduce undesirable vocal behaviors and to promote healthy vocal behaviors. Finally, if the child has a structural deviation or neurologic condition that interferes with normal voice production, the speech-language pathologist can help the child learn to produce the best voice possible without developing harmful compensatory habits that can lead to laryngeal hyperfunction.

After a careful consideration of all assessment data, make a recommendation, which might include one or more of the following:

1. The child's voice appears to be within normal limits and, therefore, therapy is not recommended at this time.

2. The child has a voice disorder, but needs to be referred to an otorhinolaryngologist, before initiating voice therapy.

3. The child needs to be referred to other professionals such as an audiologist, neurologist, psychologist, or counselor. The clinician would explain why such referrals are necessary and what the referred-to professional will do.

4. Voice therapy is recommended and will include direct therapy and behavior modification and general parent and child education on healthy vocal

behaviors. The family may seek services at his or her facility or, if they prefer, seek help from another professional in the community. If they prefer to seek help at another facility, the clinician would give them a list of clinics in the area and offer to send reports to the clinician who would be serving the child.

5. Voice therapy is not recommended because the child has velopharyngeal insufficiency or incompetence (VPI) and the necessary medical intervention has not been completed. The child may be re-evaluated after the medical intervention is completed.

Suggest Prognosis

With treatment, prognosis is generally good for improved voice; however, several prognostic indicators should be considered. Such factors as the type of voice disorder, the severity of the voice disorder, the need for medical management, the motivation of the client and parents, and stimulability or response to trial therapy may all affect the final outcome of treatment.

- Functional voice disorders with no associated medical pathology have a very good prognosis for improvement with voice therapy.

- Chronic functional voice disorders with associated medical pathology such as nodules, polyps, or contact ulcers may require medical intervention, voice therapy, or both. The prognosis for improvement in voice is very good with an effective combination of medical management and voice therapy.

- The prognosis for improved voice in children with organic or neurologic voice disorders will vary depending on the severity of the medical condition, the need for medical management, and the severity of the voice disorder. There may be times when the prognosis of achieving a normal voice may not be realistic. For example, a young child with laryngeal papilloma may not have vocal folds capable of normal vibration, or a child with cerebral palsy may not have the neuromuscular control needed for normal respiration, phonation, and resonance. In most cases, however, improvements in voice can often be achieved with the combination of competent medical management and sustained voice therapy.

- The prognosis for improved voice in VPI is dependent on the success of medical intervention. Voice therapy, following successful medical or prosthetic management, may be beneficial in facilitating the best voice possible given the child's structural deviations.

Answer Frequently Asked Questions

Most parents of children with voice disorders ask clinicians questions about voice disorders and their treatment. The clinician should give answers that are honest and scientifically justifiable. Some commonly encountered questions and their answers follow. You may need to modify the terms you use to suit the age and educational level of the child or family members you are speaking to.

What Causes Voice Disorders in Children?

Most childhood voice disorders are associated with laryngeal hyperfunction related to vocal abuse or misuse. [*Provide an explanation of vocal abuse and misuse, as appropriate.*] This vocal abuse and misuse can actually lead to structural changes in the larynx, such as swelling, nodules, or polyps. These changes affect the sound of the voice. It has been estimated that 45 to 80% of childhood dysphonia cases are the result of vocal nodules due to vocal abuse. The elimination of vocal abuse and misuse should help to improve your child's voice and may help reduce or eliminate a laryngeal pathology. The diagnosis of these types of laryngeal pathologies cannot be done simply by listening to the voice. A medical doctor will need to examine the larynx to determine if they are present.

Gastroesophageal reflux disease and laryngopharyngeal reflux may also contribute to hoarse voice. These problems must also be diagnosed and treated by a medical doctor. [*Provide a detailed description of GERD and LPR if it has already been diagnosed as a contributing factor*].

Some children have other known physiologic, structural, or neurologic conditions that are associated with their voice disorder. These must be diagnosed by a medical doctor and often require medical management in lieu of, or in addition to, voice therapy. Examples of these types of conditions include cleft palate, cerebral palsy, and hearing loss. [*Give more details if the child has one of these conditions or any other condition in addition to a voice disorder*].

How Long Does It Take to Treat Voice Disorders Effectively?

It depends on several factors. Because many voice disorders are associated with medical conditions, prompt and effective medical intervention may be needed prior to, or in conjunction with, voice therapy. The sooner the treatment is started, the more sustained and systematic the treatment is, the faster the progress. Therapy is typically scheduled for twice a week. If parents work with their children at home, following the suggestions given to them, the progress is faster. Generally, the more severe the disorder, the greater the length of treatment. [*Address the child's specific severity of the disorder and make comments on potential duration of treatment.*] Most functional voice disorders with no associated medical pathology, or even with small, newly formed nodules, can be resolved in less than 3 months with consistent, effective therapy. A severe voice disorder or one that is associated with a significant medical condition may require a lengthier period of voice therapy.

What Are Some of the Treatment Options?

There are several treatment options available. Most treatment plans include a combination of procedures. We might offer, for example:

- Direct therapy in which we reduce the kind of voice problems your child has; we may also teach an easier and healthier way of producing voice.

- Behavior modification or changing your child's behavior. It means that we reduce or eliminate such vocally abusive behaviors as excessive talking, yelling, screaming, and talking with inappropriate pitch.

- Sometimes called vocal hygiene education, which is also behavior modification. We teach your child healthier ways of producing voice. We teach good vocal behaviors to avoid voice problems in the future.

- Airflow management, as we sometimes call it. It means that we teach the child to breathe properly during talking. Some faulty manners of breathing may be bad for healthy voice production.

- If necessary, some form of ear training or auditory monitoring of the voice. We may teach children to listen to their voice more carefully so that they can better monitor how they produce voice and talk.

When Do We Start Treatment?

We recommend that we start treatment sooner rather than later for better and lasting outcome. It is important, however, that your child is examined by an otorhinolaryngologist—an ENT specialist—before we initiate therapy. Therefore, it is recommended that you pursue a laryngeal examination as soon as possible, and once that is completed, we can set up a date to begin treatment. If the laryngeal examination has already been completed, you can set up a date to begin therapy right away. *[Depending on the service setting, the clinician offers additional information on when and how to begin a treatment program for the child.]*

CHAPTER 13

Assessment of Voice: Protocols

- Note on Common Protocols
- Note on Specific Protocols
- Interview Protocol
- Vocal Abuse and Misuse Inventory
- Child Voice Evaluation Protocol
- Resonance and Velopharyngeal Function Assessment Protocol
- Voice Stimulability Assessment Protocol

Note on Common Protocols

In completing a voice assessment, the clinician may use the common protocols given in Chapter 2, also available on the CD. To make a comprehensive assessment of voice disorders in children, the clinician may modify as needed and print for use the following common protocols from the CD:

The Child Case History Form

Orofacial Examination and Hearing Screening Protocol

Use this protocol along with the *Instructions for Conducting the Orofacial Examination: Observations and Implications*. If the preliminary findings of the orofacial examination suggest the possibility of velopharyngeal inadequacy or incompetence, use the *Resonance and Velopharyngeal Function Assessment* protocol in this chapter.

Assessment Report Outline

Expand the voice section in the outline to include all relevant information gathered through the case history, interview, assessment, and reports.

Note on Specific Protocols

This chapter contains a collection of protocols that can be used individually or combined in a variety of ways to facilitate the evaluation of a child's voice problems. Each of these protocols is also available on the CD.

The protocols on the CD may be individualized and printed out as a group and used for a complete voice assessment. Also, one or more protocols may be selectively printed out and used as needed. In assessing children with multiple disorders of communication, the clinician may combine these protocols with protocols from other chapters. For example, the clinician may combine these voice assessment protocols with speech assessment protocols (Chapter 7), language assessment protocols (Chapter 9), or fluency assessment protocols (Chapter 11).

Voice Assessment Protocol 1
Interview Protocol

Child's Name _____ DOB _____ Date _____ Clinician _____

Preparation

☐ Review the "interview guidelines" presented in Chapter 1.

☐ Make sure the setting is comfortable with adequate seating and lighting.

☐ Record the interview whenever possible.

☐ Find out if the parent is comfortable having the child in the same room during the interview. If so, have something for the child to do (toys, books, etc.). If not, make arrangements for someone else to supervise the child during the interview.

☐ Whenever possible, review the case history ahead of time, noting areas you want to review or obtain more information in.

Introduction

☐ Introduce yourself. Briefly review your plan for the day and how long you expect it to take.

Example: "Hello Mr./Mrs. [parent's name]. My name is [clinician's name] and I am the speech pathologist who will be assessing [child's name] today. I would like to start by reviewing the case history and asking you a few questions. Once we are finished talking, I will work with [child's name]. Today's assessment should take about [estimate the amount of time you plan to spend]."

Interview Questions

☐ What is your primary concern regarding your child's voice?

☐ Can you describe the problem?

☐ When did you first notice that your child's voice was different?

☐ How did the problem progress from there?

☐ Has it gotten better or worse?

☐ Have you seen your family doctor about your concerns?

☐ Did your family doctor refer you to an ear, nose, and throat specialist?

☐ What did the doctor(s) tell you?

☐ Is it hard for people to understand your child? Approximately what percent of his [her] speech do you understand? How do you respond when you can't understand?

☐ How does your child react when others don't understand him [her]?

(continues)

Interview Protocol (continued)

☐ Are there times when your child's voice is better or worse? For example, is it better in the morning than in the evening or vice-versa?

☐ Has your child ever lost his [her] voice completely? How long did it last?

☐ Do you feel that your child's voice problem is affecting his [her] social interactions?

☐ Do you feel that your child's voice problem is affecting his [her] school performance?

☐ Has anyone else in your family ever experienced a voice problem?

☐ Is anyone in your family hard of hearing?

☐ Is there anyone living in the home who smokes? Is your child exposed to second hand smoke outside the home?

☐ Are there any other children living in the home? How many? Ages?

☐ Does your child attend day care, preschool, school? Where?

☐ How does your child interact with other children?

☐ Does your child participate in sports? Which ones? How often?

☐ Is your child involved in drama?

☐ Is your child involved in debate club or public speaking?

☐ Is your child in a choir or singing group?

☐ Do you have a pet? How does your child interact with the pet?

☐ Does your child have asthma?

☐ Has your child seen any other specialists for this problem? If so, who and when? What were their recommendations? How have you followed up on this?

☐ Does your child have reflux (GERD or LPR)? [provide a brief explanation of these problems, as needed]

☐ Has your child seen any other specialists for this problem? If so, who and when? What were their recommendations? How have you followed up on this?

☐ Does your child experience frequent or chronic allergies or colds?

☐ Has your child had a history of ear infections?

☐ Has your child ever had a hearing test? If yes, when and where? What were the results?

☐ Has your child seen any other specialists for this problem? If so, who and when? What were the recommendations? How have you followed up on this?

☐ Has your child received speech or voice therapy before? If yes, when and where? What did they work on in therapy? Can you describe the types of activities that were used?

☐ How did your child respond? Do you feel the therapy was helpful? Why or why not?

☐ Is your child currently on any medications?

Review the Vocal Abuse and Misuse Inventory with the parent and identify any behaviors that might be contributing to the cause or maintenance of the voice problem.

Review the case history and follow-up with any additional questions you need clarification on. Fill in any "blanks" in the medical, developmental, social, and educational histories.

Closing the Interview

Summarize the major points that you gathered from the interview, allowing the parent or caregiver to interrupt or correct information, as needed. Close the interview with the following:

☐ Do you have any questions for me at this point?

☐ Thank you very much for you input. The information has been very helpful.

☐ Now, I will work with [child's name]. Once we are finished, I will sit down to share my findings with you.

Voice Assessment Protocol 2
Vocal Abuse and Misuse Inventory

Child's Name _____ DOB _____ Date _____ Clinician _____

Individualize this protocol on the CD and print it for your use.

Instructions: *Use the rating scale below to rate each area on the inventory as it applies to your child. Please use the lined area for any additional comments.*

0 = never   1 = occasionally   2 = frequently   3 = always

☐ yelling, screaming: _____

☐ arguing with siblings and friends: _____

☐ excessive talking: _____

☐ talking at an inappropriate pitch level: _____

☐ talking at an inappropriate loudness level: _____

☐ athletic activities that involve yelling or loud talking: _____

_____

☐ cheerleading activities: _____

☐ vocalizing toy or animal noises: _____

☐ using the telephone: _____

☐ talking in the car: _____

☐ talking in a noisy environment: _____

☐ talking in a smoky environment: _____

☐ singing: _____

☐ participation in plays, debate club or public speaking: _____

_____

☐ grunting during exercise or lifting: _____

☐ crying: _____

☐ frequent or excessive coughing: _____

☐ frequent or excessive throat clearing: _____

☐ breathing through the mouth: _____

☐ talking at an inappropriate pitch level: _____

☐ exposure to environmental irritants: _____

☐ exposure to second-hand smoke: _____

☐ upper respiratory infections: _____

☐ asthma attacks: _____

Dietary considerations:

☐ dairy products: _____

☐ caffeine products (coffee, tea, soft drinks): _____

_____

☐ mint products (gum, mints, candy): _____

☐ tomato-based products: _____

☐ citrus products: _____

☐ spicy foods: _____

Voice Assessment Protocol 3
Child Voice Evaluation Protocol

Child's Name _____ DOB _____ Date _____ Clinician _____

Individualize this protocol on the CD and print it for your use.

Physician: _____

Findings:

Description of the Problem (Summarize findings from Case History and Interview)

Description of Home and School Environments

Medical and Developmental History

Birth and Development:

Surgeries / Injuries / Accidents:

Current Medications:

☐ allergies   ☐ asthma   ☐ GERD or LPR
☐ chronic "colds"   ☐ other:

Inventory of Vocal Abuse and Misuse

Instructions: Use the rating scale below to rate each area on the inventory.

0 = never   1 = occasionally   2 = frequently   3 = always

☐ yelling, screaming   ☐ arguing with siblings and friends
☐ excessive talking   ☐ talking at an inappropriate loudness level
☐ cheerleading activities   ☐ vocalizing toy or animal noises
☐ using the telephone   ☐ athletic activities that involve yelling
☐ talking in a noisy environment   ☐ talking in a smoky environment
☐ talking in the car   ☐ singing
☐ crying   ☐ participation in plays or public speaking

☐ grunting during exercise or lifting   ☐ frequent or excessive coughing

☐ frequent or excessive throat clearing   ☐ breathing through the mouth

☐ exposure to environmental irritants   ☐ exposure to second-hand smoke

☐ Other:

Dietary considerations:

☐ dairy products   ☐ tomato-based products

☐ citrus products   ☐ caffeine products (coffee, tea, soft drinks)

☐ spicy foods   ☐ mint products (gum, mints, candy)

Instructions: Use the child's spontaneous speech sample and reading sample (if the child is able to read) to note the following:

Breathing and Breath Support (circle all that apply)

Clavicular   Thoracic   Diaphragmatic-Abdominal

Inadequate Breath Support   Irregular Breathing Rhythm   Mouth Breather

Vocal Quality (circle all that apply)

Breathy   Hoarse   Harsh   Glottal Fry

Glottal Attacks   Phonation Breaks   Pitch Breaks

Monotone   Voice Onset   Voice Termination

Strained-Strangled   Whisper Aphonia   Other:

Resonance (circle all that apply)

Hypernasality   Hyponasality   Assimilation Nasality   Nasal Emission

Note: If resonance is a concern, attach the "Resonance and Velopharyngeal Function Assessment" protocol.

Pitch (circle all that apply)

Age/sex appropriate   Too High   Too Low   Monopitch

Variable   Diplophonia   ***Habitual Pitch*** = _____ Hz.

Other:

Loudness (circle all that apply)

Appropriate   Too Loud   Inadequate Loudness   Loudness Decay

Variable   ***Average Loudness Level*** = _____ dB.

Other:

(continues)

Child Voice Evaluation Protocol (continued)

Laryngeal Tension (mark all that apply)

☐ Child complains of pain in the laryngeal area

☐ Pain upon laryngeal palpation

☐ The laryngeal position in the neck is very rigid: the clinician is not able to gently "wiggle" it back and forth.

☐ Other:

Maximum Phonation Time: /a/ = _____ seconds

s/z Ratio: /s/ = _____ seconds   /z/ = _____ seconds

_____ seconds   _____ seconds

_____ seconds   _____ seconds

s/z ratio = _____ (longest /s/) ÷ _____ (longest /z/) = _____

Other Clinical Tasks (circle tasks that were administered and note the results)

Assess nasal patency

Words per Breath

Highest Pitch (falsetto with /i/)

Lowest Pitch (glottal fry)

Pitch Range

Loudness Range

Vocal Endurance (count vigorously from 1–100)

Testing for Hard Glottal Attacks (count from 80–89)

Attach protocol for the Resonance and Velopharyngeal Function Assessment, as needed.

Stimulability (circle tasks that were administered and note the results) A separate protocol for stimulability assessment is available and can be attached, as needed.

Coughing, throat clearing, and laughing

Inhalation Phonation

Glottal Fry

Yawn-sigh

Tone Focus

Explore the pitch range, listening for improved vocal quality

Summary

Recommendations

☐ Vocal quality appears to be within normal limits, therefore therapy is not recommended at this time.

☐ Recommend evaluation and laryngoscopy by an ENT to rule out or confirm the presence of vocal pathology.

☐ Recommend a full audiologic evaluation.

☐ Voice therapy is recommended for the following goals:

Other:

Voice Assessment Protocol 4
Resonance and Velopharyngeal Function Assessment Protocol

Child's Name _____ DOB _____ Date _____ Clinician _____

Individualize this protocol on the CD and print it for your use.

If a resonance problem is suspected, additional clinical tasks may be conducted to confirm or rule out the presence of hypernasality, hyponasality, nasal emission, or assimilation nasality. Furthermore, observations made during these clinical tasks will assist in determining whether the resonance problem is the result of an organic condition, such as VPI, or the result of faulty learning. The clinician should select clinical tasks from those described below to evaluate a child's resonance further.

1. ☐ *Alternative nose holding technique*
    - Have the child say /u/ –or– alternate /a/-/i/-/a/-/i/.
    - Alternate between occluding and releasing the child's nostrils.

    Results: ☐ the child's voice changed (suspect hypernasality)
              ☐ the child's voice did not change (hypernasality is not indicated)

2. ☐ *Nonnasal words and phrases*
    - Have the child recite nonnasal words and phrases (below) (Boone, 1993):
        ○ This horse eats grass.
        ○ I saw the teacher at church.
        ○ Sister Suzie sat by a thistle.

    Results: ☐ excessive nasal pressure is felt, or a nasal snort is heard (suspect hypernasality)

3. ☐ *"Maybe-baby"* (Boone & McFarlane, 1988)
    - Have the child recite "maybe-baby-maybe-baby . . . "

    Results: ☐ it sounds like "maybe-maybe-maybe . . . " (suspect hypernasality)
              ☐ it sounds like "baby-baby-baby-baby . . . " (suspect hyponasality)

4. ☐ *"Humming"*

    Result: ☐ impaired humming (suggests hyponasality)

5. ☐ *Count from 60 to 100* (adapted from Mason & Grandstaff, 1971)
   - Have the client count from 60 to 100 while the clinician listens for the following:
     - 60 to 69 = listen for VPI and nasal emission secondary to frequent /s/ productions
     - 70 to 79 = listen for assimilation nasality secondary to the recurring /n/ phoneme
     - 80 to 89 = listen for normal or near normal resonance and articulation
     - 90 to 99 = listen for substitutions of /d/ for /n/ which would indicate hyponasality

   Results: ☐ nasal emission/VPI   ☐ assimilation nasality
   ☐ hyponasality   ☐ normal resonance

6. ☐ *"Suzy-suzy-suzy-suzy . . . "* This task can be used to determine if the child's hypernasality is the result of a physical etiology or if it is the result of faulty learning.
   - Have the child recite "suzy-suzy-suzy . . . " as you occlude their nares.
   - Suddenly release the nares.

   Results: ☐ the child immediately reverts back to their hypernasal pattern (it is likely the result of a physical, organic etiology such as VPI)

   ☐ the child has one or more normal productions before reverting to the hypernasal pattern (it is likely functional)

7. ☐ *Modified tongue anchor procedure* (Fox & Johns, 1970)
   - Tell the child to "puff up your cheeks like this" and model the behavior. Practice until the child is able to do it.
   - Tell the child to stick out the tongue. Hold the tongue tip with a piece of sterile gauze.
   - While you are holding the tongue, tell the child to puff up his or her cheeks again. At the same time, occlude the child's nares.
   - Tell the child to continue holding the air in his or her mouth. Release the nose.
   - As the nostrils are released, listen for nasal emission.
   - Repeat this procedure several times to verify your observations.

   Results: ☐ nasal emission occurs (the velopharyngeal seal is considered inadequate)

   ☐ no nasal emission occurs (the velopharyngeal seal is considered adequate)

(continues)

Resonance and Velopharyngeal Function Assessment Protocol (continued)

8. ☐ *Nasally loaded words and phrases* (Boone, 1993)
    *   Have the child recite these words, phrases, and sentences; the combination of nasal and nonnasal sounds will exaggerate the presence of assimilation nasality, making it easier to identify.
    *   During the production of some of these words, phrases, and sentences, alternately occlude and release the child's nares.

Words	Phrases	Sentences
knees	another night	Mike wants more noodles.
now	no more	Mommy made lemon jam.
mate	not again	Make my lunch.
money	more money	Jenny made me mad.
moon	man on the moon	No more singing tonight.
my	Mickey Mouse	Make noise with a drum.

Result: ☐ assimilation nasality noted   ☐ no assimilation nasality noted

☐ the occluded and unoccluded productions sound the same (hyponasality is present)

9. *Pressure consonants*
    *   Have the child produce words, phrases, and sentences that contain pressure consonants (/p/, /b/, /t/, /d/, /k/, /g/, /s/, /z/, /f/, /v/, /ʃ/, /ʒ/, /tʃ/, /dʒ/, /ð/, and /θ/) that stress a weak velopharyngeal system and reveal hypernasality or nasal emission:

Words	Phrases	Sentences
pepper	black pepper	Pass the pepper.
baby	baby bib	The baby bib is blue.
tickle	teddy bear	Tickle the teddy bear.
daddy	daddy digging	Daddy dug a deep ditch.
cake	birthday cake	Don't kick the birthday cake.
goat	big goat	Give the goat a big hug.
feather	soft feather	Find a soft feather.
vest	blue vest	The blue vest is size five.
Suzie	Suzie sews	Suzie sews zippers.
shoe	dishwasher	The shoe is in the dishwasher.
cheese	cheese sandwich	Chew the cheese sandwich.
third	third bath	Her third bath was on Thursday.
they	their father	They saw their father the other day.

Result: ☐ hypernasality or nasal emission noted (possible VPI)

Voice Assessment Protocol 5
Voice Stimulability Assessment Protocol

Child's Name _____ DOB _____ Date _____ Clinician _____

Individualize this protocol on the CD and print it for your use.

Use the boxes "□" to indicate whether a task was successful. For Part I, mark with a "+" if phonation is produced and a "–" if phonation is not produced. For Part II, mark with a "+" if the quality of phonation is improved and a "–" if the quality of phonation is not improved.

I. Tasks Used to Evoke Phonation in a Potentially *Aphonic* Patient

1. *Nonspeech acts* are sometimes useful in helping children with functional aphonia "find" their voice. Have the child do the following tasks.

   □ coughing
   □ throat clearing
   □ laughing

   If you marked a "+" for any of the tasks, try shaping that phonation into a hum or vowel production as a precursor to producing words, phrases, and conversational speech.

   Results of attempting to shape nonspeech acts into speech sounds:

2. □ *Inhalation phonation:* Have the child produce inhalation phonation if you suspect aphonia or ventricular phonation.
   - Demonstrate this technique for the child and ask the child to:
     ○ Phonate a high-pitched "humming" sound as you inhale
     ○ Try to match that phonation as you exhale
     ○ Repeat, but as you exhale glide your pitch down to a lower level
     ○ Repeat [until an acceptable pitch is produced on exhalation]
   - Shape the exhaled "hum" phonation into words, phrases, and conversational speech

3. □ *Glottal fry:* Glottal fry, produced in a relaxed manner at a low pitch with very little airflow or subglottic air pressure, is a useful stimulation technique for improving a hyperfunctional voice and it is sometimes successful in evoking voice in a child who is aphonic. Glottal fry can be attempted using both inhalation and exhalation. The desired outcome is the production of a slow series of individual "pops."

(continues)

Voice Stimulability Assessment Protocol (continued)

- Demonstrate the technique for the child and ask the child to:
  - ○ Let out about half of your air, then say /i/ softly
  - ○ Cue the child to lower the pitch or slow down the airflow, as needed
  - ○ Encourage a wider mouth opening, then shape various vowel sounds as the child is producing /i/ with glottal fry

II. Tasks Used to Assess Stimulability for the Production of a More Relaxed Phonation with Improved Vocal Quality in a Child with Dysphonia

1. ☐ *Glottal fry*: (previous section)

2. ☐ *Inhalation phonation*: (earlier section)

3. ☐ *Yawn-sigh*: The yawn-sigh is an excellent technique for minimizing laryngeal tension and is a useful stimulability technique with children who have a hyperfunctional voice disorder.
    - Explain to the child that when the mouth is opened wide during a yawn, it is very relaxing, and that the "sigh" at the end of the yawn will be the best voice
    - Demonstrate the technique for the child
    - Have the child practice producing large, relaxed, open mouth yawns that extend into a "sigh"

    Improved vocal quality during the "sigh" is a good prognostic indicator and may be helpful in shaping "h-words" or open mouth vowels.

4. ☐ *Tone focus*: Tone focus may be useful as a stimulability technique for children who have vocal hyperfunction or who have a voice that sounds as if it is being produced too low, deep down in the throat. It may help the child to resonate a little higher up, thus taking the focus off the laryngeal area.
    - Have the child "hum" and feel with their fingers for vibration around their nose and eyes. This area is called the "facial mask."
    - Once the child can feel the vibration during humming, slowly shape various vowel sounds while maintaining the vibration (resonation in the facial mask).
    - Try shaping from vowel sounds into words.

    If vocal quality improves, this is a good prognostic indicator for using tone focus or resonant voice therapy procedures.

5. ☐ *Explore the pitch range, listening for improved vocal quality*: Explore the pitch range to find out if a slight elevation or lowering of pitch improves vocal quality in a child who speaks in an inappropriate pitch.

PART VI

Assessment of Nonverbal and Minimally Verbal Children

CHAPTER 14

Assessment of Nonverbal and Minimally Verbal Children: Resources

- An Overview of Nonverbal and Minimally Verbal Children
- The Assessment Team
- Assessment of Nonverbal or Minimally Verbal Children
- Case History and Interview
- Orofacial Examination and Hearing Screening
- Standardized and Criterion-Referenced Instruments
- Systematic Quantitative and Qualitative Observations of Nonverbal Communication
- Assessment of Receptive Language
- Assessment of Verbalizations
- Analysis and Integration of Assessment Results
- Prognosis for Developing Verbal Communication
- Postassessment Counseling

The assessment of nonverbal or minimally verbal children poses a unique challenge for speech-language pathologists. A *nonverbal* child may be defined as the one that is "essentially speechless" (Hegde, 1996, p. 148), although a nonverbal child may vocalize and gesture to a limited extent. The terms *prelinguistic* or *preverbal* are also sometimes used to describe this population. A *minimally verbal* child is the one who produces "simple, isolated word responses; perhaps a few phrases; but no sentence structure" (Hegde, 1996, p. 149).

It may be noted that nonverbal and minimally verbal are not mutually exclusive categories. Children vary on the continuum of communication skills. At the one extreme of this continuum, we find children with little or no verbal behavior, but they may have some basic nonverbal behaviors that function as verbal behaviors (e.g., a child who whines or cries when something is wanted). As we move on the continuum, we find children who exhibit extremely limited verbal repertoire that may be inadequate for social communication. This chapter is about these two groups of children on the lower end of the verbal behavior continuum.

An Overview of Nonverbal and Minimally Verbal Children

Nonverbal or minimally verbal children often fall within a broader definition of *developmentally disabled* which includes children who have a severe, chronic disability attributable to an intellectual or physical impairment or a combination of these two that result in substantial functional limitations (Administration on Developmental Disabilities, US Department of Health and Human Services, 2005). Impaired speech, language, and interpersonal skills, such as those demonstrated by non-verbal or minimally verbal children contribute to significant functional limitations. Depending on the severity of physical or intellectual disabilities, some of these children may go on to develop verbal communication, whereas others may require an augmentative or alternative communication (AAC) system to support or facilitate speech production. Still others may rely on AAC as their only means of communication (Mirenda, 2003), described in greater detail in Chapter 16.

Nonverbal and minimally verbal children come from varied etiologic groups. Some will have a primary diagnosis that includes intellectual disability along with a significant communication disorder. Children diagnosed with autism may be in this group, depending on the level of their intellectual disability. The primary characteristic of autism is impairments in verbal and nonverbal communication. Overall delays in the development of expressive language vary; some children develop verbal communication whereas others do not. Approximately one third to one-half of children with autism do not develop functional speech (Mirenda, 2003; Prizant, 1983). There are also a number of syndromes characterized by intellectual disability and significant speech and language disorders. These include Down syndrome, fetal alcohol syndrome (FAS), fragile X syndrome (FXS), Prader-Willi syndrome (PWS), and Williams syndrome, among others (Hegde & Maul, 2006). Prenatal factors such as maternal exposure to Rubella, maternal anoxia, and maternal ingestion of certain pathogens or drugs may contribute to a diagnosis of intellectual disability with communication disorders. Other etiologic factors include an anoxic event or traumatic brain injury that occurs during or after delivery; endocrine and metabolic disorders such as hypothyroidism, phenylketonuria (PKU), and Tay-Sachs disease; and cranial abnormalities.

Other nonverbal or minimally verbal children may have a primary diagnosis of physical disability that is not associated with intellectual disability. Such diagnoses include spinal cord injury, traumatic brain injury, cerebral palsy, and deafness. Cerebral palsy (CP) refers to a complex set of neuromotor disorders caused by injury to the developing nervous system. It may or may not be associated with intellectual disability, visual impairments, hearing loss, seizures, and learning impairments. It is often described as a congenital disorder even though neurological deficits may not be evident at birth. Depending on the pattern of neuromotor involvement, a child may exhibit one of four types of CP: spastic, ataxic, athetoid, or mixed. Impaired neural control of the muscles causes movement disorders. When this affects the speech musculature dysarthria may be present. Dysarthria is a speech disorder characterized by muscle weakness, paralysis, or incoordination. Muscles of respiration, phonation, resonation, and articulation may be affected, causing varied and sometimes detrimental effects on speech production. Dysarthria can also be the result of traumatic brain injury or spinal cord injury.

Profound congenital or prelingual hearing loss can affect all aspects of communication, including speech production, language, and vocal quality. Typical oral language development requires adequate hearing, so these children often present as nonverbal or minimally verbal. Children who are deaf may develop verbal communication if spoken language is emphasized in their home and academic environments. Others will learn the American Sign Language (ASL), a fully developed nonoral language, as their primary mode of communication.

As described, various etiologic factors and diagnoses may apply to nonverbal and minimally verbal children. In addition, some children may experience a combination of these factors. The severity of their intellectual, physical, and communicative disabilities also varies. The heterogeneity of this population may limit the usefulness of standardized tests and requires speech-language pathologists to be creative in their use of child-specific assessment procedures. Nonverbal or minimally verbal children's communication skills or potential must be evaluated through careful observation and assessment of their facial expressions, vocalizations, gestures, and actions. Several recent studies have emphasized the importance of evaluating early gestures of very young children diagnosed with, or at risk for, communicative disorders because of their correlation with later language development (Crais, Watson, & Baranek, 2009; Flenthrope & Brady, 2010). Nonverbal and minimally verbal children should be assessed to offer early intervention services when needed. The earlier the services are provided, the more likely the children are to develop effective communication (Guralnick, 2011; National Research Council & Institute of Medicine, 2000; Paul & Roth, 2011). According to ASHA (2008), early intervention services should be family centered and culturally and linguistically appropriate; should promote children's participation in their natural environments; should be based on the highest quality of evidence available; and should be comprehensive, coordinated, and team-based.

The Assessment Team

The assessment of nonverbal or minimally verbal children requires the speech-language pathologist to participate as one member of an assessment team. Beukelman and Mirenda (2005) and Glennen and DeCoste (1997) describe several patterns of team organization that may be used in the assessment of this population. For instance, a *multidisciplinary team* includes a variety of specialists that independently complete his or her portion of the assessment, makes discipline-specific recommendations and decisions during team meetings, and often independently provides direct service to the client. An *interdisciplinary team* also includes specialists who conduct individual assessments, but the assessments are followed by a meeting in which they discuss their findings and make collaborative recommendations and decisions. The team would then continue to meet regularly to discuss client progress and update the treatment plan, as needed. In a *transdisciplinary team*, information sharing and service delivery are done in such a way that the professionals involved actually become proficient in areas other than their primary specialty. Assessment and goal setting are completed through a collaborative effort of all those involved.

The term *interdisciplinary team* will be used from this point forward; however, an assessment team may successfully work within any of these models. Depending on the setting, the interdisciplinary team may include any combination of the following professionals: speech-language pathologist, psychologists, physical therapists, occupational therapists, special education teachers, and medical personnel. In addition, family members or caregivers should also be included as members of the interdisciplinary assessment team.

The speech-language pathologist is responsible for assessing verbal and nonverbal communication skills to establish the child's current receptive and expressive language skills, evaluating the effectiveness of the child's communication strategies, and making recommendations for treatment that will promote continued development of verbal, nonverbal, or both types of functional communication. The role of the speech-language pathologist is discussed in detail throughout the remainder of this chapter.

The psychologist specializes in the assessment of behavior and intellectual skills and helps to identify any intellectual (cognitive) deficits that might affect the child's language learning or influence the selection of verbal or nonverbal treatment programs. In addition, the psychologist assists in determining the level of complexity of the nonverbal program selected for the child. The psychologist can also identify problem behaviors and design behavioral intervention for the elimination of inappropriate behaviors and establishment of appropriate behaviors.

The physical therapist (PT) is qualified to assess the physical abilities and limitations of the child, including the child's fine and gross motor abilities, strength, range of motion, coordination, and balance. Significant motor impairments may influence the effectiveness of a child's attempts at nonverbal communication. For example, it is essential to find out whether a child's inability to point to something or follow directions is due to a motor disability or poor receptive language. In addition, assessment of physical abilities is essential to recommend an augmentative and alternative communication (AAC) strategy. Physical limitations must be considered in the selection of an appropriate communication system.

The occupational therapist (OT) is qualified to assess daily living skills, sensory skills, and motor impairments in children with cognitive deficits, developmental disabilities, and physical injuries. Occupational therapists also make recommendations for, and assess the effectiveness of, adaptive equipment used during activities of daily living (ADLs). This would include recommendations for the selection of an appropriate AAC device for a nonverbal or minimally verbal child, as discussed in Chapter 16.

The special education teacher is responsible for establishing appropriate academic goals for the child and implementing strategies that will help the child meet those goals. The special education teacher can also provide the assessment team with valuable information on the child's communication needs and abilities in the classroom setting. The child's regular classroom teacher is also a valuable resource for information on the child's academic, social, and peer interaction skills.

Many other specialists may be included on the team, as needed. For example, an audiologist should be included for a child with a hearing impairment and various medical personnel might be involved for a medically complex child. Social workers, interpreters, resource specialists, behavioral specialists, or AAC consultants may also be members of the team or provide requested information or service. These professionals, and others who might be involved on an assessment team, are presented in Table 14–1.

Table 14–1. Professionals Who Might Be Involved in the Assessment of Nonverbal or Minimally Verbal Children, or AAC Assessment

Profession	Areas of Expertise as a Team Member
AAC Consultant (Many school districts, organizations, or assistive technology companies have someone designated as an "AAC expert/consultant." They may be from different backgrounds.)	• operational requirements of various AAC devices • access issues and aids • funding issues • matching child's capabilities to a specific device • selection and implementation of AAC • management of communication interventions
Audiologist	• hearing assessment • aural rehabilitation • maintenance of assistive listening devices
Behavioral Specialist	• behavioral management strategies
Computer Technology	• evaluation, development, and modification of software programs to meet the child's communication needs
Education (teachers, instructional aids, resource specialists, special educators)	• academic curriculum • social development • cognition and concept development • specific learning disabilities • vocational curriculum • integration of AAC into the classroom

(continues)

Table 14–1. *(continued)*

Profession	Areas of Expertise as a Team Member
Engineering	• implementation and maintenance of electronic or mechanical aids and devices
Interpreter	• ASL, manual communication • interpreting for clients and families when second language issues exist
Medicine	• medical management • management of medications • management of rehabilitation program
Occupational Therapist	• activities of daily living (ADLs) • adaptive equipment • upper extremity strength and range of motion (ROM) • positioning • mobility aids • occupational therapy
Physical Therapist	• mobility and ambulation • motor control • strength and ROM • positioning • physical therapy
Psychologist	• level of cognitive functioning • learning styles and strategies • specific learning disabilities • estimates of learning potential • behavior management • counseling
Social Services	• identification of family and community resources • evaluation of general living situation • funding alternatives
Speech-Language Pathologist	• assessment of speech and language • contribute to cognitive-communication evaluation • verbal and nonverbal communication strategies • specific communicative disorders • selection and implementation of AAC • management of communication interventions • speech-language therapy

Assessment of Nonverbal or Minimally Verbal Children

Much of what was discussed about language assessment in Part III of this book will apply to this population as well. Many of these children will respond to typical tasks used to assess receptive language. Therefore, several of the standardized tests discussed in Chapter 8 might be useful if they are developmentally appropriate and the procedures allow for scoring of the receptive portions only. Obviously, most standardized tests of expressive language would not be useful with these children. As we shall see later, there are, however, a few standardized and criterion-referenced instruments that might be helpful.

The primary tool for assessing nonverbal and minimally verbal children is systematic quantitative and qualitative observations of the child's communication behaviors (Hegde & Maul, 2006). These observations, along with information gathered during the interview, will tell us a great deal about a child's communication skills and potential. Therefore, a combination of the following components will make up the assessment of a nonverbal or minimally verbal child:

- Case history and interview
- Orofacial examination and hearing screening
- Standardized and criterion-referenced instruments
- Systematic quantitative and qualitative observations of nonverbal communication
- Assessment of receptive language
- Assessment of verbalizations that do occur
- Analysis and integration of assessment data
- Prognosis for developing verbal communication
- Postassessment counseling, which includes recommendations.

Case History and Interview

Information obtained from a written case history helps the speech-language pathologist plan an evaluation that includes materials appropriate to the child's developmental level and interests, and will assist in the formulation of interview questions. The case history can provide the clinician with a fairly good idea of the child's developmental history, social skills, play, motor and sensory capabilities, and communication behaviors. The case history and interview should be designed to get information on the parent's views about AAC systems, their level of knowledge and acceptance of nonverbal means of communication, family resources that are available to gain access to a system that might be expensive, and their level of motivation for learning to use the system and supporting the child. With necessary modifications, the *Case History Protocol* presented in Chapter 2 can be used with this population; an interview protocol specifically designed for parents of nonverbal children is provided in Chapter 15.

The Individuals with Disabilities Education Act (IDEA) of 1997 mandates that family members are team members who actively participate in the assessment and treatment of children with communicative disorders. The interview is often the first opportunity to make a personal connection with the parents or caregivers. It is a good opportunity to clarify any missing or contradictory information on the case history, establish rapport with the parents, and to investigate their concerns, impressions, and expectations regarding their child's communication and potential therapy plan. Interview questions will be highly individualized; however, a list of possible items is provided in the *Assessment of Nonverbal or Minimally Verbal Children: Interview Protocol* presented in Chapter 15.

Orofacial Examination and Hearing Screening

If possible, an orofacial examination and a hearing screening should be completed, as described in Chapters 1 and 2. The *Orofacial Examination and Hearing Screening* protocol presented in Chapter 2 can be used with this population. If the child is unable or unwilling to participate in these activities, then the structural and functional adequacy of the orofacial structures should be observed, as closely as possible, during informal activities. Such activities might include, but not be limited to, making funny faces in a mirror, blowing bubbles, blowing a pinwheel, blowing kisses, licking a lollipop, eating or drinking, and making a variety of vocalizations. Any indications of weakness or incoordination during these activities should be noted, and a more complete orofacial examination should be included as part of the recommendations for follow-up.

Often, it is not possible to complete a hearing screening with this population. Even if the child is cooperative, inconsistent responses may render the results inaccurate or unreliable. In this case, if it has not already occurred, a complete audiologic evaluation should be recommended. Early identification of a hearing loss or ruling it out as a contributing factor is important in the communication assessment of nonverbal or minimally verbal children.

Standardized and Criterion-Referenced Instruments

Limited verbalization and varying degrees of physical and intellectual disabilities may render most standardized tests inappropriate for nonverbal or minimally verbal children. Clinicians should carefully consider their strengths and limitations, as discussed in Chapter 3, prior to including them in an assessment. Several standardized and criterion-referenced tests have been developed specifically for use with nonverbal or minimally verbal children. These instruments may also be appropriate for assessing language abilities as part of an AAC assessment. In addition, several standardized tests designed to measure receptive vocabulary through a simple picture identification task, such as the Peabody Picture Vocabulary Test-Third Edition (PPVT-III) may be a useful component of the assessment when modified to accommodate a child's physical limitations. Bristow and Fristoe (1987) found that the response mode on the PPVT-III could easily be adapted (e.g., pointing, eye gaze, use of a head wand) to meet the individual needs of a motorically involved child without significantly compromising test validity. A summary of assessment instruments that may be appropriate for the assessment of language in nonverbal or minimally verbal children, including those being considered for AAC, are presented in Table 14–2.

Table 14–2. Instruments for Assessing Speech and Language in Nonverbal or Minimally Verbal Children, Including Those That Are Specific to AAC Assessment

Assessment Instrument	Age Range	Skills Assessed
Analysis of Communication Interaction (DynaVox Mayer-Johnson, 2009)	School-age children	Classroom communication behaviors (specific to AAC)
Augmentative and Alternative Communication Profile (Kovach, 2009)	2 to 21 years	Functional skills for developing communicative competence using AAC systems
Autism Screening Instrument for Educational Planning-3rd Edition (ASIEP-3) (Krug, Arick, & Almond, 2008)	2 to 13;11 years	Autism behaviors checklist, vocal behavior analysis, interaction assessment, and prognosis of learning rate
Bracken Basic Concept Scale–Revised (Bracken, 1998)	2;6 years to 7 years	Basic concepts and receptive language skills in individuals who are unable to speak, read, or write English; criterion referenced form available in Spanish
Child Development Inventory (CDI) (Ireton, 1995)	15 months to 6 years	Social, self-help, gross and fine motor, receptive and expressive language, letters, numbers, general development (based on parent/caregiver report)
Clinical Evaluation of Language Fundamentals, Second Edition-Preschool (CELF-Preschool) (Semel, Secord, & Wiig, 2004)	3 years to 6 years	Receptive, expressive, and pragmatic language; also available in Spanish.
Communication Assessment Record (CAR) (Silver, 2005)	All ages	Understanding of communication, social interaction, functional use of communication; specific to ASD
Communication and Symbolic Behavior Scales-Developmental Profile (CSBS-DP) (Wetherby & Prizant, 2003)	9 months to 6 years	Nonverbal and verbal communication at a functional communication age between 6 months–24 months (direct observation or parent report)
CSBS-DP Infant-Toddler Checklist and Easy Score (Wetherby & Prizant, 2003)	6 months to 24 months	Gestures, words, sounds, eye gaze, object use, other nonverbal communication behaviors
Communication Matrix-Revised (Rowland, 2004)	All ages	Communication behaviors and functions (AAC and other forms of communication)
Developmental Observation Checklist System (DOCS) (Hresko, Miguel, Sherbenou, & Burton, 1994)	Birth to 6 years	Domains: cognition, language, social, fine and gross motor skills, adaptive functioning in the environment (based on parent/caregiver report)

(continues)

Table 14–2. *(continued)*

Assessment Instrument	Age Range	Skills Assessed
Forerunners in Communication (ComFor) (Noens, van Berckelaer-Onnes, Verpoorten, & van Dujin, 2006)	Developmental level of 12 to 60 months	Perception and sense-making of nontransient forms of communication at the levels of presentation and representation; also available in French
Language Development Survey (LDS) (Rescorla, 1989)	18 months to 35 months	Vocabulary production, use of word combinations (based on parent/caregiver report)
Language Use Inventory (LUI) (O'Neill, 2009)	18 months to 47 months	A standardized measure of early pragmatic language development (based on parent/caregiver report)
MacArthur Communicative Development Inventories: Words & Gestures, 2nd Edition (Fenson et al., 1993)	8 months to 16 months	Vocabulary comprehension, vocabulary production, use of gestures (based on parent/caregiver report); now available in Spanish (Inventario I: Primeras Pulabras y Gestos) & several other languages
MacArthur Communicative Development Inventories: Words & Sentences, 2nd Edition (Fenson et al., 1993)	16 months to 30 months	Vocabulary production, grammatic development (based on parent/caregiver report); now available in Spanish (Inventario II: Pulabras y Enunciados) & several other languages
Peabody Picture Vocabulary Test-Third Edition (PPVT-III) (Dunn & Dunn, 1997)	2;3 years to 40;11 years	Comprehension of single words
Preschool Language Scale, Fourth Edition (PLS-4) (Zimmerman, Steiner, & Evatt-Pond, 2002)	Birth to 6;11 years	Receptive and expressive language: vocabulary, basic concepts, morphology, syntax
Receptive–Expressive Emergent Language Test-3rd Edition (REEL-3) (Bzoch, League, & Brown, 2003)	Birth to 3 years	Receptive and expressive language (based on parent/caregiver report)
Receptive One-Word Picture Vocabulary Test-4th Edition (ROWPVT-4) (Brownell, 2000)	2;11 years to 11;11 years	Receptive language
Sequenced Inventory of Communication Development–Revised (SICD-R) (Hedrick, Prather, & Tobin, 1995)	4 months to 4 years	Receptive and expressive language skills at a level of 4 months–48 months (direct observation or parent report)

Table 14–2. *(continued)*

Assessment Instrument	Age Range	Skills Assessed
Stages (Pugliese, 2001) [computer software]	School-age children with cognitive and language delays	Cause and effect, receptive language, basic concepts, reading and math readiness, written expression, money skills, and time skills
Test for Auditory Comprehension of Language-3 (TACL-3) (Carrow-Woolfolk, 1999)	3 years to 9;11 years	Comprehension of word categories, grammatic features, and syntax
Test of Early Communication and Emerging Language (TECEL) (Huer & Miller, 2011)	2 weeks to 24 months	Receptive and expressive language (direct observation or parent/caregiver report)
Test of Semantic Skills-Primary (TOSS-P) (Bowers, Huisingh, LaGiudice, & Orman, 2002)	4 years to 8;11 years	Receptive and expressive language: labeling, categorizing; specifying attributes, definitions, and functions
Test of Early Language Development-3rd Edition (TELD-3) (Hresko, Reid, & Hammill, 1991)	2;7 years to 7;11 years	Comprehension and production of semantic and syntactic structures
Test of Language Development-Primary (TOLD-P:4) (Newcomer & Hammill, 1997a)	4 years to 8;11 years	Comprehension and production of words; articulation; grammatic understanding

Systematic Quantitative and Qualitative Observations of Nonverbal Communication

As stated earlier, the primary tool for assessing nonverbal and minimally verbal children is systematic quantitative and qualitative observations of the child's communication behaviors (Hegde & Maul, 2006). The clinician will engage the child in a variety of structured "play" activities to gather quantitative and qualitative information regarding the child's communication behaviors. Most nonverbal children will use a combination of atypical vocalizations, gestures, facial expressions, end emotional expressions to communicate. They might also demonstrate a number of inappropriate or aggressive behaviors. Nonverbal attempts at communication may be subtle so the speech-language pathologist needs to observe carefully. Eventually, the treatment plan may include helping the parents to identify and respond appropriately to these attempts at communication. Minimally verbal children may also produce several words or word combinations.

The clinician should arrange the room in a way that encourages the child to interact, and provide access to a variety of toys and stimulus items. It may be helpful to have the parent provide several of the child's favorite toys or books. The assessment should include observations of spontaneous play as well as the child's response during various tasks designed to evoke the following:

- **Social interaction:** Throughout the assessment, the clinician should observe the child's social interaction skills. Does the child seek out the attention of the clinician, engage in isolated play, or avoid interactions? Does the child become upset when the clinician attempts to interact? Does the child make and sustain eye contact? Does the child engage in turn-taking? Are the child's facial expressions and emotional expressions appropriate to the communication context? Does the child return the clinician's smile or express pleasure? How does the child express frustration or discomfort?

- **Initiation of communication with another person:** To observe this skill, the clinician should eliminate all but one or two toys or books from the room, sit with her or his back to the child, and read the book aloud or play with the toy. Does the child attempt to initiate communication? If so, how? Typical behaviors might include such vocalizations as grunting or yelling, and such nonverbal responses as grabbing at the clinician, making eye contact, smiling, manipulating an object to get attention, or handing something to the clinician.

- **Joint attention:** Successful communication often requires joint attention in which both parties are looking at, or attending to, the same object or event. This can be assessed by playing with a toy together or looking at a book together. The clinician should point to pictures in the book and see if the child's gaze follows. Does the child engage in joint attention? If so, how long does he or she maintain it? How does the child get the clinician to attend to something?

- **Requests for a desired object or action:** The clinician should have a number of desired objects or food items in the room to evoke requests (mands). Does the child request them? If so, how? Typical behaviors might include gesturing or moving body parts to indicate "more," pointing to the desired object, moving toward the object, directing his or her eye gaze to the object, leading the clinician to the object, manipulating the clinician's hand to do something, handing the object to be manipulated to the clinician, reaching up to the adult as a request to be picked up, changing facial expressions, or vocalizing. See Behavioral Assessment in Chapter 5 and the *Behavioral Assessment Protocol* in Chapter 9 to assess requests (mands) in a functional manner. The following activities may also help evoke requests (Hegde & Maul, 2006):

  - Engage in an activity such as blowing bubbles or playing with a toy. Stop, put the item up on a shelf, and note down how the child requests that toy.

  - Activate a wind-up toy, let it run down, and see how the child requests that the toy be restarted.

  - Blow up a balloon, let it go so it flies around the room until it deflates, and note down whether the child requests in some way to re-inflate the balloon.

- ○ Engage the child in a familiar song or game such as "The Wheels on the Bus" or "Peek-a-boo," stop, and assess how the child requests that the activity be continued.

- **Declaratives:** Naming or describing (tacting) can often be stimulated by introducing a novel object or event into the environment. For example, have the child remove unseen objects from a bag. Does the child attempt to name or comment on the object? Does the child express delight or displeasure when encountering novel stimuli? Does this evoke any type of vocalization? Does the child hold an object up to show it to someone, implying joint reference skills? See Behavioral Assessment in Chapter 5 and the *Behavioral Assessment Protocol* in Chapter 9 to assess tacts in a functional manner.

- **Protest:** The clinician needs to identify ways in which the child expresses displeasure or shows that he or she does not want a particular object or activity. Nonverbal children often protest or show displeasure through such undesirable behaviors as hitting, pinching, kicking, running away, pushing objects away, pushing the clinician's hand away, crying, or verbalizing in the form of yells, grunts, or other noises. Although these behaviors are undesirable, they are still attempts at communication and need to be considered during the evaluation. For a functional analysis of why children exhibit such behaviors, see the section on Behavioral Assessment in Chapter 5.

In addition to the specific areas just described, the clinician should make observations regarding the type of play activities the child engages in. This may provide additional insight into the child's intellectual functioning and social interaction skills. The clinician should attempt to answer the following questions:

- Does the child engage in primitive play routines such as sensorimotor exploration, mouthing of objects, and shaking and banging objects?

- Does the child demonstrate such actions as pushing a car or brushing his or her hair with a brush?

- Does the child engage in symbolic play or "pretend"?

- Does the child engage in parallel play?

- Does the child participate fully as a play partner, including the demonstration of turn-taking?

A protocol designed to record both qualitative and quantitative observations of the communication behaviors described so far has been included in Chapter 15 (*Nonverbal Expressive Communication: Qualitative and Quantitative Assessment Protocol*).

If possible, systematic observation of the child's communication should also take place while watching the child interact with a familiar person, usually a parent, sibling, or other caregiver. The child's communication behaviors are likely to be more typical when he or she is interacting with a familiar person than when interacting with the clinician. Often, a child may resist interacting with a new person, and it is not unusual to have parents say that their child communicates differently at home. Observation of the parent-child interaction will also help assess the quality of the parents' language model and what they may or may not be doing to facilitate communication with their child. The treatment plan for nonverbal or minimally verbal children, particularly those that are very young, is likely to include parent education and training regarding strategies to facilitate communication and language development in their child.

A videotape of the child interacting at home in his or her natural environment might provide even more useful information than observing the parent-child interaction in the clinic setting. A protocol for documenting *Interaction Between Communicative Partners and the Child* is available in Chapter 15. This should be used in conjunction with the *Qualitative and Quantitative Assessment Protocols for Nonverbal Receptive and Expressive Communication.*

Assessment of Receptive Language

As discussed earlier, some nonverbal or limited verbal children may respond appropriately to standardized tests or test items designed to examine receptive language. In addition, receptive language skills of these children often are better than their expressive language skills. A standardized test may not, however, be appropriate for some children, and even when they are used, the results should be backed up by observations of the child's communication in natural settings or during child-specific assessment tasks.

Although commonly used, the term *receptive language* refers to an inference, not something observable. It is inferred from nonverbal responses given to verbal stimuli. Several typical activities for assessing nonverbal responses to verbal stimuli are described in this section and are also included in the *Nonverbal Receptive Communication: Qualitative and Quantitative Assessment Protocol* presented in Chapter 15. It should be noted that many of these activities can also be adapted, as needed, for incorporation into an AAC assessment. Note that in the following suggested activities designed to assess *receptive vocabulary* or *understanding* of some concepts, the clinicians offers verbal stimuli and the child responds nonverbally.

1. To assess *receptive vocabulary*, have the child identify body parts, pictures, or objects when named by the clinician. The mode of identification may include pointing to or touching the items, looking at the item (eye gaze), or handing the item to the clinician. Use this activity also to assess the child's understanding of colors, shapes, letters, and numbers. For example, "Give me the red block," "Give me 2 blocks," or "Show me the circle."

2. To assess the *understanding of pronouns,* ask the child to point to pictures representing "*He* is jumping" versus "*She* is jumping" versus "*They* are jumping," and so on.

3. To assess the understanding of singular verses plural, ask the child to give you *the block* versus *the blocks.*

4. To assess the understanding of prepositions, ask the child to put the block *in the box* versus *under the box* versus *on top of the box,* and so on.

5. Use similar strategies to assess a child's understanding of basic concepts such as *big* versus *little* or *full* versus *empty.*

6. Have the child follow simple, basic commands and gradually increase the length or complexity of these commands. To minimize the influence of contextual information, include several items which involve atypical actions such as, "Kiss the ball" or "Sit on the book."

7. Ask the child several simple, concrete *yes-no* questions to further check comprehension.

Assessment of Verbalizations

Most nonverbal children produce some type of atypical vocalizations or idiosyncratic noises, and some minimally verbal children might produce single words or even a few multiword combinations. These verbalizations should be noted, along with their potential effects on the listeners. The assessment should include an inventory of true words or word approximations. Whether verbalizations that are not word approximations are *Phonetically Consistent Forms* (PCF) should be noted (Dore, Franklin, Miller, & Ramer, 1976). A PCF is a vocalization that is stable and consistently produced under specific stimulus conditions (e.g., in relation to a certain object, person, or situation). PCFs typically consist of vowels or consonant-vowel combinations (Haynes & Pindzola, 2004). In addition to assessing the child's spontaneous verbalizations, the clinician should assess the child's imitation of nonspeech sounds, speech sounds, simple words, and phrases.

In essence, the limited amount of verbal language produced by this group of children often greatly limits the usefulness of speech and language sample analysis protocols presented in Chapters 7 and 9. Therefore, we propose a single protocol designed to assess any verbalizations that do occur, including both the speech and language aspects of those verbalizations. The *Verbalizations of Nonverbal or Minimally Verbal Children: Assessment Protocol* was designed for this purpose and is available in Chapter 15. It should be used in conjunction with the *Qualitative and Quantitative Assessment Protocols for Nonverbal Receptive and Expressive Communication* to make a complete assessment of the child's verbal, as well as nonverbal, communication skills.

Analysis and Integration of Assessment Results

The assessment of nonverbal and minimally verbal children involves the analysis and integration of assessment results from various sources. Results of such standard and common sources of information, as the case history, interview, orofacial examination, hearing screening or audiologic assessment, and standardized and criterion-referenced instruments must be integrated with unique data that emerge from specialized sources. These sources include the systematic qualitative and quantitative observation of nonverbal communication, the assessment of verbalizations that do occur, and information from a variety of other professionals and team members. Information from these varied sources will be integrated and analyzed in order to determine whether the child's lack of verbal communication is associated with a severe speech production disorder such as dysarthria or childhood apraxia of speech, with a severe language disorder, or with a combination of both. Next, the child's prognosis for developing verbal communication will be evaluated and subsequent recommendations made.

1. Draw a profile of the child and the family. Consider information provided in the case history and interview when formulating a profile of the child's and the family's communication patterns; explore the family's ethnocultural background and any bilingual or bidialectal status; describe the onset and development of the disorder, associated clinical conditions, family's reaction to the child's communication problem, ethnocultural values and factors that affect the child's communication disorder, previous assessment or treatment results, and reports from other professionals; describe the academic demands the child faces in school; describe the child's interests, hobbies, any special talents, and favorite activities.

2. Analyze the effects of the child's communication problem on academic achievement, and socialization. Use the information from the case history, interview, academic records, and information supplied from the teachers and other professionals to make this analysis.

3. To evaluate the presence of a severe speech production disorder, the clinician should:
    *   Review the orofacial examination and diadochokinetic results for signs of severe muscle weakness, incoordination, or motor sequencing deficits.
    *   Establish the child's phonetic inventory for sounds produced spontaneously.
    *   Create an inventory of additional speech sounds the child produced imitatively.
    *   Establish the intelligibility of any words or word combinations produced by the child.
    *   Make an analysis of apraxic speech, if warranted; use the *Childhood Apraxia of Speech Assessment Protocol* in Chapter 7.
    *   Make an analysis of dysarthria, if warranted; use the *Dysarthric Speech Assessment Protocol* in Chapter 7.

4. As discussed earlier, standardized language tests often are not appropriate for nonverbal or minimally verbal children. However, if they are administered, the results should be summarized and integrated into the information described below. To analyze a child's expressive communication the clinician describes any observed or reported attempts at verbal or nonverbal communication. Several of the protocols available in Chapter 15 will be helpful for organizing and documenting these communication attempts. The clinician should:
    *   Describe unintelligible vocalizations.
    *   List true words or word approximations produced by the child spontaneously.
    *   List true words or word approximations produced by the child imitatively.
    *   List PCFs used by the child.
    *   List any word combinations produced by the child.

- Describe gestures used by the child and their communicative intent.
- Describe any other non-verbal behaviors exhibited by the child in an attempt to communicate.
- Note whether the child seeks or avoids social interaction, initiates communication, establishes joint attention, or demonstrates appropriate eye contact.
- Note any unusual, stereotypic, echolalic, or idiosyncratic productions that might be characteristic of autism spectrum disorder.

5. To analyze the child's receptive language the clinician summarizes the results of any standardized receptive language tests that were administered, and describes verbal and non-verbal responses given to verbal stimuli. The clinician should:
   - Describe the child's ability to identify one or more objects, body parts, pictures, and familiar people when named.
   - Describe the child's ability to follow simple, concrete, one-step directions, with and without visual cues.
   - Describe the child's ability to follow complex or multi-part directions, with or without visual cues.
   - Describe the child's ability to follow directions that require an understanding of basic concepts, morphologic structures, or syntactic structures.

The integration and subsequent analysis of the information described above may lead to a differential diagnosis of a speech production disorder or language disorder. The clinician is directed to the *Diagnostic Criteria and Differential Diagnosis* section in Chapter 6, and the *Differential Diagnosis of Child Language Disorders* section in Chapter 8. The information and guidelines presented in these sections will assist the clinician in making a differential diagnosis of speech production or language disorders in nonverbal or minimally verbal children.

Prognosis for Developing Verbal Communication

Prior to arriving at a set of recommendations, the clinician should summarize the collected data. This summary should include a description of the child's communication strengths and weaknesses. This information will help the clinician estimate the child's prognosis for developing verbal, nonverbal, or both kinds of skills. The prognosis for developing verbal communication is highly variable because of the heterogeneity of the population. With early intervention, parent training, and family involvement, the speech and language skills of most young children will improve significantly. There are, however, several indicators that the prognosis for developing verbal communication may be limited (Hegde & Maul, 2006):

- A primary diagnosis that is typically associated with a lack of speech and language development (e.g., profound intellectual disability, severe autism, serious neuromuscular disorders, and severe expression of genetic syndromes that prevent oral language acquisition)

- A history of regression where the child once had a few words that disappeared with no development of new language skills (e.g., Childhood Disintegrative Disorder) (American Psychiatric Association, 2000b)

- Poor stimulability for oral speech as indicated by an inability to imitate verbalizations (Carr & Dores, 1981; Yoder & Layton, 1988)

- No or few canonical vocal communication acts (utterances that contain at least one C-V sequence) (Yoder, Warren, & McCatheren, 1998)

- Few nonverbal or verbal communication acts that direct the adult's attention to an object or shared event (Yoder, Warren, & McCatheren, 1998)

- The age of the child (older children are less likely to show the progress younger children might).

Postassessment Counseling

During the final phase of the assessment, the clinician counsels the parents or others who accompany the child. Although the results of the assessment may not have been fully analyzed, the clinician will have gained clinical impressions that are valid enough to summarize the results, make a tentative diagnosis, offer recommendations, describe treatment options, suggest prognosis, and answer the most frequently asked questions.

Make a Tentative Diagnosis

Summarize your observations and clinical impressions gained from the observations. To the extent the observations justify, make as clear a diagnosis as possible. Describe the main features of the child's speech production or language disorder as described in Chapters 6 and 8. Speech and language disorders that are severe enough to render a child nonverbal or minimally verbal are often associated with other clinical conditions. Point out typical associations while avoiding any implication that one clinical condition may be the cause of the other clinical condition. For example, you might say that children with autism typically have language disorders, but do not imply that autism is the cause of the language disorder.

Suggest Prognosis

As discussed earlier, the prognosis for these children to develop verbal communication is highly variable because of the heterogeneity of the population. The clinician should summarize the child's strengths and weaknesses as they relate to the indicators described in the section titled *Prognosis for Developing Verbal Communication*. Information presented in the *Suggest Prognosis* sections of Chapters 6 and 8 may also be helpful here. Estimate the child's prognosis for developing verbal communication, nonverbal communication, or both kinds of skills. With early intervention, parent training, and family involvement, the speech and language skills of some of these children will improve significantly. If the prognosis for developing verbal communication is poor, early intervention focused on the development of AAC strategies may greatly improve their functional communication skills.

Make Recommendations

If the child's diagnosis and prognosis are favorable for the development of functional verbal communication, then the parents may be counseled as per the *Postassessment Counseling* outlined in Chapter 8 for children with language disorders and in Chapter 6 for children with severe speech production disorders. If the assessment resulted in a guarded or poor prognosis for the development of verbal communication, then parents should be counseled to consider AAC assessment, as discussed in Chapter 16.

Answer Frequently Asked Questions

Frequently asked questions associated with severe speech and language disorders are addressed in Chapters 6 and 8. Frequently asked questions regarding AAC are addressed in Chapter 16. Clinicians are directed to these chapters for information that will assist them in answering questions that are commonly asked by parents or caregivers of nonverbal and minimally verbal children.

CHAPTER 15

Assessment of Nonverbal and Minimally Verbal Children: Protocols

- Note on Common Protocols
- Note on Specific Protocols
- Assessment of Nonverbal and Minimally Verbal Children: Interview Protocol
- Verbalizations of Nonverbal or Minimally Verbal Children: Assessment Protocol
- Nonverbal *Expressive* Communication: Qualitative and Quantitative Assessment Protocol
- Nonverbal *Receptive* Communication: Qualitative and Quantitative Assessment Protocol
- Interaction Between Communicative Partners and the Child: Assessment Protocol

Note on Common Protocols

In completing a speech and language assessment for a nonverbal or minimally verbal child, the clinician may use several of the common protocols given in Chapter 2, also available on the CD. To make a comprehensive assessment, the clinician may modify as needed and print for use the following common protocols from the CD:

The Child Case History Form

Orofacial Examination and Hearing Screening Protocol

Use this protocol along with the *Instructions for Conducting the Orofacial Examination: Observations and Implications.* If the preliminary findings of the orofacial examination suggests the possibility of velopharyngeal inadequacy or incompetence, use the *Resonance and Velopharyngeal Function Assessment* protocol in Chapter 13. Often, it is not possible to complete a hearing screening with this population. In this case, if it has not already occurred, a complete audiologic evaluation should be recommended.

Assessment Report Outline

Expand the language section to include relevant information gathered through the observations of nonverbal and verbal communication strategies. Include information relevant to AAC if it was included in the assessment. Recommendations should include referral for an AAC assessment, as appropriate.

Note on Specific Protocols

This chapter contains a collection of protocols that can be used individually or combined in a variety of ways to facilitate the evaluation of a child's communication disorder. Each of these protocols is also available on the CD.

The protocols on the CD may be individualized and printed out as a group and used for a complete assessment. Also, one or more protocols may be selectively printed out and used as needed. In assessing children with multiple disorders of communication, the clinician may combine these protocols with protocols from other chapters. It should be noted that nonverbal and limited verbal children are extremely heterogeneous, representing a wide range of ages, cognitive abilities, and motor abilities. Therefore, specific protocol items may need to be eliminated or adjusted, as needed for a specific child. For example, the interview protocol includes a wide array of questions that may not apply to all children. If the child is not in a school setting, or if AAC is not a consideration, then those questions can be eliminated during the interview.

Nonverbal and Minimally Verbal Children Assessment Protocol 1
Interview Protocol

Child's Name _____ DOB _____ Date _____ Clinician _____

Individualize this protocol on the CD and print it for your use.

Preparation

☐ Review the "interview guidelines" presented in Chapter 1.

☐ Make sure the setting is comfortable with adequate seating and lighting.

☐ Record the interview whenever possible.

☐ Find out if the parent is comfortable having the child in the same room during the interview. If so, have something for the child to do (toys, books, etc.). If not, make arrangements for someone else to supervise the child in a different room during the interview. If it is not too distracting, it might be valuable to have a nonverbal or minimally verbal child in the same room, as there may be opportunities to observe communication attempts at this time (e.g., trying to get mom's attention).

☐ Review the case history ahead of time, noting areas you want to review or obtain more information about.

Introduction

☐ Introduce yourself. Briefly review your plan for the day and how long you expect it to take.

Example: "Hello Mr. /Mrs. [parent's name]. My name is [clinician's name] and I am the speech-language pathologist who will be assessing [child's name] today. I would like to start by reviewing the case history and asking you a few questions. Once we are finished talking, I will spend some time observing [child's name] as he interacts with you. I may also spend some time working with [child's name] individually. Today's assessment should take about [estimate the amount of time you plan to spend].

☐ Who is the person(s) being interviewed?

Name(s):

Relationship(s) to child:

(continues)

Interview Protocol (continued)

Interview Questions

These questions may need to be individualized, depending on the child's age, communication abilities, cognitive abilities, motor abilities, and living situation. If it is decided to use a standardized measurement instrument based on parent or caregiver report, those questions may be integrated into, or used in lieu of, all or some of the questions listed below.

☐ Review the Case History and ask follow-up questions, as needed, regarding the child's medical, developmental, educational and social history.

☐ Has anyone else in your family had communication problems?

☐ Has [child's name] ever had his [her] hearing tested? If yes, what were the results? If no, do you suspect any hearing problems?

☐ Has [child's name] ever had his [her] vision tested? If yes, what were the results? If no, do you suspect any vision problems?

☐ Has [child's name] ever had his [her] speech or language assessed before? If yes, when and where was this done? What were the results? How did you feel about that?

☐ Has your child received speech-language therapy before? If yes, when and where? What did they work on in therapy? Can you describe the types of activities that were used? How did your child respond? Do you feel the therapy was helpful? Why or why not?

☐ Has your child seen any other specialists for this problem? If so, who and when? What were their recommendations? How have you followed up on this?

☐ Does [child's name] have any physical problems? Can you describe them to me?

☐ Do you have any concerns about [child's name] fine motor or gross motor skills?

☐ Please describe a typical day in the life of your child. (Note information regarding the child's routine; opportunities for cognitive, speech, and language stimulation; opportunities for socialization and communication; communication partners; household rules; behavioral problems; etc.)

☐ With whom does [child's name] communicate with throughout the day?

☐ Does [child's name] attend any type of school or preschool? When? Where? How does he [she] communicate there?

☐ How are your child's preacademic or academic skills?

☐ What is your child's primary method of communication?

☐ How does [child's name] communicate with you?

☐ How does [child's name] communicate with other family members?

☐ How does [child's name] communicate with other children?

☐ How does [child's name] communicate with strangers?

☐ How does [child's name] tell you he [she] wants or needs something? (points, gestures, vocalizes, pulls on you, etc.)

☐ Does [child's name] make eye contact when he [she] tries to communicate with you?

☐ Does [child's name] try to say words?

☐ Does [child's name] have any true words that you and others understand? If yes, what are they?

☐ About what percent of your child's speech is understood by you? By others?

☐ Does [child's name] ever combine words together? If yes, can you give me some examples?

☐ How does [child's name] react when others do not understand?

☐ What does [child's name] do when he is upset or does not get what he [she] wants? How do you react to this?

☐ Does your child exhibit any specific behavior problems that you are concerned about? How do you handle these?

☐ Does your child exhibit any antisocial or socially inappropriate behaviors? How do you handle these?

☐ Does [child's name] exhibit any self-stimulating behaviors (e.g., rocking, flapping arms, spinning, etc.)? If yes, when do they occur?

☐ Does [child's name] seem to understand what you say to him [her]? Can you give me an example?

☐ Does your child respond to his [her] name? How?

☐ Does [child's name] answer questions? How?

☐ Does [child's name] follow directions? Can you give me an example?

☐ Does [child's name] attempt to imitate others? Can you give me some examples?

☐ What types of play activities does your child engage in?

☐ Does [child's name] play with objects appropriately?

☐ Does [child's name] use objects to pretend? For example, does he [she] pretend to talk on a toy phone or pretend to drink from a cup?

☐ Does your child use toys for banging, mouthing, spinning, manipulating, or exploring in other ways?

☐ Does [child's name] play with other children? Does [child's name] play with other adults? If yes, does your child take turns, share toys, or make eye contact when playing with others?

☐ Is English your child's first language? If not, what other language(s) is he [she] exposed to?

☐ What language is spoken most often in the home?

(continues)

The following questions are more specific to AAC. They can be selected and added as part of any assessment where there is a possibility that AAC might be considered.

☐ What types of verbal or nonverbal communication strategies have you tried with your child? (The clinician may need to provide examples of verbal and nonverbal communication strategies.)

☐ Have you ever considered nonverbal communication strategies such as sign language, gestures, pictures, electronic devices or other things that might help your child communicate?

☐ These are also sometimes called augmentative or alternative communication (AAC) systems or devices. Which ones have you tried or considered?

☐ Have you ever seen or known anyone else who used a nonverbal communication system?

☐ Do you have specific concerns regarding nonverbal communication strategies? (If yes, address their concerns here. They can also be addressed as part of the postassessment counseling if AAC is recommended.)

☐ I'm not saying that [child's name] will need a nonverbal communication system, but if we think it would help him [her] to communicate would you be open to trying it or learning more about it?

☐ How do you think other family members will feel about this? Will they be supportive? Will they use the system to communicate with [child's name]?

☐ At home, who will be the primary person responsible for helping [child's name] use the AAC system, and for helping others learn to communicate with [child's name]?

☐ At school, who will be the primary person responsible for helping [child's name] use the AAC system, and for helping others learn to communicate with [child's name]?

☐ At [other environments the child is in], who will be the primary person responsible for helping [child's name] use the AAC system, and for helping others learn to communicate with [child's name]?

☐ Some AAC systems or devices don't cost anything, others may have a minimal cost involved, and still others are relatively expensive. Can you tell me about any financial resources or limitations that we should consider as we move forward with our assessment? Once we complete our assessment and make our recommendations, we will also provide you with additional information regarding costs and possible funding resources.

Closing the Interview

☐ Summarize the major points that you gathered from the interview, allowing the parent or caregiver to interrupt or correct information, as needed.

☐ Is there anything else you would like me to know about [child's name] communication?

☐ Do you have any questions for me at this point?

☐ Thank you very much for you input. The information has been very helpful.

☐ Now, I want to observe the different ways that [child's name] communicates with you. I would like you to spend a few minutes playing with him [her]. I may ask you to do some specific things with [child's name], but other than that, just interact as you normally would. At some point, I may ask you to sit off to the side or leave the room so that I can work individually with [child's name] for a few minutes. Once we are finished, I will sit down to share my findings with you.

Nonverbal and Minimally Verbal Children Assessment Protocol 2
Verbalizations of Nonverbal or Minimally Verbal Children: Assessment Protocol

Child's Name _____ DOB _____ Date _____ Clinician _____

Individualize this protocol on the CD and print it for your use.

Typical Vocalization	Communicative Context

Atypical Vocalizations List phonetically transcribed or described atypical vocalizations or idiosyncratic noises:

_____

_____

_____

_____

_____

_____

True Words and Word Approximations

List true words and word approximations below. Word approximations should be phonetically transcribed. Circle "O" if you observed the child using the word, and "R" if it was reported by a family member or caregiver.

True Word or Approximation	Phonetic Transcription	Observed or Reported	Communication Context
		O R	
		O R	
		O R	
		O R	
		O R	
		O R	
		O R	
		O R	
		O R	
		O R	
		O R	
		O R	
		O R	
		O R	
		O R	
		O R	
		O R	
		O R	
		O R	
		O R	
		O R	
		O R	

(continues)

Verbalizations of Nonverbal or Minimally Verbal Children: Assessment Protocol (continued)

Word Combinations

Word Combinations (transcribe, as needed)	Observed or Reported	Communication Context
	O R	
	O R	
	O R	
	O R	
	O R	
	O R	
	O R	
	O R	
	O R	
	O R	
	O R	
	O R	
	O R	
	O R	
	O R	
	O R	
	O R	
	O R	
	O R	
	O R	
	O R	
	O R	
	O R	
	O R	

Phonetically Consistent Forms (PCFs)

A PCF is a vocalization that is stable and consistently produced in the context of certain objects, persons, or situations. PCFs usually consist of vowels or consonant-vowel combinations.

Phonetically Consistent Forms (transcribe, as needed)	Observed or Reported	Communication Context
	O R	
	O R	
	O R	
	O R	
	O R	
	O R	
	O R	
	O R	
	O R	
	O R	
	O R	
	O R	
	O R	
	O R	
	O R	

Add additional rows, as needed.

(continues)

Verbalizations of Nonverbal or Minimally Verbal Children: Assessment Protocol (continued)

The Child's Imitative Phonetic and Basic Language Skills

1. Did the child imitate nonspeech sounds, such as that of a car,
    a bell, or animal sounds?   No   Yes

    If yes, provide examples:

2. Did the child imitate speech sounds?   No   Yes

    If yes, provide examples:

3. Did the child imitate simple words?   No   Yes

    If yes, provide examples:

4. Did the child imitate simple phrases?   No   Yes

    If yes, provide examples:

Comments on the child's verbal speech and language skills:

Nonverbal and Minimally Verbal Children Assessment Protocol 3
Nonverbal *Expressive* Communication:
Qualitative and Quantitative Assessment Protocol

Child's Name _____ DOB _____ Date _____ Clinician _____

Individualize this protocol on the CD and print it for your use.

Prior to initiating the assessment, arrange the room in a way that encourages the child to interact. Provide access to a variety of age-appropriate toys, books, and stimulus items. The assessment should include observations of spontaneous play as well as the child's responses during various tasks designed to evoke social interaction, initiation of communication, joint attention, requests, declaratives, and protest. This protocol is worded to document the child's interaction with the clinician; however the same activities and protocol can be used to observe the child's interaction with others. This assessment is based on observation of the child while interacting with: (circle all that apply)

      the clinician   parent(s)   sibling(s)

      other children   other: _____

Expressive Communication			
Communication Skill	**Child-Specific Strategy**	**Behavior**	**Scoring**
Social Interaction During Play Activities	1. Engage the child in spontaneous play activities.	Does the child become upset when the clinician attempts to interact?	Y N
		Does the child avoid interacting or prefer to play by him or herself?	Y N
	2. After a few minutes, turn away and play with something by yourself.	Does the child seek out the attention of the clinician?	Y N
		How does the child get the clinician's attention?	

(continues)

*Nonverbal **Expressive** Communication: Qualitative and Quantitative Assessment Protocol (continued)*

Communication Skill	Child-Specific Strategy	Behavior	Scoring	
Social Interaction During Play Activities *(continued)*	3. Spend several minutes playing. Include activities that require "turn-taking."	Does the child make eye contact?	Y	N
		Does the child sustain eye contact appropriately?	Y	N
		Does the child engage in turn-taking?	Y	N
		Are the child's facial expressions and emotional responses appropriate to the context/activity?	Y	N
		How does the child express frustration, anger, or discomfort?		
		Other Comments:		
Initiation of Communication	Eliminate all but 1 or 2 toys or books from the room. Sit with your back to the child and read the book or play with the toy.	Does the child attempt to initiate communication?	Y	N
		If yes, how? (quantify these behaviors by tallying the number of times each one occurs)	☐ vocalizing, such as grunting or yelling	
			☐ grabbing	
			☐ hitting	
			☐ making eye contact	
			☐ smiling	
			☐ moving an object or handing something to the clinician to get attention	
			☐ other:	

Communication Skill	Child-Specific Strategy	Behavior	Scoring
Joint Attention	Joint attention means that both parties are looking at or attending to the same object or event. Engage in one or more of the following activities together: ☐ play with a toy ☐ look at a book ☐ work on a puzzle	When pointing to pictures in a book, does the child's eye gaze follow? Does the child engage in joint attention during these activities? If yes, for how long is it maintained? How does the child get the clinician to attend to something? (quantify these behaviors by tallying the number of times each one occurs)	Y N Y N ☐ vocalizing ☐ pointing ☐ moving the clinician's hand ☐ physically turning the clinician's head ☐ moving an object toward the clinician ☐ other:
Request for a Desired Object or Action (Imperative)	1. Place a number of "desired toys" or a "desired food item" in the room, but out of the child's reach. 2. Engage in an activity such as blowing bubbles or playing with a toy. Stop and put the item up on a shelf. How does the child react? 3. Activate a wind-up toy and then let it run down. How does the child react?	Does the child request something? If yes, how? (quantify these behaviors by tallying the number of times each one occurs)	Y N ☐ vocalizing ☐ crying ☐ pointing ☐ gesturing an action or "more" ☐ moving toward the object ☐ manipulating the clinician's hand to do something

*Nonverbal **Expressive** Communication: Qualitative and Quantitative Assessment Protocol (continued)*

Communication Skill	Child-Specific Strategy	Behavior	Scoring
Request for a Desired Object or Action (Imperative) *(continued)*	4. Blow up a balloon or throw a paper airplane. Let it fly around the room. How does the child react when it stops? 5. Engage in a familiar song/game, such as "peek-a-boo" or "wheels on the bus." Stop. How does the child react?		☐ reaching to be picked up ☐ other:
	6. For one or more of the activities above (1–5), model a correct verbal response, such as "bubble," "go," or "more." 7. For one or more of the activities above (1–5), model a correct gestural response or "sign," such as "want," "bubble," or "more." Use hand-over-hand modeling to help the child gesture, then reinforce by responding positively to it.	How does the child respond to clinicians' modeling? (quantify these behaviors by tallying the number of times each one occurs)	☐ attempts to imitate verbalizations ☐ attempts to imitate gestures ☐ other:

Communication Skill	Child-Specific Strategy	Behavior	Scoring
Declaratives	Attempt to evoke by presenting a novel item or event into the environment. For example, have the child remove an unseen object from a bag. How does the child react?	Does the child attempt to name or comment on the object? Is there a verbal response? Is there a gestural response? Other:	Y　　　N Y　　　N Y　　　N
Protest	During the previously described activities identify ways in which the child expresses displeasure or shows that they do not want a particular toy or activity.	How does the child show displeasure? (quantify these behaviors by tallying the number of times each one occurs)	☐ says "no" ☐ shakes head to indicate "no" ☐ vocalizes (yells, grunts, other noises) ☐ cries ☐ turns away, moves away, or runs away ☐ hits, pinches, kicks ☐ pushes objects away ☐ pushes clinician's hand away ☐ other:

(continues)

*Nonverbal **Expressive** Communication: Qualitative and Quantitative Assessment Protocol (continued)*

Communication Skill	Child-Specific Strategy	Behavior	Scoring
Types of Play the Child Engages In	Use the activities described above to assess the types of play the child engages in.	Does the child engage in primitive play routines? (quantify these behaviors by tallying the number of times each one occurs)	Y N ☐ engaging in sensorimotor exploration ☐ mouthing objects ☐ shaking or "spinning" objects ☐ banging objects
		Does the child demonstrate functional use of an object such as pushing a car, flying an airplane, or brushing his/her hair with a hair brush?	Y N
		Does the child engage in symbolic play or "pretend"?	Y N
		Does the child participate appropriately as a play partner, including the demonstration of turn-taking? Other:	Y N

Nonverbal and Minimally Verbal Children Assessment Protocol 4
Nonverbal *Receptive* Communication:
Qualitative and Quantitative Assessment Protocol

Child's Name _____ DOB _____ Date _____ Clinician _____

Individualize this protocol on the CD and print it for your use.

Receptive Communication		
Communication Skill	**Child-Specific Strategy**	**Scoring**
Comprehension of Single Words	1. Have the child identify people or objects in the environment. "Where is mommy/daddy/ name of sibling or other person who accompanied the child?" "Where is the window/chair, etc.?" 2. Have the child identify body parts named by the clinician. "Where is your nose?" "Show me your eyes." 3. Place several common objects or toys on the table (e.g., ball, car, cup, doll teddy bear, etc.). "Where is (name toy/object)?" "Show me (name toy/object)." "Give me (name toy/object)." 4. Repeat #3 using age-appropriate picture stimuli of common objects, or family members. This activity can also be used to assess the child's understanding of shapes or colors. 5. Look at a book together and ask the child to identify pictures in the book.	*Qualitative Analysis:* What was the child's mode of response? ☐ pointing ☐ eye gaze ☐ other: Does the child's accuracy improve with repetition? Y N Does the child's accuracy improve with cueing? Y N ☐ visual cuing ☐ tactile cuing ☐ other: *Quantitative Analysis:* Quantify the child's receptive vocabulary by tallying a "+" every time the child correctly identifies the stimulus item, and a "−" every time the child is incorrect. The clinician may choose to list the actual stimulus words, as appropriate. ☐ body part identification ☐ identification of objects or toys ☐ identification of pictures

(continues)

*Nonverbal **Receptive** Communication: Qualitative and Quantitative Assessment Protocol (continued)*

Communication Skill	Child-Specific Strategy	Scoring
Understanding of Basic Concepts (these words are often used as modifiers)	1. Utilize several contrasting objects or pictures to represent all or some of the following concepts: big/little, long/short, empty/full, happy/sad, rough/smooth, soft/hard, hot/cold, high/low, tall/short, fast/slow. For example: • Place a large ball and a small ball on the table and ask the child: "Show me the big one." or "Show me the little one." • Place pictures on the table representing a full glass and an empty glass and ask the child: "Show me the full glass." or "Show me the empty glass." 2. Assess number concepts by placing several objects (e.g., blocks) on the table and tell the child: "Give me one block." "Give me two blocks." "Give me [number] blocks."	Quantify the child's understanding of basic concepts by tallying a "+" every time the child correctly identifies the stimulus item, and a "–" every time the child is incorrect. ☐ big ☐ little ☐ long ☐ short ☐ empty ☐ full ☐ happy ☐ sad ☐ rough ☐ smooth ☐ soft ☐ hard ☐ hot ☐ cold ☐ high ☐ low ☐ tall ☐ short ☐ fast ☐ slow ☐ numbers: ☐ other: total % correct =

Communication Skill	Child-Specific Strategy	Scoring

Understanding Singular Versus Plural	1. Place several of the same object on the table (e.g., balls, blocks, cars, etc.). Say to the child:
	"Give me the ball."
	"Give me the balls."
	Repeat with different objects.
	
	2. Place pictures showing a singular form (e.g., cat) and a plural form (e.g., cats) on the table and say to the child:
	"Show me the cat."
	"Show me the cats."
	Repeat with different objects.
		Quantify the child's understanding of singular and plural by tallying a "+" every time the child correctly identifies the stimulus item(s), and a "−" every time the child is incorrect.
		
		☐ singular form
		  • pictures
		  • objects
		  total % correct
		  for singular forms =
		
		☐ plural form
		  • pictures
		  • objects
		  total % correct
		  for plural forms =

Understanding of Pronouns	Display pictures of children and animals performing various actions, such as a boy jumping, a girl jumping, a horse jumping, and a group of children jumping. Say to the child: "Show me *he* is jumping." "Show me *she* is jumping." "Show me *it* is jumping." "Show me *they* are jumping." Repeat with different pictures.	Quantify the child's understanding of pronouns by tallying a "+" every time the child identifies the correct picture and a "−" every time the child is incorrect. ☐ he ☐ she ☐ it ☐ they total % correct for pronouns =
Understanding of Prepositions	1. Ask the child to move object, such as: "Put the block *in* the box." "Put the block *under* the box." "Put the doll *on* the chair." "Put the doll *behind* the chair." "Put the block *beside* the box." Repeat with different objects. 2. Display pictures that represent the various prepositions and ask the child to identify the correct one, such as: "Show me the dog is under the table."	Quantify the child's understanding of prepositions by tallying a "+" every time the child correctly places an object or identifies the correct picture and a "−" every time the child is incorrect. ☐ in ☐ under ☐ on ☐ behind ☐ beside total % correct for prepositions =

(continues)

*Nonverbal **Receptive** Communication: Qualitative and Quantitative Assessment Protocol (continued)*

Communication Skill	Child-Specific Strategy	Scoring
Comprehension of Simple Questions	If the child has a verbal or gestural strategy for indicating "yes" and "no," ask several simple, concrete questions. Intermix the questions so both "yes" and "no" responses are required. Ask questions such as: • Is your name _____? (ask with correct and incorrect name) • Do you have a brother/sister? • Do you have a dog/cat? • Is this a ball? (hold up a ball or something other than a ball) • Is this your shirt? (point to child's shirt or a different clothing item) • Is this my nose? (point to your nose or other body part)	What was the child's mode of response? Quantify the child's understanding of questions by tallying a "+" every time the child correctly responds with "yes" or "no" and a "–" every time the child is incorrect. total % correct for yes-no questions =
Comprehension of Basic Commands	1. These tasks may need to be adjusted depending on the child's physical capabilities. Ask the child to follow some simple directions, such as: • stand up • sit down • raise your hand • stomp your feet • throw the ball • kiss the baby (doll) • tickle the teddy bear 2. Note the child's ability to follow directions during the previous tasks: Understanding of Basic Concepts, Understanding Singular Versus Plural, and Understanding of Prepositions.	Quantify the child's understanding of basic commands by tallying a "+" every time the child responds correctly and a "–" every time the child is incorrect. ☐ simple, concrete directions total % correct for simple, concrete directions =

Communication Skill	Child-Specific Strategy	Scoring
	3. If the child does well on 1 & 2, try some complex or multiple-part commands, such as: • Stand up and raise your hand. • Go get the book and put it in the box. • Pick up the bear and put it on your head. • Give me the ball and the truck. • Kiss the baby and tickle the bear.	☐ complex and multipart directions total % correct for complex and multipart directions =

Nonverbal and Minimally Verbal Children Assessment Protocol 5
Interaction Between Communicative Partners and the Child: Assessment Protocol

Child's Name _____ DOB _____ Date _____ Clinician _____

Communicative Partner (CP):   Relationship:

Individualize this protocol on the CD and print it for your use.

Observe the parent or communicative partner (CP) as they interact with the child. Identify the communicative behaviors that are demonstrated by the CP. This information can be helpful in assessing the communication strategies being used, and in identifying areas that need to be addressed in the intervention plan. In order to quantify these behaviors, place a tally mark in the "Yes" column each time the behavior occurs. Place a tally mark in the "No" column each time there is an opportunity for the given behavior to occur, but it does not.

Communicative Behavior	Was the behavior demonstrated?	
	Yes	No
The parent/CP encourages communication by looking at the child expectantly.		
The parent/CP reinforces communication through action or verbalization.		
The parent/CP talks at the child's eye level.		
The parent/CP successfully interprets the child's verbalizations.		
The parent/CP successfully interprets the child's nonverbal communicative intent.		
The parent/CP creates communication opportunities.		
The parent/CP does not reduce communication opportunity by anticipating the child's needs ahead of time.		
The parent/CP attempts to establish joint reference with the child.		
The parent/CP talks about present context (here and now).		
The parent/CP reduces his or her sentence length when speaking to the child.		
The parent/CP reduces his or her sentence complexity when speaking to the child.		

Communicative Behavior	Was the behavior demonstrated?	
	Yes	No
The parent/CP uses a slower speech rate when speaking to the child.		
The parent/CP repeats frequently (redundancy).		
The parent/CP paraphrases utterances in different ways.		
The parent/CP uses exaggerated intonation patterns.		
The parent/CP places stress on important words.		
The parent/CP uses concrete, high-frequency vocabulary.		
The parent/CP does not dominate the conversation.		
The parent/CP avoids excessive questions and commands.		
The parent/CP demonstrates self-talk.		
The parent/CP demonstrates parallel talk.		
The parent/CP demonstrates expansion.		

Other Observations or Comments:

CHAPTER 16

Assessment for Augmentative and Alternative Communication Systems

- The Three Phases of AAC System Assessment
- The Role of Speech-Language Pathologists
- Resources for the Clinician
- Historical Perspective
- Revised Participation Model
- Analysis and Integration of Assessment Results
- Postassessment Counseling

As described in Chapter 14, the prognosis for a nonverbal or minimally verbal child to develop verbal communication will vary depending on the severity of his or her physical or intellectual disabilities. When the assessment results indicate a poor prognosis for the development of oral speech, the clinician should consider an augmentative or alternative communication (AAC) system. Demographic studies indicate that approximately two million Americans (between 0.8% and 1.2% of the U.S. population) are unable to speak or write to meet their daily communication needs (ASHA, 2004a). In an urban area of Washington state, Matas, Mathy-Laikko, Beukelman, and Legresley (1985) found that 0.3 to 0.6% of school-age children and 3 to 6% of children receiving special education services were unable to communicate through speech. Burd, Hammes, Bronhoeft, and Fisher (1988) found that 2% of all students receiving special education services in the state of North Dakota were "nonverbal." Binger and Light (2006) reported that 12% of preschoolers receiving special education services required AAC. They also reported that 71% of the AAC users in their study were male, and 29% were female. A 2002 survey of speech-language pathologists revealed that 45% of those surveyed indicated they regularly serve individuals with AAC needs (ASHA, 2002).

The inability to speak or write without assistance can result from a variety of congenital or acquired conditions, many of which were described in Chapter 14. The most common congenital conditions associated with severe communicative disorders include autism, intellectual disability, cerebral palsy, several genetic syndromes, and severe apraxia of speech. Acquired impairments that might result in a need for AAC in children include traumatic brain injury, hypoxia, or spinal chord injury. Such conditions may be chronic in some individuals, resulting in a long-term need for AAC. In some cases, the need for AAC is temporary. For instance, people after laryngeal surgery or temporary tracheotomy may need AAC for a short duration. Most AAC assessments are done with a long-term perspective, however.

The Three Phases of AAC System Assessment

The underlying clinical conditions that necessitate an AAC system for a child may change over time. The child's capabilities may improve or deteriorate. Consequently, communication needs and skills of AAC users may change as they get older. This will in turn require changes in the system initially selected for the child. Therefore, AAC assessment is a dynamic process. Beukelman and Mirenda (2005) describe this process as having three phases: the initial assessment for today, the detailed assessment for tomorrow, and the follow-up assessment.

Phase I: Initial Assessment for Today involves completing the initial assessment to design an intervention that matches the child's communication needs and capabilities. It also includes refining the intervention as needed and developing a basic communication system to facilitate interactions with family members, friends, teachers, and others who are familiar to the child.

Phase II: Detailed Assessment for Tomorrow involves developing a communication system that will support the individual user in a variety of environments that reflect his or her lifestyle (home, school, work, social settings). It may also involve attempts at expanding the AAC system to include both basic conversational communication and specialized communication that is needed for each environment.

Phase III: Follow-Up Assessment is needed to ensure that the AAC system continues to meet the needs of the individual. It involves maintaining a comprehensive AAC system that meets the changing communication needs, capabilities, and lifestyles of the individual.

The Role of Speech-Language Pathologists

According to the American Speech-Language-Hearing Association's (2004a) *Scope of Practice for Speech-Language Pathologists*, clinicians are responsible for "developing, selecting, and prescribing multimodal augmentative and alternative communication systems, including unaided strategies (e.g., manual signs, gestures) and aided strategies (e.g., speech-generating devices, manual communication boards, picture schedules)" (p. 6). AAC is a set of procedures and processes by which an individual's communication skills (production and comprehension) can be maximized for functional communication (American Speech-Language-Hearing Association, 2002, 2004a; Beukelman & Mirenda, 2005). It involves supplementing or replacing natural speech or writing with aided or unaided symbols. Symbols may be graphic, auditory, gestural, or tactile. Aided symbols require some type of transmission device such as objects, pictures, or line drawings. Unaided symbols are those that require only the body to produce (e.g., sign language, gestures, or facial expressions). Four critical components that comprise all AAC interventions are: (1) symbol types, (2) AAC aids, (3) AAC techniques, and (4) AAC strategies (American Speech-Language-Hearing Association, 2004a; Beukelman & Mirenda, 2005).

Symbol types include aided or unaided, as described previously. The term *AAC aid* refers to any device (electronic or not) that helps a person convey or receive messages. The term *AAC technique* refers to the various ways a message can be transmitted. This includes ways in which messages are selected or identified (direct selection or scanning), and the types of displays (fixed or dynamic). *AAC strategy* refers to a plan or process for conveying symbols in the most efficient and effective way and includes strategies to enhance message timing, communication rate, and grammatic formulation.

In 2002, the American Speech-Language-Hearing Association (ASHA) published a statement specifying the knowledge and skills needed for AAC service delivery. It emphasized that AAC is a multidisciplinary field that requires skills beyond the typical discipline-specific training received by most speech-language pathologists, physical therapists, occupational therapists, educators, or others involved in AAC assessment and intervention. In this sense, it is a specialty area within several professions and requires a team approach to assessment and intervention, as described in Chapter 14. Not all speech-language pathologists are expected to engage in all areas of AAC practice; however, they are expected to recognize situations in which consultation or referral to another professional is necessary to provide quality services to someone who may benefit from AAC. The information and protocols presented in Chapters 14 and 15 will be helpful in determining when to refer a child for AAC assessment.

Resources for the Clinician

A speech-language pathologist planning to participate as a member of an AAC team should go beyond this information to develop the knowledge, skills, and competencies needed to provide AAC assessment and intervention services. The specific proficiencies, knowledge, and skills needed to provide AAC assessment and intervention services are available in the ASHA document entitled "Augmentative and Alternative Communication: Knowledge and Skills for Service Delivery" (American Speech-Language-Hearing Association, 2002).

In addition to the ASHA website, several other excellent resources also offer detailed information on AAC assessment and intervention:

- AAC Institute. This is a nonprofit, charitable organization dedicated to the most effective communication for people who rely on AAC (http://www.aacinstitute.org).

- AAC-RERC. This is a subgroup of collaborative researchers from the Rehabilitative Engineering Research Center that are dedicated to the development of effective AAC technology. Their Web site (http://www.aac-rerc.psu.edu/) contains information on reimbursement for services, research, and other resources.

- AAC Tech Connect. This online resource (http://www.aactechconnect/freetools/?forms) contains a dynamic list of forms and templates currently being used clinically to gather information, record data, and assist with device decision making for AAC systems.

- American Speech-Language-Hearing Association (ASHA) Web site (http://www.asha.org) contains multiple documents, position statements, papers, and technical reports on AAC service delivery.

- Assistivetech.net is an online resource for assistive technology and contains links to other disability related information and vendors that sell AAC products.

- Beukelman, D. R., and Mirenda, P. (2005). *Augmentative and Alternative Communication: Supporting Children and Adults with Complex Communication Needs* (3rd ed.). Baltimore, MD: Paul H. Brookes Publishing Co.

- Cress, C. and Marvin, C. (2003) "Common questions about AAC services in early intervention." *Augmentative and Alternative Communication, 19,* 254–272. This article contains excellent information for parents who are considering AAC for their children, and the professionals who support them. A summary of the research related to commonly asked questions about AAC and other valuable AAC information is available at http://www.unl.edu/barkley/present/cress.shtml

- International Society of Augmentative and Alternative Communication (ISAAC) is located in Toronto, Ontario, Canada (http://www.isaac-online.org).

- Light, J. C., Beukelman, D. R., and Reichle, J. (2003). *Communicative Competence for Individuals Who Use AAC.* Baltimore, MD: Paul H. Brookes Publishing.

- Parette, P., VanBiervliet, A., and Hourcade, J. (2000). *Families, cultures and AAC.* An interactive multimedia education tool that focuses on AAC as it relates to children from diverse cultural backgrounds. Available in English and Spanish from Program Development Associates (http://www.pdassoc.com).

- Quality Indicators for Assistive Technology (QIAT) Consortium Web site contains guidelines that can be used for service delivery of assistive technology in the schools (http://www.natri.uky.edu/assoc_projects/qiat).

- Rehabilitation Engineering and Assistive Technology Society of North America (RESNA) is a professional organization dedicated to promoting the health and well-being of people with disabilities through increasing access to technology systems (http://www.resna.org). The RESNA Catalyst Project site contains links to statewide programs across the U.S. that focus on AT resources and information (http://www.resnaprojects.org/allcontacts/statewidecontacts.html).

- Trace Center: University of Wisconsin. This site contains a searchable inventory of assistive technology products, manufacturers, and information. It also contains links to other informative sites (http://www.trace.wisc.edu).

Historical Perspective

AAC assessment procedures were being pioneered during the 1970s and early 1980s, (Goosens & Crain, 1985; Shane, 1980). At that time, assessment guidelines recommended the evaluation of perceptual skills, motor abilities, cognitive abilities, academic skills, communication skills, psycholinguistic abilities, access issues, seating, and positioning. Early on, AAC was often considered a "last resort" in communication options, offered only when all other attempts at developing intelligible speech had failed (Silverman, 1980). Therefore, early AAC assessment models often focused on evaluating the prognosis for developing speech; if this prognosis was judged good, the child was not considered for AAC on the assumption that it might inhibit speech and language development. Consequently, children often spent years making little to no progress in traditional speech therapy before AAC was considered. It is now believed that the use of AAC does not inhibit speech and language development, and that in some cases it might even facilitate it (Balandin, 2007; Blischak, Lombardino, & Dyson, 2003; Carr & Felce, 2007; Charlop-Christy, Carpenter, Le, LeBlanc, & Kellet, 2002; DiCarlo, Stricklin, Banajee, & Reid, 2001; Frost & Bondy, 2002; Ganz & Simpson, 2004; Kravits, Kamps, Kemmerer, & Potucek, 2002; Millar, Light, & Schlosser, 2006; Mirenda, Wilk, & Carson, 2000; Romski & Sevcik, 1993; Schlosser & Wendt, 2008; Sigafoos, Didden, & O'Reilly, 2003; Silverman, 1995).

According to Glennen and DeCoste (1997), early assessment procedures also emphasized the evaluation of certain cognitive skills, on the assumption that they are prerequisites for AAC use. AAC services were often withheld from a child who had not yet mastered presumed cognitive prerequisites (Chapman & Miller, 1980; Cress & Marvin, 2003). Later in the 1980s, evidence emerged that challenged the need to base AAC decisions on cognitive criteria (Kangas & Lloyd, 1988; Notari, Cole, & Mills, 1992; Reichle & Karlan, 1985; Romski, Sevcik, & Pate, 1988). Investigators examined the relationship between nonlinguistic concepts and language in typically developing children (Goldfield & Reznick, 1990; Gopnik & Meltzoff, 1986; Rice, 1989), language and cognition in developmentally delayed individuals (Abbeduto, Davies, & Furman, 1988; Abbeduto, Furman, & Davies, 1989; Atlas & Lapidus, 1988; Rast & Meltzoff, 1995), and language development and Piagetian stages in typically developing children (Lifter & Bloom, 1989; McCune, 1995; Shore, 1986). These studies demonstrated a correlational relationship between language and cognition for children with and without disabilities. They did not, however, support a causal relationship or provide evidence supporting the use of cognitive prerequisites.

Romski and Sevcik (1993) assert that there are no clear prerequisite skills for AAC use, and that certain milestones are not necessary to begin developing an AAC system for functional communication. The "candidacy" or "eligibility" criteria for AAC services is no longer considered the best practice, and should not be used. Children should not be eliminated from consideration for AAC because they do not meet some pre-established cognitive criteria; that some presumed cognitive processes cause behavioral skills has never been experimentally demonstrated anyway. Speech-language pathologists do not need to waste months or even years teaching prerequisite skills such as visual tracking, attending, matching, and imitation prior to introducing an AAC system. Instead, it is proposed that children with severe communication impairments learn communication skills and any other needed skills (such as attending or visual tracking) through the actual use of AAC strategies (Glennen & DeCoste, 1997).

In the mid-1980s assessment theory shifted to a focus on the child's *need* for improved functional communication, called the *communication needs model* (Beukelman, Yorkston, & Dowden, 1985). This model involves an evaluation of children's communication needs within their natural environments (e.g., home, preschool, school). If there are unmet communication needs, then an AAC system might be considered.

In 2004, ASHA endorsed the *participation model* as a framework for implementing AAC assessment and intervention. Beukelman and Mirenda (1988) have revised the participation model to include their communication needs model. Several other revisions or modifications have been made to this model over the past 10 years (Light, Roberts, Dimarco, & Greiner, 1998; Schlosser et al., 2000). We use the *Revised Participation Model* as a framework for describing the components of AAC assessment.

Revised Participation Model

Beukelman and Mirenda (2005) describe the revised participation model as a "systematic process for conducting AAC assessments and designing interventions based on the functional participation requirements of peers without disabilities of the same chronologic age as the person who may communicate through AAC" (p. 136). This model emphasizes the need for multiphase assessment and consensus building through a team approach and includes the following assessment components:

1. Conduct a *participation inventory* to identify communication patterns and needs.
2. Identify *opportunity barriers* through an assessment of policy barriers, knowledge barriers, skill barriers, and attitude barriers.
3. Identify *access barriers* through an assessment of current communication, the potential to use or increase natural speech, the potential for environmental adaptations, and the potential to use an AAC system or device.

4. Assess specific capabilities, including seating, positioning, motor capabilities, cognitive-communication capabilities, literacy, spelling abilities, and sensory-perceptual skills.

Participation Inventory

The assessment process begins by describing the participation patterns and communication needs of the child, referenced against the child's peers of the same chronologic age. This is done by completing a *Participation Inventory* (Beukelman & Mirenda, 2005) of regularly occurring activities that the child participates in at home, school, or other settings. The inventory should include the following:

- The activity being assessed
- The goal of the activity
- The steps needed to meet the activity goal
- The level of independence demonstrated by an age-matched peer with no disabilities participating in the activity (independent, independent with setup, requires verbal assistance, requires physical assistance, does not participate)
- The level of independence being targeted as a goal for the child using AAC (independent, independent with setup, requires verbal assistance, requires physical assistance, does not participate)
- Opportunity barriers (policy, practice, knowledge/skill)
- Personal barriers (physical/motor, cognitive, expressive communication, literacy, visual, auditory).

Opportunity Barriers

Opportunity barriers are defined as obstacles imposed by people other than the individual with the communicative disorder that cannot be eliminated simply by providing an AAC system. Beukelman and Mirenda (2005) describe the following types of opportunity barriers: policy barriers, practice barriers, knowledge barriers, skill barriers, and attitude barriers.

Policy barriers result from legislative or regulatory decisions. In the case of a child, policy barriers might result from rules set by parents or guardians in the home, or written policies that have been established for the governance of a preschool, school, or hospital. An example of a policy barrier might be a school district that segregates disabled students from their nondisabled peers.

Practice barriers result from procedures that have become common in a family or school even though they are not an actual policy. An example of a practice barrier would be a school that restricts students from using district-funded AAC devices outside of the school setting even though this is not an established districtwide or statewide policy.

Knowledge barriers result when someone other than the AAC user lacks information regarding specific aspects of AAC intervention or technology, and that lack of information results in limited opportunities for participation. This can occur with potential communication partners or even members of the AAC team.

Skill barriers can occur when communication partners or supporters have difficulty actually implementing the AAC technique or strategy. Finally, *attitude barriers* occur when an individual's attitudes or beliefs keep an AAC user from participating in activities with his or her same-age peers who do not have disabilities.

Access Barriers

Access barriers occur as the result of limitations in the current capabilities of the child, or limitations in the communication system currently being used. For example, an access barrier might result from an AAC system that has inadequate vocabulary storage for a specialized class or club the child attends. Access barriers may also result from a lack of mobility, literacy problems, sensory-perceptual impairments, or intellectual limitations. Beukelman and Mirenda (2005) recommend the following steps for assessing access barriers:

1. Assess current communication.
2. Assess the potential to use or increase natural speech.
3. Assess the potential for environmental adaptations.
4. Assess the potential to utilize an AAC system.

Current Communication

The child's current communication is assessed in terms of operational and social competence. Operational competence refers to the child's ability to use specific techniques such as eye gaze, gestures, pointing, writing, and so forth. Social competence refers to the child's ability to use any communication strategy in a socially appropriate way. Informal procedures that can be used to assess these skills were discussed in Chapter 14 under the heading *Systematic Quantitative and Qualitative Observations of Nonverbal Communication*. One formal assessment tool that can be used to assess current communication is the *Communication Matrix* developed by Rowland (2004). This matrix is used to document the communication techniques being used, the body part or parts used for each technique, and any adaptations needed for the technique to be used (e.g., a particular sitting position). In addition, the clinician rates the child's operational and social competence in using each technique. Several other observation or interview-based instruments are available to help the AAC team assess the child's current communication. These are included in Table 14-2, in Chapter 14.

Potential to Use or Increase Natural Speech

Most children with severe communication disorders are able to produce some types of vocalization or speech. The potential for natural speech to improve or to be used for communication should be assessed. A number of the formal and informal assessment resources and protocols described, respectively, in Chapters 6 and 7 can be used to evaluate the child's speech sound production and overall intelligibility. In addition, the information presented earlier in Chapter 14 under the section entitled *Assessment of Verbalizations* is applicable here. Robbins and Osberger (1992) described 10 levels of communication effectiveness with natural speech. These levels are included in their *Meaningful Use of Speech Scale* (MUSS):

1. Vocalizes during communicative interactions
2. Uses speech to attract other people's attention
3. Varies vocalizations with content and intent of messages
4. Is willing to use speech primarily to communicate with familiar people or on known topics
5. Is willing to use speech to communicate with unfamiliar people on known topics
6. Is willing to use speech primarily to communicate with familiar people on novel topics or with reduced contextual information
7. Is willing to use speech primarily to communicate with unfamiliar people on novel topics or with reduced contextual information
8. Produces messages understood by people familiar with his or her speech
9. Produces messages understood by those unfamiliar with his or her speech
10. Uses appropriate repair and clarification strategies.

The MUSS is used via observation and family interview to rate each level on a scale of 0 to 4, with 0 indicating that the behavior never occurs and 4 indicating that it always occurs. The information gathered regarding the child's ability to produce natural speech will help to determine whether AAC is needed to augment existing speech that is insufficient for functional communication, or to replace natural speech as the primary mode of communication.

Potential for Environmental Adaptations

The AAC team should also consider any environmental adaptations that might be made to facilitate communication and reduce the impact of access barriers. Environmental adaptations include changes that are made to physical spaces, locations, or physical structures. These adaptations often occur as common-sense solutions to specific situations that might arise. For example, a customized or slanted work space may help a child who depends on writing or uses a communication device.

Potential to Use an AAC System

According to Beukelman and Mirenda (2005), the fourth step in assessing access barriers is to assess the potential to utilize an AAC system. They describe three profiles that can be used to do this: (1) the operational requirements profile, (2) the constraints profile, and (3) the facilitator skills profile. The final component of the participation model, the assessment of specific capabilities, will also contribute to determining the potential to use an AAC system.

The AAC team will need to identify which of the many AAC systems or device options may be appropriate for a given child. The operational requirements profile will assist in matching the needs and capabilities of the child with the operational requirements of a specific system or device. Devices can be low-tech (nonelectronic) or high-tech (electronic). Therefore, team members will need to familiarize themselves with the operational requirements of various AAC options. Operational requirements may include the following:

- Display requirements (number of items, size of display, layout of items)
- Skills needed to use selected output modalities
- Alternative access system requirements regarding motor and sensory interface between the child and the device.

The constraints profile is used to identify constraints other than those directly related to the child or AAC techniques and is associated with family preferences, the preferences and attitudes of other communication partners, the skills and abilities of communication partners, and funding issues. Beukelman and Mirenda (2005) emphasize the importance of identifying these constraints early in the process so that subsequent decisions do not conflict with them, and so that efforts can be made to establish consensus regarding the acceptability of various systems or devices. Typical areas of concern include system portability, durability, and appearance; the time and skills needed to learn a system; the quality and intelligibility of speech output in speech-generating devices (SGDs); and the naturalness of communication exchange achieved with the system.

The cultural background of families and communication partners can also influence their preference of certain systems and their acceptance of AAC in general. Different cultures have different views of disability, attitudes toward technology, and expectations of their children. Speech-language pathologists should implement culturally and linguistically appropriate AAC programs that take into consideration the cultural and social communities, interaction patterns, and customs in which the AAC user participates, or hopes to participate. Therefore, AAC team members involved in the assessment of children from diverse cultural backgrounds should take the time to learn about their values, expectations, child rearing practices, and communication styles; guidelines offered in Chapter 4 on assessing ethnoculturally diverse children are generally useful. They may also consider using an assessment instrument such as the *Protocol for Culturally Inclusive Assessment of AAC* by Huer (1997). Bilingual children should be assessed in both languages because an assessment for AAC includes an evaluation of existing receptive and expressive language skills. Similarly, an assessment of a bidialectical child should include both variations of English (Hegde, 2008a). Finally, any recommendations for a specific AAC system must take the child's needs regarding multiple languages or dialects into consideration.

The skills and abilities of communication partners and facilitators must also be taken into consideration. The term *facilitator* refers to a family member, professional, or frequent communication partner who assumes responsibility to teach the child the skills needed to use the AAC system or device effectively, for introducing new communication partners to the system, and for keeping the selected AAC system up-to-date and operational (Beukelman & Mirenda, 2005). Therefore, if a high-tech device is being used, the facilitator must be competent in programming, maintaining, and using it. With either a high-tech or low-tech device, the facilitator must be competent in the social and strategic use of the system to provide adequate instruction and good modeling for the user and new communication partners. Not having a knowledgeable and competent facilitator available may limit the AAC choices.

Assessment of Specific Capabilities

The assessment of specific capabilities involves the identification of a child's level of performance critical to AAC intervention, such as language, literacy, cognition, and motor control (Yorkston & Karlan, 1986). The goal is to develop a profile of the child's capabilities that can be matched to the operational requirements of one or more AAC options. A capability profile should emphasize the child's strengths and skills, rather than his or her impairments (Beukelman & Mirenda, 2005).

The assessment of specific capabilities needed for AAC is not generally well-served by the use of norm-referenced tests. The limits imposed by the speech-language, intellectual, or motor disabilities of a potential AAC user often make it impossible to administer the test in the standardized manner. Some professionals, however, may administer norm-referenced tests that contain appropriate content with modifications, as needed. For example, they might allow the child to use an eye gaze response instead of pointing. The administration of norm-referenced tests with modifications may be useful in gathering general information about a child's capabilities, but should not be used to obtain scores that are converted to mental age or developmental equivalencies.

Due to the limitations of norm-referenced tests, AAC professionals often rely on criterion-based assessment procedures. The goal of these procedures is to determine whether the child can demonstrate the skills and abilities needed to successfully implement a particular AAC device or system. Therefore, the assessment team will often begin by administering a series of carefully selected, criterion-referenced tasks. The child's performance on these tasks, as well as any adaptations or assistance that facilitates success, are observed and recorded. Based on these results, a prediction is made as to one or more AAC devices or techniques that the child might be able to use efficiently and effectively. This approach is called *predicative assessment* or *feature matching* (Glennen, 1997; Yorkston & Karlan, 1986). Ideally, the child is then allowed to use the selected device or system for a designated trial period. This trial may last several weeks, or even months, depending on the AAC system selected. This approach requires members of the team to be knowledgeable about the AAC devices that are available and their specific operational needs. It also requires availability of AAC devices for trial usage. Table 16–1 summarizes a list of instruments designed specifically for AAC assessment and feature matching.

Assessment of Seating and Positioning

The assessment of seating and positioning is typically carried out by a physical therapist or occupational therapist, often with input from an AAC consultant or wheelchair consultant. Many AAC users have disabilities that severely restrict movement or require the use of a wheelchair. Child safety should always be a priority. In addition, the child's seating and positioning may need to be adjusted to best facilitate motor control, reduce discomfort or distraction, maximize access to an AAC device, or facilitate efficient use of an AAC system. Consideration should also be given to the child's ability to access and use the AAC system in multiple places, such as from a chair as well as a bed.

Table 16–1. Instruments to Assist with *Feature Matching* and the Selection of an Appropriate AAC System or Device

Assessment Instrument	Age Range	Skills Assessed
Assistive Technology Screener (Judd-Wall, 1995)	school-age	Documents past and current AT/AAC use and degree of success; the need for additional supports in nine areas, including AAC
AAC Feature Match (Dodgen and Associates, 1996) [computer software: CD-ROM]	school-age and adult	Identifies a client's needs with regards to symbols, encoding technique, selection technique, microswitch type(s), feedback, display characteristics, output, mounting, and other features; results in recommendations of potential AAC devices that match the identified features, along with a report and vendor request letters; requires that an AAC assessment has already been completed
AAT Assessment Tool (Dodgen & Associates, 1998) [computer software: CD-ROM]	school-age and adult	Communication goals and needs: vision, hearing, fine motor, and gross motor abilities (upper and lower limbs); and cognitive, expressive language, literacy, and oral-motor skills
Augmentative Communication Assessment Profile (Goldman, 2002)	children, ages 3 to 11, with ASD	Skills that are related to manual signing (Makaton), low-tech communication displays that require pointing, and low-tech communication displays that require picture exchange
Augmentative Communication Evaluation Summary (Georgia Project for Assistive Technology)	all ages	Access evaluation, symbol evaluation, use of devices, system recommendations
EvaluWare (Assistive Technology, Inc., 1999) [computer software: CD-ROM]	school-age	Interactive tasks designed to assess motor access skills (e.g., input method and settings), looking skills (e.g., symbol type and size of visual arrays and targets), listening skills (e.g., preferred feedback and type of voice output) and ability to use an on-screen keyboard and word prediction software
Matching Assistive Technology and Child (MATCH) (Scherer, 1997)	infants and young children	Helps parents and team members determine a child's functional limitations and related goals, family considerations that may impact technology use, and appropriate technologies and training strategies

Table 16–1. *(continued)*

Assessment Instrument	Age Range	Skills Assessed
Observing the Classroom Environment (DynaVox Mayer-Johnson, 2008)	school-age children	Classroom communication behaviors (specific to AAC)
Preschool AAC Checklist (Henderson, 1995)	developmental level of 3 to 9 years	Checklist designed to monitor a child's development of AAC skills & technology use; includes information on AAC system descriptions, AAC skills, strategies, and resources
Social Networks: A Communication Inventory for Individuals with Complex Communication Needs and Their Communication Partners (Blackstone & Hunt-Berg, 2003)	all ages	Communication skills, communication partners, modes of expression representational and selection strategies, topics of conversation, types of communication (specific to AAC)
UKAT Toolkit (University of Kentucky, 2002)	school-age	Summarize assessment data, document the results of equipment/device trials, plan implementation, monitor student progress, and complete professional self-assessment of AT knowledge and skills

Assessment of Motor Capabilities

The physical therapists and occupational therapists are primarily responsible for assessing the child's motor capabilities. Initially, they may need to identify a motor technique that allows the child to participate in the assessment process. Ultimately, they will identify a motor technique or techniques that the child can use to access his or her AAC system or device. One goal is to identify motor capabilities that can be used to facilitate such nonverbal communication as gesturing or manual signing. Another goal is to identify motor capabilities that will allow the child to access an AAC device. Examples might include head movements needed to control a wand or activate a switch, or hand movements needed to activate a switch or point to a selected item.

Assessment of Language

If not yet completed, the child's receptive and expressive language needs to be evaluated as part of the AAC assessment. The assessment of existing oral speech and language skills, and comprehension of spoken language, even in severely impaired individuals, is essential because any selected nonverbal means of communication will build on the child's existing language skills, including single-word receptive vocabulary, as well as morphologic and syntactic knowledge. Many of the principles and procedures presented in Chapter 14: Assessment for Nonverbal or Minimally Verbal Children, particularly those in Standardized and Criterion-Referenced Instruments, Systematic Quantitative and Qualitative Observations of Nonverbal Communication, Assessment of Receptive Language, and Assessment of Verbalizations, apply here. Therefore, a combination of appropriate informal and formal procedures should be selected, adapted as needed for the individual child, and used to assess the receptive and expressive language abilities of a child being considered for AAC.

Assessment of the Ability to Use Symbols

One goal of the assessment is to select the types of symbols that will meet the child's current communication needs and match his or her current abilities. Throughout these assessment activities, the mode of response will need to be adjusted so that it is appropriate to the child. Some children will communicate by pointing, whereas others may do so by an eye gaze, head movement, object or picture manipulation, or other established response mode. Beukelman and Mirenda (2005), suggest that this assessment include the following components:

1. Assess whether the child understands the functional use of the object. For this task, the team, with input from family members or caregivers, selects 10 familiar, functional items, such as a cup, toothbrush, spoon, and so forth. These are the *referents*. The team also compiles a variety of *symbols* (e.g., photographs, line drawings, miniature objects, etc.) that represent the selected referents. The clinician then should:
    a. Give an object to the child and see if he or she can show how it is used. This can be done in a play format.
    b. Tell the child, "Show me what you do with this."
    c. Ask family members to provide examples of the child's understanding of the use of an object (e.g., pointing to or reach for the juice when a cup is presented).
    d. Demonstrate correct use (e.g., use of a spoon to eat) and incorrect use (e.g., use of a spoon to brush hair) of an object, and note how the child reacts. Does the child's reaction consistently suggest a correct understanding of the object's function?

2. Assess the child's receptive labeling ability. For this task, the clinician should:
    a. Present two or more pictures or items and ask the child, "Show me/Give me/Point to the _____".
    b. Ask *Yes-No* questions if the child can consistently indicate "yes" and "no;" ask, "Is this a [incorrect label]?" and "Is this a [correct label]?"
    c. Use a matching format in which the child is asked to match an object to a symbol or a symbol to an object.

3. Assess whether the child can use symbols to answer questions. This is an example of symbol use in context, which is a higher level skill than those described previously. A question and answer format can be used; the clinician should:

    a. Identify items and concepts that are familiar to the child; family and caregiver input may be sought for this purpose.

    b. Present two or more symbols and ask such questions as: "Which one do you use to brush your teeth?" or "What is your favorite food?"

4. Assess whether the child can use symbols to make requests: another example of symbol use in context; the clinician may:

    a. Create opportunities for the child to request specific items. For example, create a "play time" with several toys or activities to choose from, or "snack time" with several foods or drinks to choose from.

    b. Make a list of items that the child knows and that are available in that particular context or situation.

    c. Provide symbols representing two or more of the available options.

    d. Structure the interaction to provide an opportunity for the child to request a specific object or action by selecting one of the symbols. As needed, use such indirect cues as: "I don't know what you want." or "Can you show me what you want?"

5. Assess advanced symbol sequences that might represent different syntactic elements. Children who use single symbols may use symbols for words other than simple nouns. They may also be able to chain symbols together to construct a message; for this assessment, the clinician should:

    a. Select a simple, repetitive game or activity (e.g., such card games as "Go Fish") or such board games as "Candy Land").

    b. Design an *activity board* which displays symbols that represent various syntactic elements: nouns, verbs, adjectives, and so forth, that is *specific to the selected activity*.

    c. Play the game. The clinician models by producing multiple one- and two-symbol messages using the display. For example: GO + FISH, MY + TURN, YOU + TURN, and GO + BLUE.

    d. Note whether the child learns to use the display quickly and how often the child chains the symbols together when given the opportunity to do so.

6. Assess symbol categorization. Some AAC systems depend on various symbol categorization strategies. For this task, the clinician may:

    a. Ask the child to sort symbols into various categories

    b. Suggest such common semantic categories as foods, clothing, animals, and so forth.

7. Assess association skills because several AAC devices require this skill; the clinician may:

    a. Provide the child with a small set of colored symbols that the child recognizes by name (e.g., toothbrush, banana, house, chair, etc.).

    b. Ask the child to use the symbols to answer questions that require different types of association (Glennen, 1997). For example, the child may be asked such questions as, "What do you use to clean your teeth?" "What goes together with table?" "Find something made of wood."

The results of the procedures described in this section will help determine whether or not the child:

- Understands the functional use of objects
- Recognizes verbal labels for symbols and their referents
- Can use symbols to answer questions or make requests
- Can use symbols representing different syntactic elements
- Can sequence or chain symbols to create a message
- Can use an AAC system that incorporates categorization or association skills.

These procedures are not standardized protocols. They consist of various activities that can be altered in a variety of ways to meet the individual child's needs and abilities. For example, some activities might require a brief period of teaching prior to the actual assessment. This "teach-test" format would fall within the realm of dynamic assessment, discussed in Chapter 5. In addition, the team can use these assessment activities to experiment and adjust the size, configuration, and spacing of symbols on an array in order to meet the individual needs of the child. The goal here is to make systematic adjustments that facilitate the child's use of symbols to communicate.

Assessment of Literacy

Several professionals, including a reading specialist, classroom teacher, or speech-language pathologist, may help assess literacy. Any reading skills identified during the assessment can be incorporated into an AAC system at a level that is appropriate for the child. In addition, the information gathered during the literacy assessment may be used to design an appropriate reading instruction program for the child. Table 16–2 summarizes a list of literacy assessment instruments that can be used with nonverbal or minimally verbal children. In addition, information provided in Chapter 17 regarding the assessment of emergent and early reading and writing skills may be helpful.

Depending on the child's age and skill level, a literacy assessment may include all or some of the following components:

1. *Letter recognition by name or sound:* This can be assessed by having the child identify with any means (e.g., pointing, eye gaze, or writing) letters on a display board or keyboard as the clinician says the name of the letter or produces the sound it makes.

2. *Phonological processing skills:* Phonological processing is thought to include *phonological awareness* (ability to recognize and manipulate the phonemes of spoken words) and *phonological recoding* (ability to use graphemes of written language to read unknown printed strings, or to spell) (Vandervelden & Siegel, 1999). This assessment often involves the use of nonword tasks, but an accurate assessment of phonological processing is difficult in children who do not speak.

3. *Word recognition and reading comprehension:* These skills may facilitate the use of a variety of AAC systems or devices. Word recognition can be informally assessed using printed words. The clinician may ask the child to identify words

Table 16–2. Instruments for Assessing Literacy Skills in Nonverbal or Minimally Verbal Children

Assessment Instrument	Age Range	Skills Assessed
Gates-MacGinitie Reading Tests-Fourth Edition (MacGinitie, MacGinitie, Marie, & Dreyer, 2000)	kindergarten to adult	Basic literacy concepts, phonological awareness, letter-sound correspondence, word decoding, reading comprehension, vocabulary
Group Reading Assessment and Diagnostic Evaluation (GRADE) (Williams, 2001)	pre-kindergarten to adult	Phonological awareness, visual skills, concepts, early literacy skills, word reading, comprehension, and vocabulary
Peabody Individual Achievement Test-Revised-Normative Update (Markwardt, 1998)	kindergarten to adult	Recognition of printed letters, reading comprehension, spelling comprehension
Test of Reading Comprehension-4th Edition (Brown, Wiederholt, & Hammill, 2009)	7 years to 17 years	General vocabulary, syntactic similarities, paragraph comprehension, sentence sequencing, and following written directions
Woodcock-Johnson III (Woodcock, McGrew, & Mather, 2007)	preschool to adult	Visual matching, reading fluency, spelling, writing, and listening comprehension

that are said, match words to symbols, match words to pictures, or match words to objects. Reading comprehension can similarly be assessed using printed phrases, sentences, or paragraphs.

4. *Spelling assessment:* Several AAC options require some level of spelling skills; therefore, an assessment of the child's spelling skills will be essential if one of these is going to be considered. According to Beukelman and Mirenda (2005), the three aspects of spelling that should be assessed are spontaneous spelling, first-letter-of-the-word spelling, and recognition spelling. *Spontaneous spelling* requires the child to spell words letter by letter. A child can demonstrate spelling skills with activities such as identifying letters to spell a word on a display or keyboard, sequencing cut out or magnetic letters, writing the word, or fingerspelling. *First-letter-of-the-word spelling* is needed for AAC devices that utilize word prediction. Therefore, it is important to assess how well a child can indicate the first letter of a word even if the child cannot spell the whole word. *Recognition spelling* means that the child can recognize words that are spelled correctly, even though he or she cannot spontaneously spell the words or their first letters. This is sometimes called a *sight word vocabulary,* and it only needs to be assessed if the child cannot demonstrate correct spontaneous spelling or first-letter-of-the-word spelling. Spelling can be assessed informally or by using spelling subtests from measures such as those listed in Table 16–2.

Assessment of Visual and Auditory Skills

A clear understanding of the child's visual skills and hearing capabilities is important for the AAC team. Hearing acuity is assessed by an audiologist, who may consider auditory brainstem response procedures for a child who cannot participate in traditional audiologic assessment procedures. Auditory AAC systems may be particularly important for children who have severe visual impairments, so it is important that steps are taken to make sure the child can hear and understand auditory information to the best of his or her ability. Some AAC systems utilize an auditorily displayed selection set (i.e., auditory scanning). It is also important for the child to understand any auditory feedback or speech output that might be incorporated into the system. Information gathered during the hearing assessment may influence decisions regarding recommendations for aural rehabilitation, the volume levels used in the AAC system, the use of synthesized or digitized speech, and the degree to which auditory and/or visual information is incorporated into the system.

Many developmental and acquired disabilities that necessitate the use of AAC also are associated with impaired vision. Therefore, an accurate and comprehensive vision assessment should be conducted by an optometrist or ophthalmologist and should include an evaluation of visual acuity, visual field problems, oculomotor functioning, light sensitivity, and color perception. It is also important to determine whether vision problems are likely to progressively deteriorate, and if so, what the time line is. Information gathered during the vision assessment can help the AAC team answer the following questions (Beukelman & Mirenda, 2005):

- What can the child see accurately?
- How should displays be sized and positioned to allow for maximal visual efficiency?
- How can oculomotor problems be minimized or accommodated for?
- Which colors can be seen and how they might accommodate for contrast problems?
- What lighting is required for optimal vision?

Analysis and Integration of Assessment Results

The assessment for AAC systems involves the analysis and integration of assessment results from various sources. Information gathered by the speech-language pathologist during administration of the orofacial examination, standardized and criterion-referenced instruments, systematic qualitative and quantitative observation of nonverbal communication, and the assessment of verbalizations that do occur, must be integrated with unique data that emerge from other specialized sources, professionals, and team members. In completing the analysis, the clinician may need to integrate the results of the current AAC assessment with those of any previous assessments completed by various members of the AAC assessment team. The main concern of this analysis and integration is to understand the overall strengths and limitations of the potential AAC user. These will include current speech and language abilities; barriers to participation; physical limitations; cognitive and neuromotor limitations; sensory-perceptual skills; financial resources; motivation to learn and use a new system of communication; and family, teacher, or caregiver support. In addition, the child's communication needs and goals will be summarized from information gathered on the participation inventory, the case history, and the interview.

The assessment team will consider all of these factors when assessing the child's candidacy for AAC, and a specific system or device will then be selected. After this selection, the cost of the device may need further consideration. Devices can be as inexpensive as a notebook and pencil, or as expensive as a speech synthesizing computer. The goal is to select one that is most affordable to the parties involved, yet is capable of meeting the communication needs of the child and promoting optimal family, academic, and social participation (Hegde, 2008a). Once all of these factors are taken into consideration, a final recommendation or set of recommendations will be made by the team in the postassessment counseling of the family and the child.

Postassessment Counseling

During the final phase of the AAC assessment, a representative of the assessment team counsels the parents or others who accompany the child. Depending on the age, the child may be part of this postassessment counseling. A set of recommendations will be made to include an appropriate AAC device or system and subsequent training that will be needed to facilitate its implementation. Additional treatment options may be presented and frequently asked questions will be addressed.

Make Recommendations

Based on a comprehensive AAC assessment, the AAC team will make a number of recommendations. Recommendations may include, but not be limited to the following:

1. If the prognosis is favorable for the development of functional verbal communication, then language intervention should be recommended. A recommendation may be made for speech-language therapy to improve verbal and nonverbal communication skills with an emphasis on functional communication. Parent training may be provided on how to stimulate and facilitate language development. If the child is very young, early intervention may be recommended within the framework of a family service plan. Temporary use of an appropriate AAC device may be a part of the verbal communication training program.

2. If the prognosis for verbal communication is unfavorable, a specific communication system, device, or both are recommended to meet the communication needs of the child, family, and educational personnel. The system and the device should also facilitate increased family, academic, and social participation and communication.

3. A trial period is established for use of the selected system to further evaluate the appropriateness and effectiveness of the system. Based on the results of this evaluation, a final decision is made to either continue using the selected system or possibly try something else.

4. Training is provided for the child, family members, educators, and peers on making good use of the selected method, and in maintaining any AAC device.

5. Periodic reassessment is recommended to maintain a comprehensive AAC system that meets the changing communication needs, capabilities, age, and lifestyles of the individual.

6. Periodic examination of any communication equipment is conducted to detect any needs for repairs or replacements.

7. Additional recommendations may be made for individual services (e.g., speech-language therapy, physical therapy, occupational therapy) designed to further improve the child's motor or communication abilities. This may facilitate a continued or expanded use of AAC, or may actually reduce the child's dependence on AAC. Referrals to other professionals are made, as needed (e.g., audiologist, psychologist, neurologist, physical therapist, occupational therapist).

Suggest a Prognosis for Functional Communication with AAC

As noted, the prognosis for successful, functional communication using AAC is highly variable because the population for which AAC is appropriate is extremely heterogeneous. Prudent prognostic statements may be delayed until the results of a trial treatment program with the selected device are clear.

Most children will benefit from a method that has been carefully selected based on a comprehensive assessment of the needs, strengths, and preferences of the client and family. Benefits will be further enhanced and sustained with continuous professional support for the child and the family, and continued support from the child's educators.

Answer Frequently Asked Questions

When a recommendation is made for an AAC assessment, or for AAC as part of an intervention plan, parents and family members often have questions. The clinician should give answers that are honest and scientifically justifiable. Some commonly encountered questions and their answers follow; the clinician may need to modify the terms to suit the age, education, and general judged sophistication of clients and families in formulating the answers.

What Is AAC?

AAC stand for augmentative and alternative communication. It refers to any device, system, or method that improves the child's ability to communicate effectively. AAC may include sign language, communication boards, or specialized and computerized instruments. Even facial expressions, simple sounds we call vocalizations or gestures that a child has learned to say something may all be a part of AAC. An AAC system often includes more than one means of communication, so the child can communicate in any effective way possible. Natural speech, even if limited, may also be a part of AAC.

Who Uses AAC and How Do I Know If It Is Right for My Child?

AAC is used when a child does not develop communication in the normal fashion. The American Speech-Language-Hearing Association estimates that there are well over two million people worldwide who use AAC because they cannot fully communicate verbally. AAC users have difficulty communicating verbally because of congenital or acquired disabilities, including cerebral palsy, genetic syndromes, intellectual disabilities, hearing impairment, head injury, or multiple disabilities. AAC is probably right for your son [daughter] if he [she] cannot effectively communicate with the typical oral language. The recommendation to use AAC is made by a team of professionals. [*briefly describe the assessment process, as appropriate*].

Will the Use of AAC Interfere with My Child's Verbal Development?

This is a fear that even researchers had many years ago. Recent research indicates that AAC facilitates spoken language and speech skills by increasing interaction, improving language and social communication, or providing a voice output model for speech. Because AAC includes all communication methods, including oral language skills even if they are limited, intervention often results in improved functional verbal skills. The child's speech may become clearer, so people can understand better. Also, children will use the quickest, most effective, and easiest communication method available to them. They generally will use verbal speech as their first choice if they can manage that; and they do become more proficient in expressing themselves verbally.

Why Not Wait and See If My Child's Verbal Communication Will Improve?

It is not a good idea, mostly because the use of AAC may actually facilitate speech and language development in your child. If you simply wait, you will only prolong the child's communication difficulty. A child who is unable to communicate effectively cannot participate in many social activities and is at greater risk for delays in social and emotional development. Such a child is more likely to develop academic and behavior problems as time goes on.

Are There Prerequisites to Use AAC?

There are no prerequisites to use AAC in the sense that we have to wait for some skills to develop. If there is a particular skill that is needed to use an AAC system, we can teach it during training. AAC is an intervention approach that can be the beginning of communication development for a child. There are a number of AAC options available to begin this process. [*Provide explanations, as appropriate and answer any additional questions the caregivers may have*].

PART VII

Literacy

CHAPTER 17

A Primer on Literacy Assessment

- Language Disorders and Literacy Problems
- Emergent Literacy
- Emergent Literacy Skill Acquisition
- Assessment of Emergent Literacy Skills
- Assessment of Reading and Writing

The American Speech-Language-Hearing Association's (2001a) position paper expanded the scope of practice of speech-language pathologists (SLPs) to include literacy assessment and intervention. Because of their sophisticated understanding and expertise in language and remediation of language disorders, SLPs are capable of making significant contributions to improving any form of communication, especially if it is a form of oral language, as literacy skills are.

Literacy skills are communicative and interactive. Talking and writing are communicative behaviors. Reading is communicative in a special sense: a writer will have affected a reader. People accomplish similar goals by talking, reading, and writing: they affect other people by their verbal actions.

Oral language skills, reading, and writing are interrelated verbal skills (Catts & Kamhi, 1999; Goldsworthy, 1996). Problems of literacy may have their origin in poor language skills, although additional variables may contribute to the maintenance of those problems. Good oral language skills may not automatically ensure good literacy skills, however. Some individuals with excellent oral language skills may have no or poor literacy skills. In the historical past, people have had good oral language skills with no or limited reading and writing skills; in some societies, people still do. This suggests that oral language skills are more essential for social survival than literacy skills and that the former do not naturally lead to the latter. Reading and writing need more formal instruction than speaking.

With their expertise in language skills, it is clear that SLPs can make significant contribution to promote literacy in children. Some SLPs have begun to specialize in literacy assessment and treatment; a certain number of clinicians in public schools may devote some of their time to contribute to the school's overall program of literacy improvement; other clinicians probably resist involvement in literacy programs because of their burgeoning caseloads of children with traditional communication disorders. Another reason for limited involvement of some SLPs in literacy programs is their lack of training in assessing and treating reading and writing disorders. Traditional SLP academic programs have not offered substantial coursework or clinical practicum in literacy. Moreover, there are specialists to deal with them in the public schools.

It is expected that SLPs will always be more concerned with the traditional oral speech, language, voice, and fluency disorders than literacy skills in public schools although some clinicians may defy this general observation and devote their professional time to literacy assessment and intervention. There is no certainty that school districts will hire additional SLPs to manage literacy problems so that children with oral communication disorders are not short-changed.

Language Disorders and Literacy Problems

It is often stated that children with early language problems are at risk for developing literacy problems in the grade school. Reportedly, almost 60% of children who have a history of language disorders may have a reading disability (Lewis, O'Donnell, Freebairn, & Taylor, 1998). The actual figure may be higher because it is difficult to imagine a child with limited oral language skills learning to read (or write) normally or sustaining reading and writing skills at his or her grade level. A child's difficulties in such contexts go hand-in-hand; it is not clear how empirically useful it is to distinguish early language problems with limited emergent literacy skills, because they may belong to the same response class. The child with early language difficulties is likely to have limited emergent literacy skills and both will have a negative effect on later language skills as well as conventional literacy skills acquired during the elementary grades.

The term *literacy* means reading and writing skills. In the context of present research on literacy, the term also includes preschool children's skills that are related to reading and writing but are not yet conventional reading and writing skills. See Table 17–1 for definitions of literacy terms.

Research suggests that a child who reads poorly at first grade may remain a poor reader (Catts, Fey, Tomblin, & Zhang, 2002; Flax et al., 2003; Justice, Chow, Capellini, Flanigan, & Colton, 2003; Whitehurst & Fischel, 2000), but it is not clear why. There should be no expectation that maturation alone will somehow solve a child's reading difficulties.

Table 17–1. Definition of Literacy Terms

Literacy skills. Fully mastered reading and writing skills; also called conventional literacy skills.

Emergent literacy skills. Early skills that precede or are presumed to be prerequisites for later developing reading and writing skills; include alphabet awareness, print awareness, and phonological awareness.

Alphabet knowledge. Emerging knowledge of the alphabet; observed during the first three years; a child may name a letter in his or her name; may begin to write some of the letters of the alphabet.

Print awareness. A child's interest in printed material, understanding that printed material is organized (moves from left to right); understanding that printed words and letters have their names.

Phonological awareness. Awareness of phonemes, and awareness and manipulation of sounds, syllables, words, rhyme, and onsets and rimes; begins around 2 years.

Phonics. A method of reading instruction that emphasizes sound-letter correspondences and skills in "sounding out" words; described as "decoding."

Phoneme. The smallest part of *spoken* language that affects word meaning.

Grapheme. The smallest part of *written* language; letters of the alphabet that represent phonemes; a grapheme may be a single letter or a combination of letters (e.g., *c* for /k/ or /s/; *ng* for /ŋ/; *ough* for /o/, /u/, or /au/).

Phonemic awareness. Skill in discriminating, identifying, and manipulating individual phonemes or sounds in spoken words.

Syllable. Part of a word containing a vowel; the vowel can stand alone or be surrounded by one or more consonants (e.g., *ba-by; re-frig-er-a-tor*)

Onset and rime. Every word has an onset and a rime. The *onset* is the initial consonant(s) sound of the syllable. A *rime* is the part of the syllable that contains the vowel and all that follows it (e.g., the onset of the word *dog* is *d-*, the rime is *–og*; the onset of the word *bring* is *br-* and the rime is *–ing*)

One would expect that a poor reader at grade one will receive additional help to overcome the deficiency. But it is not clear whether children who read poorly at first grade: (a) do not receive prompt additional intervention they need, (b) the intervention they do receive is ineffective, or (c) the effects of prompt and effective intervention are countered by some unknown variables.

Deficiencies in both oral language and literacy skills need planned and effective intervention. Good oral language skills may make it somewhat easier to teach reading and writing skills to children but even excellent oral language skills will not automatically ensure literacy skills. Literacy skills must be explicitly *taught*. Because of their technical training in assessing and treating language disorders, SLPs can play several useful roles in promoting improved literacy skills in children. The American Speech-Language-Hearing Association (2001b) recommends that SLPs may design and implement programs to:

1. Prevent literacy problems by promoting home environments that stimulate better language acquisition and emergent literacy skills

2. Identify children at risk for reading and writing problems

3. Help assess reading and writing problems; be a part of the multidisciplinary assessment teams in schools

4. Provide intervention and document outcomes for reading and writing intervention programs

5. Provide assistance to general education teachers, parents, and students; act as consultants

6. Advocate effective literacy practices, and advance the knowledge base.

In addition to the listed roles, clinicians can integrate literacy skills into their speech-language assessment and treatment of children. Selection of speech-language treatment targets may be based on the literacy demands made at different grade levels.

Emergent Literacy

The concept of *emergent literacy* has played an important role in promoting the involvement of SLPs in literacy assessment and intervention. The concept contrasts with the earlier view of *reading readiness*. It was thought that reading (and writing) skills could not be taught to a child who was not ready for it. Among other factors, a mental age of 6.5 years, measured on IQ tests, was considered a part of this presumed reading readiness. In addition, children needed to acquire various auditory or motoric skills before they could be taught literacy skills (Erickson, 2000; Polloway & Smith, 1992). An unfortunate consequence of this readiness concept was that many children, especially those with slightly below average intellectual skills, were not offered reading and writing instruction. Even normally developing children who could have learned to read and write at a younger age were not taught the skills because they were presumed *not ready* (Erickson, 2000). This educational practice persisted for many years in spite of no demonstrated evidence of readiness as a prerequisite for learning to read and write. This dogmatic practice may have been responsible for low literacy skills in many children.

The more recently advocated *emergent literacy* view suggests that young children exhibit a variety of unconventional literacy behaviors that may be precursors to later and conventional literacy skills (Justice, 2006). Long before they enter the first grade, children show an awareness of printed material and learn rudimentary literacy skills (Gillam & Johnston, 1985; Justice, 2006; Snow, Burns, & Griffin, 1998; Sulzby, 1985; van Kleeck, 1990, 1998; Whitehurst & Lonigan, 1998). For example, children younger than 5 react to labels or logos on products, signs on the road or around the house, the printed alphabet, printed pages, and other graphic signs in their environment. Children like to hold and look at books even when they cannot read and even when the pages contain only printed text with no pictures. They may pretend to read a letter, even when they cannot recognize the alphabet. Young children may hold pens or crayons and scribble or draw. They may sit at a desk like adults do and pretend-write. Children may vocally play with rhyming words. These are among the emergent literacy skills observed in children who cannot yet read or write.

Early literacy skills greatly vary across preschoolers. This variation is due largely to differences in the home environment of young children. Studies have shown that the home *literacy environment* of young children may vary on a continuum of impoverished to enriched literacy resources. A literacy-enriched home contains plenty of books, magazines, and other printed materials for both the adults and children to read. Children have ready access to printed materials and are reinforced for looking at them and handling them. Writing materials and supplies also are plentiful, and children have easy access to them. The home contains a preschool child's writing chair and a desk, pens, crayons, coloring books or sheets, blank paper, storybooks with large pictures, pictures with words printed under them, charts of the alphabet or days of the week, and maps of the country or the world, all freely available for the child to see, hold, and handle. In addition, a literacy-enriched environment contains educational toys. For example, wooden blocks with the letters of the alphabet, beads to help count the numbers, toys that talk and help learn words, and so forth. Most homes have more or fewer of such literacy materials for the child to learn from. At the other extreme is the literacy-impoverished home environment that contains very few or no such materials.

Home literacy environment also differs in the degree to which the parents, other caregivers, and older siblings stimulate, prompt, and reinforce literacy skills in preschoolers. *Role-modeling of literacy skills*, as it is often described, is thought to encourage emergent (as well as more conventional) literacy skills in children; the absence of which may be partly responsible for lack of emergent literacy skills in children. Family members who read and write regularly when the child is around are more likely to stimulate emergent and later literacy skills than those who typically do not read or write at home. Some highly literate parents who extensively read and write at home may recall their young children who wanted to "compete" with them with pretend-writing or reading. In the experience of one of the authors, a boy who, at age 3, seeing his father pointing out an article published in a scientific journal, scribbled something on a sheet of paper, inserted it into another issue of the same journal, and showed it off to his mother by saying, "Mom, I have an article published here!"

A well-established fact of emergent literacy stimulation is story book reading to children. There is no age that is too young to be read to. A parent's expressive storytelling will bring smiles to the face of wide-eyed infants who do not understand the words read aloud to them. Storybook reading to young children is not only good for stimulating emergent literacy skills, but also to enrich or enhance their oral language skills (Snow, Burns, & Griffin, 1998; Whitehurst & Lonigan, 1998). Once again, family environments vary in the extent to which the young children are regularly read to, creating some differences in emergent literacy skills across children.

In essence, presence of varied literacy materials, parental and older sibling literacy role models, and storybooks being read aloud, are the three most important variables that seem to stimulate early and emergent literacy skills in children. When these variables are operative, the child is likely to exhibit more advanced emergent literacy skills than when those variables are absent.

A literacy-rich home is also an environment that reinforces more advanced oral language skills in children of all ages. Children in such environments may acquire more words, more advanced or abstract words, and begin to speak in more complete sentences sooner than those who live in homes with limited literacy materials (Teale & Sulzby, 1986; Whitehurst & Lonigan, 1998).

A child with good emergent literacy skills is likely to learn conventional literacy skills faster than one with limited emergent skills. Good emergent literacy skills make it easier for the child to benefit from formal instruction in conventional reading and writing skills. (Hart & Risley, 1995, 1999; Whitehurst & Fischel, 2000). Generally, research has shown that emergent literacy skills are correlated with more conventional literacy skills in school-age children (Justice, 2006; Pence, 2007). This positive correlation is neither surprising nor remarkable because emergent literacy skills and conventional literacy skills probably belong to the same or similar response class. Emergent literacy skills are rudimentary literacy skills that are shaped into more complex (and conventional) reading and writing skills. It would be remarkable and surprising if they did not correlate.

A clear description of emergent literacy skills gives the educators and SLPs an opportunity to intervene at an early age to prevent potential reading and writing disabilities later in the child's life. SLPs in schools and pediatric clinics have an opportunity to serve on preschool assessment teams that evaluate both language skills and emergent literacy skills. Clinicians who serve children at early elementary grades can integrate assessment of literacy skills as well as home literacy environment with oral language assessment. Whenever practical, SLPs can integrate literacy intervention with oral speech and language treatment.

Emergent Literacy Skill Acquisition

Generally, SLPs have paid greater attention to emergent literacy skills than to conventional reading and writing skills. Literature on emergent literacy skills is expanding in speech-language pathology (e.g., see Justice, 2006; Pence, 2007). Development of emergent literacy skills and their relation to later language and literacy problems have been especially important for SLPs. There is extensive literature on conventional literacy skills (mastery of reading and writing skills) in education and other disciplines. In this chapter, space permits only a brief sketch of major trends in children's literacy acquisition.

In an effort to understand emergent literacy skill development, *phonological awareness* and *print awareness* have been studied extensively. Emergent literacy skill learning precedes more conventional reading and writing. That there are significant individual differences in acquiring oral language skills is well known; one can expect similar individual differences in the acquisition of literacy skills: both emergent and conventional. Different children will acquire various emergent and conventional literacy skills at different age levels. Therefore, an understanding of a general sequence that most children follow may be more important than specific ages at which particular skills emerge or are mastered. Specific-age based literacy acquisition norms can be completely altered by an exceptionally enriched literacy environment and early stimulation of reading and writing with positive reinforcement. Although one might expect simpler skills to be acquired sooner than complex skills, children have defied this expectation. Children may learn a skill experts consider complex before they learn a skill considered simple (Schuele, Skibbe, & Rao, 2007). This finding cautions clinicians to be skeptic about categorization of skills as *simple* or *complex* based on the topographic features of skills. Such findings, combined with individual differences in literacy skills that may be due to environmental variations, also should prompt clinicians to question age-based norms on literacy skill acquisition.

Nonetheless, research has identified a general sequence in the acquisition of **emergent literacy skill development**:

- **Phonological awareness:** This is a set of skills in understanding how meaningful words, phrases, and sentences are created by blending sounds or phonemes (Robertson & Salter, 1997). Simpler phonological awareness skills are acquired earlier than more complex skills; generally, the order of acquisition, from the simplest to the most complex, is as follows (Pence & Justice, 2008; Schuele, Skibbe, & Rao, 2007):
  - Awareness of syllable segments (the child can clap once for each part or segment in a word); possibly, 2- to 3-year-olds can do this
  - Awareness of rhyme (the child can correctly answer such questions or requests as "Do *hat* and *rat* rhyme?" "Tell me a word that rhymes with *Tim*"); beginning at age 2; 3- to 4-year-olds may be proficient in this skill
  - Awareness of initial sounds in words (the child can correctly answer such questions as, " What sound does *Daddy* start with?" "Find another picture whose name starts like *dog*."); late preschool children can do this
  - Awareness of final sounds in words (the child correctly can answer such questions as, "Do *bats* and *cats* end with the same sound?" "Do *dog* and *mat* end with the same sound?"); late preschool and early kindergarten children can do this
  - Skills in blending sounds (combining phonemes to achieve words); early kindergarten children can do this
  - Skills in segmenting words into sounds (can break a word into its specific phonemes); middle to late kindergarten children can do this
  - Skills in deleting, adding, or substituting sounds in words; elementary grade children can do this.

- **Alphabet knowledge.** Naming the letters of the alphabet is an important early skill in learning to read and write. Once again, individual differences in learning this skill are significant, and depend on the home literacy environment (Pence & Justice, 2008). Some milestones in achieving this skill include:
  - Awareness of the alphabet. Most children become aware of their alphabet by age 3; some at 18 months may recognize a few letters whereas some 3-year-olds may not, however.
  - Awareness of the letter in one's own name. Preschool children begin to recognize the letters in their names.
  - Printing the letters of the alphabet. Some preschool children begin to print the letters of the alphabet.
  - First the beginning letters, then the subsequent letters. Children seem to master the beginning letters of the alphabet before they master the subsequent, and especially the final, letters. A possible exception is the letters in one's own name, which may be learned relatively early, regardless of the position of those letters in the alphabet string.
  - First the letters for which the name and its pronunciation are identical (e.g., the name of the letter B is Bi) and then the letters whose names are different (e.g., the letter X is pronounced ɛks).
  - First the letters that stand for consonants the child learns earlier in oral language than those that stand for consonants that are learned later (e.g., the child will learn to recognize the letters B and M—corresponding to early sounds acquired—than the letters T and V—corresponding to the later sounds acquired).

- **Print knowledge (awareness).** Children's varied and relevant reactions to printed materials is called *print knowledge* or *awareness* (Whitehurst & Lonigan, 1998). Though described separately, alphabet knowledge is part of print awareness. Children acquire skills in describing and reacting to printed materials in a certain sequence (Justice & Ezell, 2004). Children learn many of the following skills between the ages of 3 and 5 years:
  - Print interest, an early skill. The child finds looking at printed material reinforcing; interested in handling printed materials (e.g., printed sheets and books).
  - Print sequence, a subsequent skill. The child knows that a printed sentence is "read" from left to right; perhaps can move his or her finger on the printed line from left to right.
  - Book handling, an intermediate skill. The child can hold a book upright, turn the pages from left to right, point to the top of the page, begin pretend-reading from the top of the page and from the left, and so forth.
  - Print elements, a later skill. The child can correctly point to a letter, a word, and a sentence.
  - Combinations of print elements, a later skill. The child recognizes that print elements may be combined to produce larger units (e.g., sentences from words).

○ Emergent writing, 3 years of age or younger. These are child's scribbles, drawings, and marks on paper; they are not yet conventional writing skills, although some may resemble letters of the alphabet and show directionality because the child scribbles from left to right; these early skills may lead to more organized printing of alphabets, and eventually, words.

Assessment of Emergent Literacy Skills

Emergent literacy skills may be assessed by several commercially available instruments or through clinician-generated materials that are more like criterion-referenced materials than normatively standardized tests. It is generally recommended that clinicians assess phonological awareness, print awareness, and home literacy environment. Of these, there is justification for being skeptical about the usefulness of phonological awareness as an essential skill to be assessed, in spite of its heavily favored status.

Assessment of Phonological Awareness

According to research data, phonological awareness is correlated with speech and language skills and literacy in children (Schuele, Skibbe, & Rao, 2007). Absent or limited phonological awareness is also correlated with speech-language disorders and literacy problems. However, such correlations do not suggest that the presence of phonological awareness is causal to normal speech and language skills or its absence is causal to speech and language disorders. That the normally developing child "knows that words are made up of *linguistic segments*" is a theoretical claim, not an empirically established fact. Most children who learn to speak their language cannot describe linguistic segments, onset, rime, or coda. Such terms are linguists' analytical tools, not empirical realities for the child.

Some clinicians believe that it is essential to assess phonological awareness problems because such problems should be treated to promote literacy skills and to remediate articulation and phonological disorders. However, assessment of phonological skills should be justified by treatment research, not by pointing out a correlation between poor phonological awareness on the one hand and poor literacy skills and speech disorders on the other. That phonological awareness skills can be taught to children who lack them is no justification that they should be taught. There should be evidence that (a) treatment of phonological awareness results in improved literacy skills or speech production skills, or (b) that without phonological awareness skills, literacy and speech production problems cannot be remediated. Unfortunately, there is no such evidence. In fact, there is contradictory evidence. Studies have shown that (a) teaching phonological awareness has no effect on later literacy skills (Nancollis, Lawrie, & Dodd, 2005) and (b) children who receive articulation treatment show improvement in articulation, but those who receive phonological awareness training show no such improvement (Hesketh, Adams, Nightingale, & Hall, 2000). Critical reviewers of phonological treatment studies have concluded that there is no causal link between phonological awareness skills and literacy skills (Castle &

Coltheart, 2004) and that phonological awareness is not a sufficient condition for literacy skills (Bus & van IJzendoorh, 1999). Therefore, it is more efficient and effective to directly assess early literacy skills and later reading and writing skills and offer direct intervention for noted deficiencies (Hegde & Maul, 2006).

Assessment of phonological awareness is still popular in speech-language pathology. Therefore, SLPs who wish to assess phonological awareness skills now have a variety of instruments marketed for that purpose. A few tests of phonological awareness are listed in Table 17–2.

Table 17–2. Tests of Phonological Awareness

Name of Test	Age Range in Years	Skills Assessed
Abecedarian Reading Assessment (Wren & Watts, 2002)	Kindergarten and first grade	Rhyming, phoneme awareness and production, first and last sound, segmentation
Get Ready to Read! Screening Tool (Whitehurst & Lonigan, 2001)	Pre-Kindergarten	Phonological awareness screening too; available in English and Spanish
Comprehensive Test of Phonological Processing (Wagner, Torgesen, & Rashotte, 1999)	5;0 through 24;11	Phoneme manipulation, including sound deletion, sound and word blending, and segmentation of sounds, words, and syllables; includes assessment of "rapid naming"
Test of Phonological Awareness (Torgensen & Bryant, 2004)	5;0 through 8;0	Phonological awareness skills; includes a kindergarten version and an early elementary version
Test of Phonological Awareness Skills (Newcomer & Barenbaum, 2003)	5;0 through 8;0	Most phonological awareness skills
Test of Phonological Awareness in Spanish (Riccio, Imhoff, Hasbrouck, & Davis, 2004)	4;0 through 10;11	Most phonological awareness skills in Spanish
Phonological Awareness Test (Robertson & Salter, 1997)	5;0 through 9;0	Rhyming, sound/letter association, word decoding, syllable segmentation, and phoneme manipulation, and "invented spelling"
Test of Preschool Early Literacy (Lonigan, Wagner, Torgesen, & Rashotte, 2007)	3;0 to 5;0 yrs	Print knowledge, oral vocabulary, and phonological awareness

Assessment of Alphabet and Print Knowledge

Although described separately, alphabet and print knowledge seem to belong to the same general response class. Therefore, these skills may be assessed together. Both include rudimentary skills from which conventional reading and writing may be shaped. The same basic set of skills of alphabet and print knowledge may lead to two sets of eventually differentiated skills of reading and writing.

Two general methods help assess alphabet and print knowledge. Clinicians can either use one of several available assessment instruments or client-specific measures they develop themselves. Both criterion-referenced and norm-referenced instruments are available for selection. Table 17–3 lists some of the published tools for assessing alphabet and print knowledge. It may be noted that a few are norm-referenced, but most are criterion-referenced.

Child-specific procedures to assess alphabet and print knowledge may be integrated with language assessment. Clinicians may use a variety of print stimuli that are also used during language sampling to assess basic print awareness skills. An advantage of child-specific materials over standardized test materials is that the clinician can take into

Table 17–3. Tests of Alphabet and Print Knowledge

Name of Test	Age Range in Years	Skills Assessed
Developing Skills Checklist: Print Concepts (CTB/McGraw-Hill, 1990)	4;0 to 6;0	Print-picture differentiation, book conventions, identification of letters, words, sentences, punctuation
Early Reading Diagnostic Assessment-Revised: Concept of Print Observation Checklist (Psychological Corporation, 2002)	Kindergarten through grade 3	Letter name identification in name, print directionality, matching speech to print, pausing between sentences
An Observational Survey of Early Literacy Achievement: Concepts About Print (Clay, 2005)	5;0 through 7;0	Print directionality, book organization, punctuation, letter and word concepts, relationship between letters and words
Emergent Literacy Screening: Print Awareness Section (Paulson et al., 2001)	3;0 to 6;0	Emergent writing skills, written name identification, book convention
Preschool Word and Print Awareness (Justice et al., 2006)	3;0 to 5;0	Letter concepts, print meaning, book and print organization
Test of Early Reading Ability-3: Conventions (Reid et al., 2001)	3;0 to 8;0	Print forms, print meaning, punctuation marks, book and print organization

consideration the child's verbal skill level and the ethnocultural background. The child-specific materials the clinician develops will be the most appropriate to assess a child's language as well as literacy skills:

- Under each picture shown to the child during language sampling, the clinician may print words that correspond to the pictures; pictures and words will be client-specific; relevant to the child's verbal skills and cultural background

- Clinician may select simple storybooks that are relevant to the child and have parents bring the child's favorite storybooks that will be used during language sampling

- Have a collection of words, phrases, and sentences that are expected to be at the child's skill level

- Have the printed alphabet available during assessment

- With such materials, the clinician may obtain child-specific measures of alphabet and print awareness skills, by asking the child to:
  - point to printed individual words and sentences
  - point to given letters of the alphabet within words or sentences (e.g., "Show me /s/ in this word.")
  - point to various named letters on the printed alphabet (e.g., "Show me /b/.")
  - name the letters of the alphabet pointed to (e.g., "What is this?" while pointing to the alphabet A.)
  - make the sound of the pointed alphabet (e.g., "What sound does this make?" while pointing to /s/.)
  - point to the letter when an alphabet-related sound is made (e.g., "Show me which letter makes sound like *sssss*.")
  - point to the letter the child's name starts with (e.g., "Show me the letter your name starts with.")
  - point to the letters that are in the child's name (e.g., "Show me all the letters in your name.")
  - recite the alphabet (e.g., "Can you say a-b-c-d?" "Can you keep going all the way to z?"
  - differentially point to upper and lower case letters of the same alphabet
  - name products by looking at their logos and signs (e.g., showing the logo of the child's favorite food product and asking, "What do you think of when you see this picture?")
  - Tell the meaning of such commonly encountered signs as *stop, exit, enter, men's room, women's room*, and so forth (e.g., showing a stop sign and asking, "What does your Mom do when she is driving you to school and sees this sign?")
  - hold a storybook to assess book orientation
  - turn pages in a book
  - point to the top, bottom, front, and back of the book

- o show how a book is read (e.g., "How do you read the book? From this side to that side or that side to this side?" while moving a finger on a line from left to right and right to left, alternately)
- o show a word, any word (e.g., "Can you point to a word on this page?")
- o point to a particular word on the page (e.g., "Show me the word *cat* on this page.")
- o show where one should start reading (e.g., "Show me where I begin reading.")
- o show a sentence ("Point to a whole sentence on this page.)
- o count the number of words in a sentence (e.g., "Tell me how many words you see in this sentence.")
- o point to a paragraph (e.g., "Show me a paragraph on this page.")
- o count sentences in a paragraph (e.g., "Tell me how many sentences you see in this paragraph.")
- o point to various and specific punctuation marks on printed pages (e.g., "Show me a full stop on this page.").

Obviously, not all children will respond correctly to all the sample strategies just listed. Some preschoolers are much more advanced than others. Therefore, instead of prejudging the child's level of alphabet and print knowledge, the clinician should test the limit by presenting progressively more difficult stimulus items. Some of the same and expanded stimulus materials and strategies may be used to assess early reading and writing skills as described in a later section.

Assessment of Home Literacy Environment and Behavioral Support

As noted earlier, home literacy environment and literacy-related actions of family members have a significant positive or negative effect on a child's emergent and subsequent literacy skills. Therefore, an assessment of the home literacy environment and literacy-related behaviors of parents and others is valuable in understanding literacy problems in children and in suggesting preventive or remedial steps.

More than just the presence of literacy materials at home, how the parents, other family members, and such caregivers as babysitters use the available resources will have a positive or negative effect on children's literacy skills. Furthermore, the family's cultural background, emphasis placed on literacy skills, any bilingual status also will influence the child's literacy skills. Cultures with strong oral traditions (e.g., many Native American tribes) may not necessarily place a great value on the printed word, but such cultures may promote excellent oral language skills (Kay-Raining Bird & Vetter, 1994). An Asian immigrant group in the United States, the Hmong people from Laos, did not have a written language until the 1950s (Lindsay, 2004). Also, some families with extremely low income may be forced to forego literacy resources in favor of essentials (Koppenhaver, Evans, & Yoder, 1991; Marvin & Mirenda, 1993).

The main objective in assessing home literacy environment is to judge the kinds of support the child receives for learning to read and write. The environmental and caregiver support should be such that the child enjoys emergent, developing, and fully developed literacy skills because of the positive behavioral support. The child should be engaged in literacy activities because they have been positively reinforced (and thus enjoyable to the child) and not because the child is trying to escape from negative consequences of *not being* engaged in such activities. Although the kinds of behavioral support the child receives is difficult to observe, the results of such support can often be judged. The frequency with which the child engages in literacy activities, the child's verbally stated likes and dislikes of literacy activities, the physical (environmental) support for such activities, and the parents' own literacy behaviors all give a good indication of the amount and nature of family support for literacy skills in a child. A final indication of past support is the child's current level of literacy skill: expected or even advanced.

Several methods are available to assess home literacy environment and caregiver support and behaviors. Direct observations of the child's home environment through home visits, parent or caregiver interviews, and various questionnaires that parents and caregivers fill out are all methods of making this assessment (Zucker & Grant, 2007). Measured skill levels themselves help validate some of the observations or raise questions about information parents give through interviews and questionnaires.

If a home visit is practical, the clinician will gain some first-hand knowledge of the literacy-related conditions that prevail at the child's home. Home visits, interviews, and questionnaires are a means to obtain answers to the following kinds of questions:

- Are there literacy materials in the household? Are there books, newspapers, and magazines?

- Are literacy materials easily accessible to the child, especially to a preschooler? Can the child easily reach them?

- Are there children's storybooks that seem to be appropriate for the child's age? Are there children's books that seem to be advanced considering the child's age? Do the books appear too simple for the child's age?

- Are there children's encyclopedias, dictionaries, books on fairy tales, and children's science books?

- Are there writing materials, such as paper, pens, blackboards, dry erase boards, easels, color crayons, markers, chalk, and so forth? Can the child easily reach them?

- Is the child's room or a place in the house set up for reading and writing? Is there furniture suitable for the child's reading and writing activities?

- Are the parents, caregivers, and older siblings good role models of literacy for the child to emulate?

- Do parents regularly read aloud storybooks to the child? How often in a week? For what duration? What kinds of books do they read to the child?

- How do parents read aloud stories to their child? Do they let the child see the text they are reading? Do they sit side-by-side with the child? Do they point to words and sentences as they read aloud? Is the storybook reading interactive? Do they frequently ask the child to point to letters, words, or sentences as they read? Do they invite comments from the child about what is being read?

- Is there evidence that parents and older siblings read and write regularly?

- Does the child receive cards from the parents (e.g., birthday card with the child's name on it)

- Do parents ask the child to print his or her name on birthday cards given to other members of the family?

- Do parents ask the child to help make a grocery list?

- Do parents take the child to the local library? Does the child borrow books from the library?

- Are there examples of the child's written or drawn products displayed at the child's room or other areas of the home?

- Does the child have educational play materials? Are thee magnetic letters and numbers? Are there maps of the country and the world hung on the walls?

- What kind of programs does the child watch on television? Do parents watch educational programs with the child?

- Do they have audio- or video-records of classic stories or nursery rhymes? Do parents and children together listen to them periodically?

The list suggested several sample questions, but it can be expanded to include additional resources and caregiver behaviors that support literacy (Pence, 2007). Zucker and Grant (2007) not only provide an exhaustive discussion of assessing home and family support for literacy, but also describe a variety of assessment questionnaires that can be administered to family members.

In addition to assessing the general literacy resources and behavioral support for literacy activities at home, the clinician may seek information on whether the parents or other caregivers have made a systematic effort to teach reading and writing to a preschooler. Many parents who think that a preschool child is not ready for reading and writing may refrain from direct instruction. But others who do not subscribe to the readiness notion may be willing to teach the child how to print the alphabet, read printed words, and eventually read simple books. The clinician may try to answer the following kinds of questions:

- Have the family members made any specific efforts to teach reading and writing to their child?

- How old was the child when they started teaching literacy skills to their child?

- Did they start with reading or printing the letters of the alphabet?

- What methods did they use to teach the literacy skills?

- What kind of materials did they use to teach reading or writing? Commercially available or parent-prepared?

- How did they react to the child's success or failure?

- Are the efforts to formally teach reading and writing systematic and continuous?

- Have they made systematic efforts to teach number concepts? How have they done it? What has the child learned?

- Are there child's progressive writing samples (including words, numbers, drawing) that could be copied for the child's academic or clinical file?

Clinicians should note that although home environments of children in the lower socioeconomic levels may not contain much literacy materials, including child's furniture and other physical support, they may still receive much behavioral support for reading and writing with the few materials that they may have. Parents may teach reading and writing with minimal materials; it is the systematic positive reinforcement for reading and writing that constitutes *behavioral support*. Literacy skill acquisition may be significantly hampered only when neither material nor behavioral support is evident. Similarly, some middle or upper class parents may not necessarily provide a literacy-enriched environment for their children or if they provide environmental (physical) support, may fail to provide behavioral support for reading and writing. Therefore, the clinician should avoid stereotypes about socioeconomic classes, and make objective assessments (Hegde & Maul, 2006).

Assessment of Reading and Writing

Unlike reading and writing specialists in schools, SLPs may take a slightly different approach to assessing emergent or conventional literacy skills in children. SLPs may make literacy assessment a part of the larger language assessment. Because of the likely coexistence of literacy and oral language problems in children, SLPs are better equipped than other professionals to make a comprehensive assessment of all language and language-based skills.

To what extent SLPs would conduct literacy assessment is likely to be a function of their (a) training in literacy assessment and intervention and (b) available professional time. As noted previously, many clinicians may not be equipped to make a thorough literacy assessment; such clinicians will depend on the expertise of their colleagues, including SLPs who do have the training and experience, and reading and writing specialists. Regardless of an expanded professional practice, a desire to help, and newly acquired expertise in literacy assessment and intervention, many SLPs in public schools may find it difficult to devote time to exhaustive assessment of literacy problems and intensive and direct literacy intervention. Clinicians who have specialized themselves in literacy problems may do more than those who have not specialized and whose caseload is full of children with more conventional communication disorders of oral language, speech, fluency, and voice. Nonetheless, all SLPs can integrate certain important elements of literacy skills into their traditional assessment (and treatment) of speech and language problems.

A complete assessment of verbal and nonverbal language skills should precede a full-fledged literacy assessment. Therefore, oral language assessment procedures described in Chapters 8 and 9 and assessment of nonverbal skills described in Chapters 14 and 15 are relevant to assess literacy skills.

Administration of available standardized tests to assess reading and writing skills in children is now within the scope of SLPs. As a matter of ethical principles, clinicians should obtain proper training in the administration and scoring of these tests. Table 17–4 presents selected standardized tests of reading and writing skills in children of different

Table 17–4. Tests of Reading and Writing Skills

Name of Test	Age Range in Years	Skills Assessed
Test of Early Written Language-2 (Hresko, 1996)	3;0 through 10;11	Emergent writing skills; spelling, capitalization, punctuation, sentence construction, writing stories about a picture prompt
Test of Written Language (Hammill & Larsen, 1996)	7;6 through 17;11	Capitalization, punctuation, spelling, vocabulary, grammar, and composition
Test of Reading Comprehension (4th edition) (Brown, Hammill, & Widerholt, 2009)	7;0 through 17;11	Comprehension of general vocabulary, syntactic similarities; answering questions regarding "story-like" paragraphs
Test of Written Expression (McGhee, Bryant, Larsen, & Rivera, 1995)	6;6 through 14;11	Writing skills, including essay writing in response to a "story starter" (e.g., student is required to continue a story to a conclusion)
Test of Written English (TWE) (Anderson & Thompson, 1988)	6;0 through 17;11	Screens for skills in written expression and paragraph writing; also assesses capitalization and punctuation
Test of Early Reading Ability (Reid, Hresko, & Hammill, 2001)	3;6 through 8;6	Alphabet knowledge, print conventions, and meaning from print
Standard Reading Inventory (Newcomer, 1999)	Preprimary to grade 8	Silent reading and comprehension and oral reading skills; contains 10 graded passages
Gray Diagnostic Reading Tests (Bryant, Widerholt, & Bryant, 2004)	6;0 through 13;11	Letter/word identification, reading vocabulary, subtests for reading comprehension, "rapid naming," and phonological awareness
Woodcock Language Proficiency Battery-Revised (Woodcock, 1991)	2;0 through adult	Oral language, reading, and written language; includes English and Spanish forms

age groups. Some may be appropriate to assess literacy skills in adults as well, as noted in the description.

As with emergent literacy skills, we recommend *child-specific* measures to assess reading and writing skills. They may be used in addition to standardized tests or by themselves especially in case of ethnoculturally diverse children. Reading and writing skills are on a continuum of development and progressively more advanced skills may be acquired throughout a life span. According to the American Speech-Language-Hearing Association (2001b), child-specific methods may be used to assess reading and writing skills at three developmental levels: (1) the preschool emergent level; (2) kindergarten through grade 3 early elementary level, and (3) grade 4 and above later level. It should be noted that the different skill levels are not discrete and adjacent levels may overlap. In addition, several skills may be assessed at multiple levels because skills are cumulative in their complexity; the same skills are assessed at increased complexity at progressively higher levels.

Assessment of Reading and Writing at the Preschool Emergent Level

If the clinician wants to gain a basic understanding of a child's literacy skills at the emergent level, then integrating literacy assessment with either speech or language assessment is a practical choice. Suggestions offered earlier about assessing print awareness may be used in the context of speech-language assessment. Perhaps in most cases, emergent reading and writing skill assessment should follow an emergent literacy skill assessment (e.g., alphabet and print knowledge, as described in the previous section).

If a more thorough literacy assessment is planned, the clinician may first assess the child's receptive and expressive language skills with procedures described in Chapters 8 and 9. After this language assessment, the clinician may concentrate on literacy assessment. The procedures would depend mostly on the age and the literacy skill level of the child.

Assessment of Reading and Writing at the Early Elementary Level (Kindergarten through Grade 3)

Children in kindergarten through grade 3 are a diverse group and may have varied skills. Some highly literate parents or other caregivers may have taught their child reading and writing skills by the time the child enters first grade. Children can be taught to read first-grade books by age 5 or 6; they can be taught to write sentences or more by that age. By the time they are 5 years of age, some children will have advanced literacy skills. Other children may not have mastered the alphabet recitation or printing when they enter the first grade. Therefore, it is appropriate for the literacy experts in schools to keep the options open of assessing early, intermediate, and relatively advanced literacy skills when working with children up to grade 3. On the other hand, SLPs, by the very nature of their work, are more likely to evaluate deficient oral language and literacy skills in children than advanced language and literacy skills. When SLPs evaluate children with language disorders, they are likely to be assessing impaired reading and writing skills.

At kindergarten through the early elementary level, the clinician should assess: (1) letter identification, (2) early reading skills, and (3) elementary writing skills. Within a somewhat extended language assessment session, the clinician may integrate language and literacy assessment procedures. If not, additional session would be needed to complete the literacy assessment.

Assessment of Letter Identification

Not surprisingly, a child's knowledge of letter name is highly correlated with later literacy skills (Kaminski & Good, 1996; Scarborough, 1998; Stevenson & Newman, 1986). Alphabet letter identification by their names is an early skill necessary for both writing and reading. Therefore, during assessment, the clinician may seek answers to the following kinds of questions with the procedures described:

- Can the child name the letters of the alphabet shown? Is the child fluent and correct in naming the letters? The clinician presents the letters of the alphabet and asks, "What letter is this?" "What do you call this?"

- Can the child recite the entire alphabet? Is the recitation fluent and correct? The clinician requests the child to recite the alphabet; prompts, if necessary.

- Can the child make the *sound* each letter represents? The clinician presents various letters of the alphabet and asks, "Do you know what sound it makes?"

Assessment of Early Reading Skills

Oral and silent reading may not necessarily mean that the read material is comprehended. Some people with and without reading disabilities may read printed material with little or no understanding of what is read. Therefore, both reading and reading comprehension should be assessed.

Early reading skills may be assessed either through clinician-prepared or through standardized assessment tools. Several standardized tests are available to assess phonological awareness, early literacy skills, and more advanced reading and writing skills. Depending on the age of the child, the clinician may administer one or more standardized tests listed in Table 17–4.

A good starting point is to find out what school curricula demand of children ready to leave kindergarten and enter the first grade. For instance, a literacy skill required of children leaving kindergarten is "sounding out" simple three-letter words or nonsense syllables. Clinicians may assess this and other early reading skills as follows:

- *Spell-and-say the word (sounding-out words).* To assess this skill, the clinician may select three-letter printed words that are appropriate for the child and the family cultural background. The clinician may ask the child to "sound out" each word and then say it (e.g., the child will spell /c/ - /a/ - /t/ and then say "cat")

- *Oral reading.* The clinician should select graded reading material that is suitable for the child's age and the reading skill level suggested from observation and parental information. Perhaps three passages, slightly increasing in the difficulty level, may help assess the child's range of reading skill. Tape recording the child's reading samples will assist in later analysis of reading errors. Omission, misreading, or addition of words, and failure to read words and sentences may all be noted during analysis.

- *Fluency in oral reading.* The same recorded reading samples will help assess fluency in reading. The clinician may count the number of words correctly read per minute (e.g., 100 words read correctly in 5 minutes = 20 words correctly read per minute). Fluency also may be judged by counting the frequency of false starts, repetitions in reading, interjections of extraneous phrases, and unusually long pauses (hesitations) at various junctures.

- *Comprehension of read material.* At the completion of each oral reading sample, the clinician should ask a series of questions to assess the child's comprehension of read material. The clinician also may have the child read a new and brief paragraph and ask questions about the information.

A child who has difficulty comprehending oral language may have difficulty understanding what is silently read. Silent reading skill cannot be directly assessed simply because it is a covert behavior. It can be assessed only through responses given to questions about the read material. That the child has difficulty reading certain words would not be evident as the child is silently reading a passage; the clinician would not know whether the child simply skipped difficult words. Generally, the words the child does not understand in oral conversation would not be understood in silent reading.

Assessment of Early Writing Skills

Assessment of early writing skills in kindergarten through grade 3 children may be accomplished in several ways. A few writing tasks can be included in the standard speech-language assessment. For example, the child may be asked to:

- Connect dots to form the letters of the alphabet
- Trace the letters of the alphabet faintly printed on paper
- Print the letters of the alphabet
- Copy a few simple printed words the clinician points to in storybooks
- Draw a face, a flower, and simple environmental objects
- Write his or her name, address, phone number, and the names of family members; may spell words phonetically (e.g., a child might write "tek" for *take,* "lern" for *learn*)
- Write to dictation
- Spontaneously write on a topic, one's experience, or write a brief story.

Obviously, the complexity of the task presented will depend on the skill level of the child. Although some advanced third grade students may write to dictation if the dictated material is from their grade level, younger children with lower skills may stop at some point in the hierarchy of skills they are asked to perform. As suggested earlier, it is always a useful strategy to plan for a range of tasks to be presented, knowing well that a given child will not perform all of them, instead of accepting the stereotypes that young children can only perform this or that skill. If the child is not requested to perform a more complex skill, the clinician would never know the child's limits.

A good approach is to ask the parents to bring writing or drawing samples to the session when the appointment is made for assessment. The parents should be requested to bring samples from different time periods. Such samples brought from home will better illustrate the progress the child has made over a period of time in learning to write. The most recent writing sample will help gauge the writing assessment entry level.

As the child writes, copies, or draws, the clinician should take notes on how well the child performs. The child may attend to the task with good concentration or may be distracted. The child may initiate writing impulsively or may pause, plan, and start in a methodic manner. A child who does not plan or has poor writing skills is likely to hesitate, erase, or cross out what has been written. There may be repeated false starts. Spelling errors may be common and letter formation may be poor.

When the child has produced more advanced writing, such as a prose paragraph, the clinician can analyze mechanics and content of writing. The clinician should analyze such writing mechanics as sentence formulation, word usage, spelling, punctuation, grammar, margins, and spacing. In analyzing the content of writing, the clinician evaluates cohesiveness, logical sequence, clarity of expression, and a good beginning and an end to the narration.

Assessment of Reading and Writing at the Later Level

Children in fourth grade and beyond (the later level) are expected to have wider and more complex literacy skills than children in the younger age levels. Reading and writing skills may achieve a degree of independence that the children can continue to make further progress on their own or with limited direction.

Older children (in fourth grade and beyond) who have literacy problems are also likely to have less severe language disorders than those in the earlier grades. By this time, their language skills may have improved because of language intervention. Also, they may have received intervention for their reading and writing problems in earlier grades. Nonetheless, those children may experience difficulties in advanced language skills, including comprehension and production of figurative and abstract language. Consequently, the children may have difficulty with advanced reading and writing tasks.

Both child-specific procedures and standardized tests may be used to assess reading and writing skills at the later level. Clinicians may prepare child-specific tasks and present them during language assessment. If more detailed assessment is needed, the clinician may devote additional time for it. The clinician may administer one of the standardized tests listed in Table 17–4 to assess reading and writing skills.

Assessment of Reading at the Later Level

Normally, children in the fourth grade and beyond will have learned to read to an extent that they can make systematic progress in reading and in handling more complex material. Learning to read will not be the main concern, unless the child still has significant reading problems; reading to learn progressively more complex information will be the main concern. Some educators have described this as a shift in the emphasis from *learning to read* to *reading to learn* (Snow, Scarborough, & Burns, 1999). A child who has made that shift will continue to make good academic progress.

Children with reading problems, however, will not make that shift easily. Their efforts to master the reading skills will continue. Consequently, these children will have difficulty in making academic progress, because much of the academic work will require good reading skills. Regardless of the age and grade, a child with significant reading problems may exhibit a range of strengths and limitations. Therefore, assessment planning should include a range of tasks to capture the child's difficulties at simpler levels as well as to test the limit of the child's reading skills. Generally, in assessing older children with mild reading problems, the clinician should be prepared to assess reading and writing at higher levels than when assessing children with severe reading and writing problems.

Some of the complete reading diagnostic tests listed in Table 17–4 allow assessment of advanced reading skills. For instance, the *Gray Diagnostic Reading Test* (Bryant, Widerholt, & Bryant, 2004) may be used to assess reading skills in children 6 years through 13;11 years. The *Standard Reading Inventory* (Newcomer, 1999) also helps assess children in that age group; in addition, it provides 10 graded passages for assessing progressively more complex reading skills.

The clinician also may select reading passages from the child's academic books that are appropriately graded. Assessment of both fluent reading and comprehension of passages that contain abstract terms, figurative language (e.g., proverbs, idioms, similes, and metaphors), special academic and scientific terms (e.g., describe versus discuss, infer, hypothesize, explain, evaluate, conclude, criticize) would be especially targeted. Whether the child can fluently read and understand technical definition of terms would be a useful assessment target. Finally, whether the child can understand as well as critically evaluate what is read should also be an assessment target.

Passages that contain complex and less frequently used sentence structures may be especially difficult for the child to understand. The child may find it difficult to understand the multiple meanings of terms in printed passages. Such literacy pieces as a short story or a poem included in the curriculum may pose special difficulties for the child. These skills should be assessed with the help of materials selected from the child's curricula or standardized tests.

Assessment of Writing at the Later Level

Assessment of writing skills of children in grades 4 and higher will concentrate more on connected, expository writing. The clinician may obtain samples of child's writing from the classroom teacher for analysis; it is essential to sample different kinds of writing (e.g., descriptions, narrative writings, cause-effect analysis, comparing or contrasting). The clinician also may dictate a passage for the child to write. In addition, the child may be asked to write a brief story and describe a familiar event (e.g., birthday party or a visit to a theme park). The child might be also asked to copy a printed paragraph; this task will be useful in assessing how well a child writes when following a written model.

In completing all assignments, the child should be encouraged to write as clearly and neatly as possible and to give as much detail as possible. The child may be allowed some time to think and plan the writing. The child should be free to make outlines or drafts. A dictionary may be made available to the child. Any written notes the child prepares before writing should be collected as well for analysis. All writing should be done in ink so the child's writing shows the errors and revisions.

An analysis of child's writing skills and problems may include a variety of measures derived from the samples. The types and varieties of errors will vary across the tasks. For example, the child may make more spelling errors while writing to dictation than copying printed paragraphs; the former requires a more rapid writing than copying or spontaneous writing on a given topic. A piece of writing may be more or less productive; a basic measure of quantitative productivity (not necessarily of quality) is the number of words in a sample of writing. Quality of writing is judged not from the number of words, but how effectively and clearly it says what it purports to say. Some verbose writing may not say much but some cryptic writing may say much more.

Easier to judge than the quality of writing are the spelling accuracy, syntactic accuracy and variety, and correct use of morphologic features. Spelling errors that are commonly found in school-age children include various kinds of omissions, substitutions, and other kinds of deviations (Moats, 1995; Nippold, 2007). The child may omit one or more sound in a consonant cluster:

- **Omissions:** The child may omit liquids or nasals in positions other than the initial (e.g., *sef* fo *self* or *ret* for *rent*); a sound in a consonant cluster (e.g., *bet* for *best*); unstressed vowels (e.g., *telphone* for *telephone*); grammatical morphemes (e.g., omission of the plural morpheme, possessive, and past-tense inflections)

- **Substitutions:** The child may substitute vowels (e.g., *bi* for *buy*); consonants (e.g., *t* for *d* or *m* for *n)*

- **Word substitutions:** Certain common words that sound similar may be substituted with each other (e.g., *there* for *their* or vice versa; *to* for *two* or vice versa)

- **Errors in derivational morphologic features:** Prefixes and suffixes that help derive other forms of the stem-words may be especially difficult (e.g., *determined-predetermined; author-coauthor; space-spatial; nature-natural; enjoy-enjoyable; happy-happiness*)

Syntactically acceptable writing should include correct sentences, both simple and complex sentences, embedded clauses, and varied types of sentences. The sentence length should vary within a piece of writing. Repetitive use of short sentences suggests a lack of syntactic complexity and variety. Other syntactic features that improve during the later period and may be missed or misused by children with writing problems include (Nippold, 2007):

- Low-frequency syntactic features. These include elaborated subjects (e.g., *animals, such as dogs, pigs, cows, and chickens were exhibited*); modal auxiliary verbs (e.g., *we should have studied harder*); the passive (e.g., *the boy was brought to the school by his mother*); appositives (e.g., *John, the weatherman, made an agreeable prediction*); the perfect aspect (e.g., *he had been doing this for many years*)

- Use of subordinating, coordinating, and correlative conjunctions that increase sentence length; although no detailed normative data are available, it is expected that school-age children (as against preschoolers) begin to use conjunctions and continue to master them throughout the elementary and high school years:
  - subordinating conjunctions (e.g., *when, although, unless*) that introduce a dependent clause (e.g., *unless he is tired*) and are attached to independent clauses (e.g., *he won't go to bed*).
  - Coordinating conjunctions (*and, but, so*) that join two independent clauses (e.g., "Chad likes to read *and* Lance likes to play.")
  - Correlative conjunctions (*both, either, neither*) that suggest symmetrical relations (e.g. "*Both* Beth and Leticia scored 100%").

Adverbial conjuncts (intersentential cohesion devices that connect sentences), are essential in more advanced writing. There are many adverbial conjuncts in English; children in the elementary grades may use only a few common conjuncts in their speech and writing; even 12- to 15-year-olds may achieve only 50% accuracy in their production. Advanced adverbial conjuncts only older students and adults use, especially in persuasive writing, include *essentially, eventually, technically, literally, unfortunately, normally,* and so forth. Some of the common adjuncts that 8- to 12-year-olds may correctly use include (Nippold, 2007):

- *then, so, though*
- *anyway, by the way*
- *even so, on the other hand*
- *however*

Mechanics of writing refer to a variety of skills that need to be assessed for acceptability. Some of the common mechanics of writing include:

- Correct use of capitalization
- Correct use of various punctuation marks including the comma, period, semicolon, exclamation marks, quotation marks, and so forth
- Giving correct margins
- Giving appropriate titles for essays and headings and subheadings within them
- Citing and referencing authors and sources of information.

Assessment of writing skills at the later level goes hand-in-hand with an evaluation of the child's advanced language skills. Any deficiency in orally producing sentences of increasing syntactic complexity and variety, academic and infrequently used terms, synonyms and antonyms, and figurative language may be reflected in the child's writing samples. Generally, significant deficiencies in oral language suggest a need for assessing similar deficiencies in written language. A comprehensive assessment of both written and oral language skills, along with an assessment of reading skills and home literacy environment, will help develop both speech-language and literacy intervention programs for the child.

References

AAC Feature Match. (1996). Arlington, TX: Douglas Dodgen and Associates.

AAT Assessment Tool. (1998). Arlington, TX: Douglas Dodgen and Associates.

Abbeduto, L., Davies, B., & Furman, L. (1988). The development of speech act comprehension in mentally retarded individuals and non-retarded children. *Child Development, 59,* 1460–1472.

Abbeduto, L., Furman, L., & Davies, B. (1989). Relation between the receptive language and mental age of persons with mental retardation. *American Journal of Mental Retardation, 93,* 535–543.

Adler, S. (1990). Multicultural clients: Implications for the SLP. *Language, Speech and Hearing Services in Schools, 21,* 135–139.

Administration on Developmental Disabilities, U.S. Department of Health and Human Services. (2005). *About ADD.* Retrieved from http://www.acf.hhs.gov/programs/add/add about.html

Agin, R. (2000). Clinical management of voice disorders in culturally diverse children: Background and definition. In T. Coleman (Ed.), *Clinical management of communication disorders in culturally diverse children.* Boston, MA: Allyn & Bacon.

Akif Kilic, M., Okur, E., Yildirim, I., & Guzelsoy, S. (2004). The prevalence of vocal fold nodules in school age children. *International Journal of Pediatric Otorhinolaryngology, 68*(4), 409–412.

Allen, K. D., Bernstein, B., & Chait, D. H. (1991). EMG biofeedback treatment of pediatric hyperfunction dysphonia. *Journal of Behavioral Therapy and Experimental Psychiatry, 22*(2), 97–101.

Allen, M. S., Pettit, J. M., & Sherblom, J. C. (1991). Management of vocal nodules: A regional survey of otolaryngologists and speech-language pathologists. *Journal of Speech and Hearing Research, 34,* 229–235.

American Academy of Pediatrics. (n.d.). *Growth and development.* Retrieved from http://www.aap.org/pubed

American Psychiatric Association. (2000a). *Diagnostic and statistical manual of mental disorders* (4th ed., Rev.). Washington, DC: Author.

American Psychiatric Association. (2000b). Childhood disintegrative disorder. In *Diagnostic and statistical manual of mental disorders* (4th ed., Rev.). Washington, DC: Author.

American Psychological Association. (1999). *Standards for educational and psychological testing.* Washington DC: Author.

American Speech-Language-Hearing Association. (n.d.). *How does your child hear and talk?* Retrieved from http://www.asha.org/public/speech/development/chart.htm

American Speech-Language-Hearing Association. (1983). Social dialects. *Asha, 25,* 23–27.

American Speech-Language-Hearing Association. (1985). Clinical management of communicatively handicapped minority language populations. *Asha, 26*(1), 55–57.

American Speech-Language-Hearing Association Ad Hoc Committee on Service Delivery in the Schools. (1993). Definitions of communication disorders and variations. *Asha, 35* (Suppl. 10), 40–41.

American Speech-Language-Hearing Association. (2001a). *Scope of practice for speech-language pathologists.* Retrieved from http://www.asha.org/docs/html

American Speech-Language-Hearing Association. (2001b). *Roles and responsibilities of speech-language pathologists with respect to reading and writing for children and adults: Practice guidelines.* Retrieved from http://www.asha.org/docs/html

American Speech-Language-Hearing Association. (2002). Augmentative and alternative communication: Knowledge and skills for service delivery. *Asha Supplement, 22,* 97–106.

American Speech-Language-Hearing Association. (2003). Code of ethics (Revised). *ASHA Supplement, 23,* 13–15.

American Speech-Language-Hearing Association. (2004a). *Roles and responsibilities of speech-language pathologists with respect to augmentative and alternative communication: Position statement.* Retrieved from http://www.asha.org/policy

American Speech-Language-Hearing Association. (2004b). *Communication facts: Incidence and prevalence of communication disorders and hearing loss in children–2004 edition.* Rockville, MD: Author.

American Speech-Language-Hearing Association. (2007). *Scope of practice for speech-language pathologists.* Retrieved from http://www.asha.org/docs/html/sp-2007-00283.html

American Speech-Language-Hearing Association. (2008). *Roles and responsibilities of speech-language pathologists in early intervention.* Retrieved from http://www.asha.org/policy

American Speech-language-Hearing Association, Working Group on Endoscopy. (2008). Position statement on endoscopy. *ASHA Practice Policy.* doi: 10.1044/policy.PS2008-00297 Retrieved from http://www.asha.org/docs/html/PS2008-00297.html

Analysis of Communication Interaction. (2009). Pittsburg, PA: DynaVox Mayer-Johnson.

Anastasi, A., & Urbina, S. (1997). *Psychological testing* (7th ed.). Upper Saddle River, NJ: Prentice-Hall.

Anderson, R. T. (2004). First language loss in Spanish-speaking children: Patterns of loss and implications for clinical practice. In B. A. Goldstein (Ed.), *Bilingual language development and disorders in Spanish-English speakers* (pp. 187–212). Baltimore, MD: Paul H. Brookes.

Anderson, V., & Thompson, S. (1988). *Test of Written English (TWE).* Novato, CA: Academic Therapy Publications.

Andrews, M. L. (1986). *Voice therapy for children.* White Plains, NY: Longman.

Andrews, M. L . (1995). *Manual of voice treatment: Pediatrics through geriatrics.* San Diego, CA: Singular.

Andrews, M. L. (2002). *Voice treatment for children and adolescents.* San Diego, CA: Singular.

Andrews, M. L. (2006). *Manual of voice treatment–Pediatrics through geriatrics* (3rd ed.). Clifton Park, NY: Thompson Delmar Learning.

Arlt, P. B., & Goodban, M. T. (1976). A comparative study of articulation acquisition as based on a study of 240 normals, aged three to six. *Language, Speech and Hearing Services in Schools, 7,* 173–180.

Arvedson, J. C., McNeil, M. R., & West, T. L. (1985). Prediction of Revised Token Test overall, subtest, and linguistic unit scores by two shortened versions. *Clinical Aphasiology, 15,* 57–63.

Atlas, J., & Lapidus, L. (1988). Symbolization levels in communicative behaviors of children showing pervasive developmental disorders. *Journal of Communicative Disorders, 21,* 75–84.

Awan, S. N., & Mueller, P. B. (1996). Speaking fundamental frequency characteristics of White, African American, and Hispanic kindergartners. *Journal of Speech and Hearing Research, 39,* 573–577.

Bach, K., McGuirt, W., & Postma, G. (2002). Pediatric laryngopharyngeal reflux. *Ear, Nose and Throat Journal* (Suppl. 2), 27–30.

Bailey, G., & Thomas, E. (1998). Some aspects of African American Vernacular English phonology. In S. Mufwene, J. R. Rickford, G. Bailey, & J. Baugh (Eds.), *African American English: Structure, history, and use* (pp. 85–109). New York, NY: Rutledge.

Bain, B., & Olswang, L. (1995). Examining readiness for learning two word utterances by children with specific expressive language impairment: Dynamic assessment validation. *American Journal of Speech-Language Pathology, 4,* 81–91.

Baker, B. M., & Blackwell, P. B. (2004). Identification and remediation of pediatric fluency and voice disorders. *Journal of Pediatric Health Care, 18,* 87–94.

Baker, M. (1984). *Voice disorders in Mexican-American and Anglo-American adolescents: A comparative study.* Unpublished doctoral dissertation, International University, Miami, FL.

Balandin, S. (2007). Unaided AAC interventions appear to facilitate the development of speech [Abstract]. *Evidence-Based Communication Assessment and Intervention, 1,* 63–64.

Bankson, N. W. (1990). *Bankson Language Test.* Austin, TX: Pro-Ed.

Bankson, N. W., & Bernthal, J. E. (1990). *Bankson-Bernthal Test of Phonology.* Chicago, IL: Riverside Press.

Barbera, M. L. (2007). *The verbal behavior approach: How to teach children with autism and related disorders.* Philadelphia, PA: Jessica Kingsley.

Battle, D. (Ed.) (2002). *Communication disorders in multicultural populations* (3rd ed.). Boston, MA: Butterworth-Heinemann.

Bayles, K., & Harris, G. (1982). Evaluating speech and language skills in Papago Indian children. *Journal of American Indian Education, 21*(2), 11–20.

Baynes, R. A. (1966). An incidence study of chronic hoarseness among children. *Journal of Speech and Hearing Research, 31,* 172–176.

Behrman, A. (2007). *Speech and voice science.* San Diego, CA: Plural.

Beitchman, J. H., Nair, R., Clegg, M., & Patel, P. G. (1986). Prevalence of speech and language disorders in 5-year-old kindergarten children in the Ottawa-Carleton region. *Journal of Speech and Hearing Disorders, 51,* 98–110.

Benedict, H. (1979). Early lexical development: Comprehension and production. *Journal of Child Language, 6,* 183–200.

Berg , B., & Eden, S. (2003). *Perceptual evaluation of voice quality in three organic voice disorders— a comparison between Consensus Auditory Perceptual Evaluation of Voice (CAPE-V) and Stockholm Voice Evaluation Approach (SVEA).* Unpublished master's thesis, Karolinska Institute, Stockholm, Sweden.

Berko-Gleason, J., & Ratner, N. N. (2009). *The development of language* (7th ed.). Boston, MA: Allyn & Bacon.

Bernthal, J., & Bankson, N. (2009). *Articulation and phonological disorders* (6th ed.). Boston, MA: Allyn & Bacon.

Beukelman, D. R., & Mirenda, P. (1988). Communication options for persons who cannot speak: Assessment and evaluation. In C. A. Coston (Ed.), *Proceedings of the National Planners Conference on Assistive Device Service Delivery* (pp. 151–165). Washington, DC: RESNA, Association for the Advancement of Rehabilitation Technology.

Beukelman, D. R., & Mirenda, P. (2005). *Augmentative and alternative communication: Supporting children and adults with complex communication needs* (3rd ed.). Baltimore, MD: Paul H. Brookes.

Beukelman, D. R., Yorkston, K. M., & Dowden, P. (1985). *Augmentative communication: A casebook of clinical management.* Austin, TX: Pro-Ed.

Bhatnagar, S. C. (2008). *Neuroscience for the study of communicative disorders* (3rd ed.). Baltimore, MD: Williams & Wilkins.

Binger, C., & Light, J. (2006). Demographics of preschoolers who require AAC. *Language, Speech, and Hearing Services in Schools, 37,* 200–208.

Bishop, D., North, T., & Donlan, C. (1996). Nonword repetition as a behavioral marker for inherited language impairment: Evidence from a twin study. *Journal of Child Psychology and Psychiatry, 36*(1), 1–13.

Blackstone, S., & Hunt-Berg, M. (2003). *Social networks: A communication inventory for individuals with complex communication needs and their communication partners.* Monterey, CA: Augmentative Communication.

Blakely, R. W. (2001). *Screening Test for Developmental Apraxia of Speech-Second Edition.* Austin, TX: Pro-Ed.

Bland-Stewart, L. M. (2003). Phonetic inventories and phonological patterns of African American 2-year-olds: A preliminary investigation. *Communication Disorders Quarterly, 24,* 109–112.

Bleile, K. (2002). Evaluating articulation and phonological disorders when the clock is running. *American Journal of Speech-Language Pathology, 11,* 243–249.

Blischak, D. M., Lombardino, L. J., & Dyson, A. T. (2003). Use of speech-generating devices: In support of natural speech. *Augmentative and Alternative Communication, 19,* 29–35.

Block, B., & Brodsky, L. (2007). Hoarseness in children: The role of laryngopharyngeal reflux. *International Journal of Pediatric Otorhinolaryngology, 71,* 1361–1369.

Bloodstein, O., & Ratner, N. B. (2008). *A handbook on stuttering* (6th ed.). Clifton Park, NY: Thomson Delmar Learning.

Bloom, L. (1970). *Language development: Form and function in emerging grammars.* Cambridge MA: M.I.T. Press. Japanese translation (1981). Tokyo, Japan: Taishukan.

Bloom, L. & Lahey, M. (1978). *Language development and language disorders.* New York, NY: John Wiley & Sons.

Bloomberg, K., & West, D. (1999). *The Triple C: Manual and video.* Bok Hill, Victoria, BC: Scope Communication Resource Center.

Boehm, (2000). *Boehm Test of Basic Concepts* (3rd ed.). New York, NY: Psychological Corporation.

Boone, D. (1993). *The Boone voice program for children* (2nd ed.). Austin, TX: Pro-Ed.

Boone, D., & McFarlane, S. (1988). *The voice and voice therapy* (4th ed.). Englewood Cliffs, NJ: Prentice-Hall.

Boone, D. R., McFarlane, S. C., & Von Berg, S. L. (2005). *The voice and voice therapy* (7th ed.). Boston, MA: Pearson Education.

Boone, D. R., McFarlane, S. C., Von Berg, S. L., & Zraich, R. L. (2010). *The voice and voice therapy* (8th ed.). Boston, MA: Pearson Education.

Boudreau, D. (2005). Use of a parent questionnaire in emergent and early literacy assessment of preschool children. *Language, Speech, and Hearing Services in Schools, 36*(1), 33–47.

Bowers, L., Huisingh, R., LaGiudice, C., & Orman, J. (2002). *Test of Semantic Skills-Primary (TOSS-P).* East Moline, IL: LinguiSystems.

Bracken, B. B. (1998). *Bracken Basic Concept Scale-Revised.* San Antonio, TX: Harcourt Assessment.

Brice, A. E. (2002). *The Hispanic child: Speech, language, culture, and education.* Boston, MA: Allyn & Bacon.

Brice, A. E., & Brice, R. G. (2009). *Language development: Monolingual and bilingual acquisition.* Boston, MA: Allyn & Bacon.

Brigance, A. (1999). *Brigance Comprehensive Inventory of Basic Skills-Revised (CIBS-R).* North Billerica, MA: Curriculum Associates.

Bristow, D., & Fristoe, M. (1987). *Systematic evaluation of the nonspeaking child.* Miniseminar presented at the annual convention of the American Speech, Language, and Hearing Association. San Francisco, CA.

Brown, R. (1973). *A first language.* Cambridge, MA: Harvard University Press.

Brown, V., Wiederholt, J., & Hammill, D. (2009). *Test of Reading Comprehension-4th Edition.* Austin, TX: Pro-Ed.

Brownell, R. (2000). *Expressive One-Word Picture Vocabulary Test: Spanish-Bilingual Edition (EOWPVT-SBE).* Novato, CA: Academic Therapy Publications.

Brownell, R. (2001). *Receptive One-Word Picture Vocabulary Test: Spanish-Bilingual Edition (ROWPVT-SBE).* Novato, CA: Academic Therapy Publications.

Brownell, R. (2011). *Receptive One-Word Picture Vocabulary Test (ROWPVT-4).* Novato, CA: Academic Therapy Publications.

Brutten, G., & Vanryckeghem, M. (2007). *Behavior Assessment Battery for children who stutter.* San Diego, CA: Plural.

Bryant, B. R., Wiederholt, J. L., & Bryant, D. P. (2004). *Gray Diagnostic Reading Tests (GDRT-2,* 2nd ed.). Austin, TX: Pro-Ed.

Budoff, M. (1987). Measures for assessing learning potential. In C. S. Lidz (Ed.), *Dynamic assessment: An interactional approach to evaluating learning potential* (pp. 173–195). New York, NY: Guilford.

Burd, L., Hammes, K., Bronhoeft, D. M., & Fisher, W. (1988). A North Dakota prevalence study of nonverbal school-age children. *Language, Speech, and Hearing Services in Schools, 19*, 362–370.

Burns, H. P., Dayal, V. S., Scott, A., Van Nostrand, A. W. P., & Bryce, D. P. (1979). Laryngotracheal trauma: Observation on its pathogenesis and its prevention following prolonged orotracheal intubation in the adult. *Laryngoscope, 89*, 1316–1325.

Bus, A. G., & van IJzendoorh, M. H. (1999). Phonological awareness and early reading: A meta-analysis of experimental training studies. *Journal of Educational Psychology, 91*, 403–414.

Bzoch, K., League, R., & Brown, V. (2003). *Receptive-Expressive Emergent Language Test (REEL-3), Examiner's manual.* Austin, TX: Pro-Ed.

Campbell, T., Dollaghan, C., Needleman, H., & Janosky, J. (1997). Reducing bias in language assessment: Processing-dependent measures. *Journal of Speech, Language, and Hearing Research, 40*, 519–525.

Campione, J., & Brown, A. (1987). Linking dynamic assessment with school achievement. In C. S. Lidz (Ed.), *Dynamic assessment: An interactive approach to evaluating learning potential* (pp. 82–115). New York, NY: Guilford.

Campisi, P., Tewfik, T., Manoukian, J., Schloss, M., Pelland-Blais, E., & Sadeghi, N. (2002). Computer-assisted voice analysis: Establishing a pediatric database. *Archives of Otolaryngology-Head and Neck Surgery, 128*(2), 156–160.

Campisi, P., Tewfik, T. L., Pelland-Blais, E., Husein, M., & Sadeghi, N. (2000). Multi-Dimensional Voice Program analysis in children with vocal cord nodules. *Journal of Otolaryngology, 29*, 302–308.

Carding, P., Roulstone, S., Northstone, K., & Team, A. (2006). The prevalence of childhood dysphonia: A cross-sectional study. *Journal of Voice, 20*(4), 623–630.

Carlson, J., & Wiedl, K. H. (1978). Use of testing-the-limits procedure in the assessment of intellectual capabilities in children with learning difficulties. *American Journal of Mental Deficiency, 82*, 559–564.

Carlson, J., & Wiedl, K. H. (1992). The dynamic assessment of intelligence. In H. C. Haywood & D. Tzuriel (Eds.), *Interactive assessment* (pp. 167–186). New York, NY: Springer-Verlag.

Carr, D., & Felce, J. (2007). Brief report: Increase in production of spoken words in some children with autism after PECS teaching to Phase III. *Journal of Autism and Developmental Disorders, 37*, 780–787.

Carr, E., & Dores, P. (1981). Patterns of language acquisition following simultaneous communication with autistic children. *Analysis and Intervention in Developmental Disabilities, 7*, 1–15.

Carr, E. G., Levin, L., McConnachie, G., Carlson, J. I., Kemp, D. C., & Smith, C. E. (1994). *Communication-based intervention for problem behavior: A user's guide for producing positive change.* Baltimore, MD: Paul H. Brookes.

Carr, M., Nagy, M., Pizzuto, M., Poje, C., & Brodsky, L. (2001). Correlation of findings at direct laryngoscopy and bronchoscopy with gastroesophageal reflux disease in children. *Archives of Otolaryngology-Head and Neck Surgery, 127*, 369–375.

Carrow-Woolfolk, E. (1998). *Test for Auditory Comprehension-3 (TALC-3).* Allen, TX: DLM Teaching Resources.

Case, J. L. (2002). *Clinical management of voice disorders* (4th ed.). Austin, TX: Pro-Ed.

Castle, A., & Coltheart, M. (2004). Is there a causal link from phonological awareness to success in learning to read? *Cognition, 91*(1), 77–111.

Catts, H. W., Fey, M. E., Tomblin, J. B., & Zhang, X. (2002). A longitudinal investigation of reading outcomes in children with language impairments. *Journal of Speech, Language, and Hearing Research, 45*(6), 1142–1157.

Catts, H. W., & Kamhi, A. G. (1999). *Language and reading disabilities.* Needham Heights, MA: Allyn & Bacon.

Cezard, J. P. (2004). Managing gastroesophageal reflux disease in children. *Digestion, 69*, 3–8.

Chapman, R., & Miller, J. (1980). Analyzing language and communication in the child. In R. L. Schiefelbusch (Ed.), *Nonspeech language and communication.* Baltimore, MD: University Park Press.

Charlop-Christy, M., Carpenter, M., Le, L., LeBlanc, L., & Kellet, K. (2002). Using the Picture Exchange Communication System (PECS) with children with autism: Assessment of PECS acquisition, speech, social-communication behavior, and problem behavior. *Journal of Applied Behavior Analysis, 35*, 213–231.

Cheng, L. L. (1991). *Assessing Asian language performance.* Oceanside, CA: Academic Communication Associates.

Chomsky, N. (1957). *Syntactic structures.* The Hague, Netherlands: Mouton.

Chomsky, N. (1965). *Aspects of the theory of syntax.* Cambridge, MA: MIT Press.

Clay, M. M. (2005). *An observation survey of early literacy achievement* (2nd ed.). Auckland, New Zealand: Heinemann.

Cline, T., & Baldwin, S. (1994). *Selective mutism in children.* London, UK: Whurr.

Cohen, J. T., Bach, K. K., Postma, G. N., & Koufman, J. A. (2002). Clinical manifestations of laryngopharyngeal reflux. *Ear, Nose and Throat Journal, 81*(9), 19–23.

Cole, P., & Taylor, O. (1990). Performance of working-class African American children on three tests. *Language, Speech, and Hearing Services in Schools, 21*, 171–176.

Collier, V. (1987). Age and rate of acquisition of second language for academic purposes. *TESOL Quarterly, 21*(4), 617–641.

Connor, C. M., & Craig, H. K. (2006). African American preschoolers' language, emergent literacy skills, and use of African American English: A complex relation. *Journal of Speech, Language, and Hearing Research, 49*, 771–792.

Connor, N., Cohen, S., Theis, S., Thibeault, S., Heatley, D., & Bless, D. (2008). Attitudes of children with dysphonia. *Journal of Voice, 22*(2), 197–209.

Conti-Ramsden, G., Simkin, Z., & Pickles, A. (2006). Estimating familial loading in SLI: A comparison of direct assessment verses parental interview. *Journal of Speech, Language, and Hearing Research, 49*, 88–101.

Cooper, E. (1999). Is stuttering a speech disorder? *ASHA, 41,* 10–11.

Cordes, A. K., & Ingham, R. J. (1998). *Treatment efficacy for stuttering: A search for empirical bases.* San Diego, CA: Singular.

Craig, H. K., Thompson, C. A., Washington, J. A., & Potter, S. L. (2003). Phonological features of child African American English. *Journal of Speech, Language, and Hearing Research, 46,* 623–635.

Craig, H. K., & Washington, J. A. (2000). An assessment battery for identifying language impairments in African American children. *Journal of Speech, Language, and Hearing Research, 43,* 366–379.

Craig, H. K., & Washington, J. A. (2002). Oral language expectations of African American preschoolers and kindergartners. *American Journal of Speech-Language Pathology, 11,* 59–70.

Craig, H. K., & Washington, J. A. (2005). Oral language expectations for African American children in grades 1 through 5. *American Journal of Speech-Language Pathology, 14,* 119–130.

Crais, E. (1995). Expanding the repertoire of tools and techniques for assessing the communication skills of infants and toddlers. *American Journal of Speech-Language Pathology, 4,* 47–59.

Crais, E., Watson, L., & Baranek, G. (2009). Use of gesture development in profiling children's prelinguistic communiation skills. *American Journal of Speech-Language Pathology, 18,* 95–108.

Crawford, J. (1996). Endangered Native American Languages: What is to be done and why? [Online]. Available FTP: ncbe.gwu.edu/misc pubs/Crawford/endangered.html

Cress, C., & Marvin, C. (2003). Common questions about AAC services in early intervention. *Augmentative and Alternative Communication, 19*(4), 254–272.

Critchlow, D. E. (1996). *Dos Amigos Verbal Language Scales-Revised.* Novato, CA: Academic Therapy Publications.

Crystal, D. (1987). *The Cambridge encyclopedia of language.* Cambridge, UK: Cambridge University Press.

CTB/McGraw-Hill. (1990). *Developing Skills Checklist.* Monterey, CA: Author.

Cummins, J. (1984). *Bilingualism and special education.* San Diego, CA: College-Hill Press.

Curlee, R. F. (1999). *Stuttering and related disorders of fluency* (2nd ed.). New York, NY: Thieme.

Dale, P. (1991). The validity of a parent report measure of vocabulary and syntax at 24 months. *Journal of Speech, Language, and Hearing Research, 34,* 565–571.

Dale, P., Bates, E., Reznick, S., & Morisset, C. (1989). The validity of a parent report instrument on child language at twenty months. *Journal of Child Language, 16,* 239–249.

Dalston, R. (1989).Using simultaneous photo-detection and nasometry to monitor velopharyngeal behavior during speech. *Journal of Speech, Language, and Hearing Research, 32,* 195–202.

Dalston, R., Warren, D., & Dalston, E. (1991). Use of nasometry as a diagnostic tool for identifying patients with velopharyngeal impairment. *Cleft Palate-Craniofacial Journal, 28,* 184–189.

Daly, D. A. (1986). The clutterer. In K. O. St. Louis (Ed.), *The atypical stutterer: Principles and practices of rehabilitation.* Orlando, FL: Academic Press.

Daly, D. A., & Burnett, M. L. (1999). Cluttering: Traditional views and new perspectives In R. F. Curlee (Ed.), *Stuttering and related disorders of fluency* (2nd ed., pp. 222–254). New York, NY: Thieme.

Darley, F. L. (1964). *Diagnosis and appraisal of communication disorders.* Englewood Cliffs, NJ: Prentice-Hall.

Darley, F. L., & Spriestersbach, D. (1978). *Diagnostic methods in speech pathology.* New York, NY: Harper & Row.

Davis, C. N., & Harris, T. B. (1992). Teacher's ability to accurately identify disordered voices. *Language, Speech, and Hearing Services in Schools, 23,* 136–140.

Dawson, J., & Stout, C (2005). *Structured Photographic Expressive Language Test (SPELT-3).* DeKalb, IL: Janelle Publications.

Dawson, J., & Tattersall, P. (2001). *Structured Photographic Articulation Test-II (SPAT-D II).* DeKalb, IL: Janelle Publications.

Deal, R., McClain, B., & Sudderth, J. (1976). Identification, evaluation, therapy and follow-up for children with vocal nodules in a public school setting. *Journal of Speech and Hearing Disorders, 41,* 390–397.

Deem, J. F., & Miller, L. (2000). *Manual of voice therapy.* Austin, TX: Pro-Ed.

DeFina, A. A. (1992). *Portfolio assessment: Getting started*. New York, NY: Scholastic Professional Books.

DeJoy, D. A., & Jordan, W. J. (1988). Listener reactions to interjections in oral reading versus spontaneous speech. *Journal of Fluency Disorders, 13*, 11–25.

Denno, D. M., Carr, V., & Bell, S. H. (2010). *Addressing challenging behaviors in early childhood settings: A teacher's guide*. Baltimore, MD: Paul H. Brookes.

de Villiers, J., & de Villiers, P. (1973). A cross-sectional study of grammatical morphemes in child speech. *Journal of Psycholinguistic Research, 2*, 267–278.

DiCarlo, C., Stricklin, S., Banajee, M., & Reid, D. (2001). Effects of manual signing on communicative verbalizations by toddlers with and without disabilities in inclusive classrooms. *Journal of the Association for Persons with Severe Handicaps, 26*, 120–126.

Dillard, J. L. (1972). *Black English: Its history and usage in the United States*. New York, NY: Random House.

DiSimoni, F. (2007). *The Token Test for Children-Second Edition*. Austin, TX: Pro-Ed.

Dobres, R., Lee, L., Stemple, J., Kummer, A., & Kretchmer, L. (1990). Description of laryngeal pathologies in children evaluated by otolaryngologists. *Journal of Speech and Hearing Disorders, 55*, 526–533.

Dollaghan, C., & Campbell, T. (1998). Nonword repetition and child language impairment. *Journal of Speech, Language, and Hearing Research, 41*, 1136–1146.

Dollaghan, C. A., & Horner, E. A. (2011). Bilingual language assessment: Meta-analysis of diagnostic accuracy. *Journal of Speech, Language, and Hearing Research, 54*, 1077–1088.

Dore, J., Franklin, M. B., Miller, R. T., & Ramer, A. L. (1976). Transitional phenomena in early language acquisition. *Journal of Child Language, 3*, 13–28.

Drumwright, A., Van Natta, P., Camp, B., Frankenburg, W., & Drexler, H. (1973). Denver Articulation Screening Test (DAST). *Journal of Speech and Hearing Disorders, 38*(1), 3–14.

Duff, M. C., Proctor, A., & Yairi, E. (2004). Prevalence of voice disorders in African American and European American preschoolers. *Journal of Voice, 18*(3), 348–353.

Duffy, J. R. (2005). *Motor speech disorders* (2nd ed.). St. Louis, MO: Mosby.

Duker, P. C. (1999). The Verbal Behavior Assessment Scale (VerBAS): Construct validity, reliability, and internal consistency. *Research in Developmental disabilities, 20*(5), 347–353.

Dunn, L., & Dunn, L. (2007). *Peabody Picture Vocabulary Test* (4th ed.). Circle Pines, MN: American Guidance Service.

Eckel, F. C., & Boone, D. R. (1981). The s/z ratio as an indicator of laryngeal pathology. *Journal of Speech and Hearing Disorders, 46*, 147–150.

Edward, H. T. (2003). *Applied phonetics: The sounds of American English* (3rd ed.). Clifton Park, NY: Thomson Delmar Learning.

Edwards, J. (1989). *Language and disadvantage* (2nd ed.). London, UK: Whurr.

Ellis-Weismer, S., Tomblin, J. B., Zhang, X., Buckwalter, P., Chynoweth, J., & Jones, M. (2000). Nonword repetition performance in school-age children with and without language impairment. *Journal of Speech, Language, and Hearing Research, 43*, 865–878.

Erickson, K. A. (2000). All children are ready to learn: An emergent versus readiness perspective in early literacy assessment. *Seminars in Speech and Language, 21*(2), 193–203.

Ervin, M. (2001). SLI: What we know and why it matters. *ASHA Leader, 6*, 4.

Esch, B. E., LaLonde, K. B., & Esch, J. (2010). Speech and language assessment: A verbal behavior analysis. *Journal of Speech-Language Pathology and Applied Behavior Analysis, 5*(2), 166–190.

EvaluWare. (1999). Retrieved from http://www.assitivetech.com/p-evaluware.htm

Fabian-Smith, L., & Goldstein, B. A. (2010a). Phonological acquisition in bilingual Spanish-English speaking children. *Journal of Speech, Language, and Hearing Research, 53*, 160–178.

Fabian-Smith, L., & Goldstein, B. A. (2010b). Early-, middle-, and late-developing sounds in monolingual and bilingual children: An exploratory investigation. *American Journal of Speech-Language Pathology, 19*, 66–77.

Fagundes, D., Haynes, W., Haak, N., & Moran, M. (1998). Task variability effects on the language test performance of southern lower socioeconomic class African American and Caucasian five-year-olds. *Language, Speech and Hearing Services in Schools, 29*, 148–157.

Fasold, R. W. (1981). The relation between black and white speech in the south. *American Speech, 56*, 163–189.

Faust, R. A. (2003, January/February). Childhood voice disorders: Ambulatory evaluation and operative diagnosis. *Clinical Pediatrics, 42*, 1–9.

Felsenfeld, S., Broen, P., & McGue, M. (1994). A 28-year follow-up of adults with a history of moderate phonological disorder: Educational and occupational results. *Journal of Speech and Hearing Research, 37*, 1341–1353.

Fendler, M., & Shearer, W. M. (1988). Reliability of the s/z ratio in normal children's voice. *Language, Speech, and Hearing Services in Schools, 19*, 2–4.

Fenson, L., Dale, P., Reznick, S., Thal, D., Bates, E., Hartung, J., . . Reilly, J. S. (1993). *MacArthur Communicative Development Inventories.* Baltimore, MD: Paul H. Brookes.

Feuerstein, R. (1979). *The dynamic assessment of retarded performers: The learning potential assessment device, theory, instruments, and techniques.* Baltimore, MD: University Park Press.

Fisher, H. B., & Logemann, J. A. (1971). *The Fisher-Logemann Test of Articulation Competence.* Boston, MA: Houghton Mifflin.

Flax, J. F., Realpe-Bonilla, T., Hirsch, L. S., Brzustowicz, L. M., Bartlett, C. W., & Tallal, P. (2003). Specific language impairment in families: Evidence for co-occurrence with reading impairments. *Journal of Speech, Language, and Hearing Research, 46*(3), 530–543.

Flenthrope, J., & Brady, N. (2010). Relationships between early gestures and later language in children with fragile X syndrome. *American Journal of Speech-Language Pathology, 19*, 135–142.

Fletcher, S. G. (1972). Time-by-count measurement of diadochokinetic syllable rate. *Journal of Speech and Hearing Research, 15*(4), 763–770.

Fluharty, N. B. (2000). *Fluharty-2: Fluharty Preschool Speech and Language Screening Test.* Austin, TX: Pro-Ed.

Forrest, K. (2003). Diagnostic criteria of developmental apraxia of speech used by clinical speech-language pathologists. *American Journal of Speech-Language Pathology, 12*, 376–380.

Fox, D. R., & Johns, D. (1970). Predicting velopharyngeal closure with a modified tongue-anchor technique. *Journal of Speech and Hearing Disorders, 35*, 248–251.

Frost, L., & Bondy, A. (2002). *Picture Exchange Communication System training manual* (2nd ed.). Newark, DE: Pyramid Education Products.

Fudala, J. B. (1974). *Arizona Articulation Proficiency Scale, Revised.* Los Angeles, CA: Western Psychological Services.

Fudala, J. B. (2000). *Arizona Articulation Proficiency Scale* (3rd ed.). Los Angeles, CA: Western Psychological Services.

Fudala, J. B., & Reynolds, W. M. (1986). *Arizona Articulation Proficiency Scale* (2nd ed.). Austin, TX: Pro-Ed.

Fujita, M., Ludlow, C., Woodson, G., & Naunton, R. (1989). A new surface electrode for recording from the posterior cricoarytenoid muscle. *Laryngoscope, 99*, 316–320.

Gallena, S., Smith, P., Zeffiro, T., & Ludlow, C. (2001). Effects of Levodopa on laryngeal muscle activity for voice onset and offset in Parkinson disease. *Journal of Speech and Hearing Research, 44*, 1284–1299.

Ganz, J. B., & Simpson, R. L. (2004). Effects on communication requesting and speech development of the Picture Exchange Communication System in children with autism. *Journal of Autism and Developmental Disorders, 34*, 395–409.

Gardner, J. W. (1961). *Excellence.* New York, NY: Harper.

Gaulin, C., & Campbell, T. (1994). A procedure for assessing verbal working memory in normal school-age children: Some preliminary data. *Perceptual and Motor Skills, 79*, 55–64.

Gauthier, S. V., & Madison, C. L. (1998). *Kindergarten Language Screening Test-Second edition (KLST-S).* Austin, TX: Pro-Ed.

Genesee, F., Paradis, J., & Crago, M. B. (2004). *Dual language development and disorders.* Baltimore, MD: Brookes.

Georgia Project for Assistive Technology. *Augmentative Communication Evaluation Summary.* Retrieved from http://www.atstar.org/docspdfs/gpat/AAC

Gerken, L. (2009). *Language development.* San Diego, CA: Plural.

German, D. J. (1991). *Test of Word Finding in Discourse.* Austin, TX: Pro-Ed.

German, D. J. (2000). *Test of Word Finding* (2nd ed.). Austin, TX: Pro-Ed.

Gherson, S., & Wilson Arboleda, M. (2010). Evaluation of the child with a vocal disorder. In C. Hartnick & M. Boseley (Eds.), *Clinical management of children's voice disorders* (pp. 31–55). San Diego, CA: Plural.

Gilbert, H. R., & Campbell, M. I. (1980). Speaking fundamental frequency in three groups of hearing-impaired individuals. *Journal of Communication Disorders, 13*, 195–205.

Gillam, R. B., & Johnston, J. (1985). Development of print awareness in language-disordered preschoolers. *Journal of Speech and Hearing Disorders, 43*, 521–526.

Gillam, R. B., & Pearson, N. A. (2004). *Test of Narrative Language*. Greenville, SC: Super Duper Publications.

Gillespie, S. K., & Cooper, E. B. (1973). Prevalence of speech problems in junior and senior high schools. *Journal of Speech and Hearing Research, 16*, 739–743.

Gillette, Y. (2003). *Achieving communication independence (ACI)*. Eau Claire, WI: Thinking Publications.

Gilliam, W. S., & de Mesquita, P. B. (2000). The relationship between language and cognitive development and emotional behavioral problems in financially-disadvantaged preschoolers. *Early Child Development and Care, 162*, 9–24.

Ginsburg, H. P. (1986). Academic diagnosis: Contributions from developmental psychology. In J. Valsiner (Ed.), *Individual subjects and scientific psychology* (pp. 253–260). New York, NY: Plenum.

Glaze, L. E. (1996). Treatment of voice hyperfunction in the pre-adolescent. *Language, Speech, and Hearing Services in Schools, 27*, 244–450.

Glennen, S. L. (1997). Augmentative and alternative communication assessment strategies. In S. L. Glennen & D. DeCoste (Eds.), *The handbook of augmentative and alternative communication*. San Diego, CA: Singular.

Glennen, S. L., & DeCoste, D. (1997). *Handbook of augmentative and alternative communication*. San Diego, CA: Singular.

Goldfield, B., & Reznick, J. (1990). Early lexical acquisition: Rate, content, and the vocabulary spurt. *Journal of Child Language, 17*, 171–183.

Goldman, H. (2002). *Augmentative Communication Assessment Profile*. Retrieved from http://www.speechmark.net/speechmark/New_Titles/acap.htm

Goldman, R., & Fristoe, M. (2000). *The Goldman-Fristoe Test of Articulation* (2nd ed.). Circle Pines, MN: American Guidance Service.

Goldstein, B. A. (2004). *Bilingual language development and disorders in Spanish-English speakers*. Baltimore, MD: Paul H. Brookes.

Goldsworthy, C. (1996). *Developmental reading disabilities: A language-based reading approach*. San Diego, CA: Singular.

Goodenough, D. R. (1949). *Mental testing: Its history, principles, and applications*. New York, NY: Rinehart.

Goosens, C., & Crain, S. (1985). *Augmentative communication assessment resource*. Wauconda, IL: Don Johnston Developmental Equipment.

Gopnik, A., & Meltzoff, A. (1986). Relations between semantic and cognitive development in the one-word stage: The specificity hypothesis. *Child Development, 57*, 1040–1053.

Gottwald, S. R., & Starkweather, C. W. (1999). Stuttering prevention and early intervention. In M. Onslow & A. Packman (Eds.), *The handbook on early stuttering intervention* (pp. 53–82). San Diego, CA: Singular.

Gray, S. D., Smith, M. E., & Schneider, H. (1996). Voice disorders in children. *Pediatric Clinics of North America, 43(6)*, 1357–1384.

Green, L. J. (2002). *African American English: A linguistic introduction*. New York, NY: Cambridge University Press.

Greene, M., & Mathieson, L. (2001). *The voice and its disorders* (6th ed) New York, NY: Thieme.

Grontved, A. M., & West, F. (2000). pH monitoring in patients with benign voice disorders. *Acta Otolaryngologica, 543*, 229–231.

Grunwell, P. (1987). *Clinical phonology*. Baltimore, MD: Williams & Wilkins.

Guess, D., & Baer, D. M. (1973). Some experimental analysis of linguistic development in institutionalized retarded children. In B. B. Lahey (Ed.), *The modification of language behavior* (pp. 3–60). Springfield, IL: Charles C. Thomas.

Guitar, B. (2006). *Stuttering: An integrated approach to its nature and treatment* (3rd ed.). Philadelphia, PA: Lippincott Williams & Wilkins.

Gupta, R., & Sataloff, R. (2009). Laryngopharyngeal reflux: Current concepts and questions. *Current Opinion in Otolaryngology-Head and Neck Surgery, 17(3)*, 143–148.

Guralnick, M. J. (2011). Why early intervention works: A systems perspective. *Infants and Young Children, 24(1)*, 6–28.

Gutierrez-Clellen, V., & Peña, E. (2001). Dynamic assessment of diverse children: A tutorial. *Language, Speech, and Hearing Services in Schools, 32*, 212–224.

Gutierrez-Clellen, V., Peña, E., & Quinn, M. (1995). Accommodating cultural differences in narrative style: A multicultural perspective. *Topics in Language Disorders, 15*(4), 54–67.

Gutierrez-Clellen, V., & Simon-Cereijido, G. (2007). The discrimant accuracy of a grammatical measure with Latino English-speaking children. *Journal of Speech, Language, and Hearing Research, 50,* 968–981.

Gutierrez-Clellen, V., Simon-Cereijido, G., & Sweet, M. (2012). Predictors of second language acquisition in Latino children with specific language impairment. *American Journal of Speech-Language Pathology, 21,* 64–77.

Hall, G., & Sundberg, M. L. (1987). Teaching mands by manipulating conditioned establishing operations. *Analysis of Verbal Behavior, 5,* 41–53.

Hall, K. D. (1995). Variations across time in acoustic and electroglottographic measures of phonatory function in women with and without vocal nodules. *Journal of Speech and Hearing Research, 38,* 783–793.

Hall, P. K. (2000). A letter to the parent(s) of a child with developmental apraxia of speech. Part I: Speech characteristics of the disorder. *Language, Speech, and Hearing Services in Schools, 31,* 169–172.

Hall, P. K., Jordan, L. S., & Robin, D. A. (1993). *Developmental apraxia of speech: Theory and clinical practice.* Austin, TX: Pro-Ed.

Haller, R. M., & Thompson, E. A. (1975). Prevalence of speech, language, and hearing disorders among Harlem children. *Journal of the National Medical Association, 67,* 298.

Halstead, L. A. (1999). Role of gastroesophageal reflux in pediatric upper airway disorders. *Otolaryngology-Head and Neck Surgery, 120,* 208–214.

Hamayan, E. V., & Damico, J. S. (1991). *Limiting bias in the assessment of bilingual students.* Austin, TX: Pro-Ed.

Hammill, D. D., & Larsen, S. (1996). *Test of Written Language.* Austin, TX: Pro-Ed.

Hanson, D. G., & Jiang, J. J. (2000). Diagnosis and management of chronic laryngitis associated with reflux. *American Journal of Medicine, 108*(Suppl.), 112–119.

Hart, B., & Risley, T. (1995). *Meaningful differences in the everyday experiences of young American children.* Baltimore, MD: Paul H. Brookes.

Hart, B., & Risely, T. (1999). *The social world of children learning to talk.* Baltimore, MD: Paul H. Brookes.

Hartnick, C., & Boseley, M. (2010). *Clinical management of children's voice disorders.* San Diego, CA: Plural.

Haynes, W. O., & Pindzola, R. H. (2004). *Diagnosis and evaluation in speech pathology* (6th ed.). Boston, MA: Pearson Education.

Heath, S. B. (1983). *Ways with words: Language, life and work in communities and classrooms.* Cambridge, UK: Cambridge University Press.

Heatley, D. G., & Swift, E. (1996). Paradoxical vocal cord dysfunction in an infant with stridor and gastroesophageal reflux. *International Journal of Pediatric Otorhinolaryngology, 34*(1–2), 149–151.

Hecht, M., Collier, M., & Ribeau, S. (1993). *African American communication.* Newbury Park, CA: Sage.

Hedrick, D., Prather, E., & Tobin, A. (1995). *Sequenced Inventory of Communication Development-Revised (SIDC-R).* Austin, TX: Pro-Ed.

Hegde, M. N. (1980). An experimental-clinical analysis of grammatical and behavioral distinctions between verbal auxiliary and copula. *Journal of Speech and Hearing Research, 23,* 864–877.

Hegde, M. N. (1987). Experimental generation of fluency [Abstract]. *Asha, 29*(10), 99.

Hegde, M. N. (1996). *A coursebook on language disorders in children.* San Diego, CA: Singular.

Hegde, M. N. (1998). *Treatment procedures in communicative disorders* (3rd ed.). Austin, TX: Pro-Ed.

Hegde, M. N. (2001). *Hegde's pocketguide to assessment in speech-language pathology* (2nd ed.). San Diego, CA: Singular.

Hegde, M. N. (2003). *Clinical research in communicative disorders: Principles and strategies.* (3rd ed.). Austin, TX: Pro-Ed.

Hegde, M. N. (2006). *A coursebook on aphasia and other neurogenic language disorders* (3rd ed.). Albany, NY: Thomson Delmar Learning.

Hegde, M. N. (2007). *Treatment protocols for stuttering.* San Diego, CA: Plural.

Hegde, M. N. (2008a). *Hegde's pocketguide to communication disorders.* Clifton Park, NY: Thomson Delmar Learning.

Hegde, M. N. (2008b). *Hegde's pocketguide to assessment in speech-language pathology* (3rd ed.). Clifton Park, NY: Thomson Delmar Learning.

Hegde, M. N. (2008c). Meaning in behavior analysis. *Journal of Speech-Language Pathology and Applied Behavior Analysis, 2.4–3.1,* 1–24.

Hegde, M. N. (2010). Language and grammar: A behavioral analysis. *Journal of Speech-Language Pathology and Applied Behavior Analysis, 5*(2), 90–113.

Hegde, M. N., & Brutten, G. J. (1977). Reinforcing fluency in stutterers: An experimental study. *Journal of Fluency Disorders, 2,* 315–328.

Hegde, M. N., Capelli, R., & De Cesari, R. (1984). Differential listener evaluations of some dysfluency forms [Abstract]. *Asha, 26*(10), 160.

Hegde, M. N., & Dansby, E. (1988). Differential listener threshold of tolerance for different forms of dysfluencies [Abstract] *Asha, 30*(10), 141.

Hegde, M. N., & Freed, D. (2011). *Assessment of communication disorders in adults.* San Diego, CA: Plural.

Hegde, M. N., & Hartman, D. E. (1979a). Factors affecting judgments of fluency: I. Interjections. *Journal of Fluency Disorders, 4,* 1–11.

Hegde, M. N., & Hartman, D. E. (1979b). Factors affecting judgments of fluency: I. Word repetitions. *Journal of Fluency Disorders, 4,* 13–22.

Hegde, M. N., & Maul, C. A. (2006). *Language disorders in children: An evidence-based approach to assessment and treatment.* Boston, MA: Allyn & Bacon.

Hegde, M. N., & McConn, J. (1981). Language training: Some data on response classes and generalization to an occupational setting. *Journal of Speech and Hearing Disorders, 44,* 301–320.

Hegde, M. N., & Stone, D. M. (1991). Listener tolerance thresholds for phrase repetitions and part-word repetitions [Abstract]. *Asha, 33*(10), 118.

Helm-Estabrooks, N. (1992). *Test of Oral and Limb Apraxia.* Austin, TX: Pro-Ed.

Heman-Ackah, Y. D., Kelleher, K., & Sataloff, R. T. (2002). Inferior glottis ridges that prevent vocal fold closure. *Ear, Nose, and Throat Journal, 81*(4), 207–209.

Henderson, J. (1995). *Preschool AAC Checklist.* Manukau City, New Zealand: Spectronics.

Herrington-Hall, B. L., Lee, L., Stemple, J. C., Nieme, K. R., & McHone, M. M. (1988). Descriptions of laryngeal pathologies by age, sex, and occupation in a treatment-seeking sample. *Journal of Speech and Hearing Disorders, 53,* 57–64.

Hesketh, A., Adams, C., Nightingale, C., & Hall, R. (2000). Phonological awareness therapy and articulation training approaches for children with phonological disorders: A comparative outcome study. *International Journal of Language and Communication Disorders, 35*(3), 337–354.

Hickman, L. A. (1997). *The Apraxia Profile.* San Antonio, TX: Psychological Corporation.

Highwater, J. (1975). *Indian America.* New York, NY: David McKay.

Hillman, R. E., Holmberg, E. B., Perkell, J. S., Walsh, M., & Vaughan, C. (1989). Objective assessment of vocal hyperfunction. *Journal of Speech and Hearing Research, 32,* 373–392.

Hirano, M. (1981). *Clinical examination of voice.* Vienna, Austria: Springer-Verlag.

Hodson, B. W. (1986). *Assessment of Phonological Processes-Revised (APP-R).* Greenville, SC: Super Duper Publications.

Hodson, B. W. (2004). *Hodson Assessment of Phonological Patterns* (3rd ed.). Austin, TX: Pro-Ed.

Hodson, B. W., Scherz, J. A., & Strattman, K. H. (2002). Evaluating communicative abilities of a highly unintelligible preschooler. *American Journal of Speech-Language Pathology, 11,* 236–242.

Hoffman, P. R., & Norris, J. A. (2002). Phonologic assessment as an integral part of language assessment. *American Journal of Speech-Language Pathology, 11,* 230–235.

Hooper, C. R. (2004, October). Treatment of voice disorders in children. *Language, Speech, and Hearing Services in Schools, 35*(4), 320–326.

Hresko, W. (1996). *Test of Early Written Language-2.* Austin, TX: Pro-Ed.

Hresko, W. P., Miguel, S. A., Sherbenou, R. J., & Burton, S. D. (1994). *Developmental Observation Checklist System (DOCS).* Austin, TX: Pro-Ed.

Hresko, W. P., Reid, D. K., & Hammill, D. D. (1999). *Test of Early Language Development-Third Edition (TELD).* Austin, TX: Pro-Ed.

Huer, M. B. (1997). Protocol for culturally inclusive Assessment of AAC. *Journal of Children's Communication Development, 19*(1), 19–34.

Huer, M. B., & Miller, L. (2011). *Test of Early Communication and Emerging Language (TECEL).* Wauconda, WI: Don Johnston.

Huilit, L. M., Howard, M. R., & Fahey, K. R. (2011). *Born to talk: An introduction to speech and language development* (5th ed.). Boston, MA: Allyn & Bacon.

Huisingh, R., Bowers, L., LaGiudice, C., & Orman, J. (2003). *Test of Semantic Skills-Intermediate (TOSS-I)*. East Moline, IL: LinguiSystems.

Hunter, E. Halpern, A., & Spielman, J. (2012). Impact of four non-clinical speaking environments on a child's fundamental frequency and voice level: A preliminary case study. *Language, Speech, and Hearing Services in Schools*. Online publication. doi:10.1044/0161-1461(2011/11-0002)

Hutchinson, B., & Hanson, M. (1979). Voice disorders. In B. Hutchinson, M. Hanson, & M. Mecham (Eds.). *Diagnostic handbook of speech pathology* (pp. 206–239). Baltimore, MD: Williams & Wilkins.

Hutchinson, T. (1996). What to look for in the technical manual: Twenty questions for users. *Language, Speech, and Hearing Services in Schools, 27*, 109–121.

Ireton, H. R. (1995). *Child Development Inventory (CDI)*. San Antonio, TX: Pearson.

Iwata, B. A., Vollmer, T. R., & Zarcone, J. H. (1990). The experimental (functional) analysis of behavior disorders: Methodology, applications, and limitations. In A. C. Repp & N. N. Singh (Eds.), *Perspectives on the use of aversive and nonaversive interventions for persons with developmental disabilities* (pp. 301–330). Sycamore, IL: Sycamore.

Johnson, T. S., & Child, D. R. (1988). Voice disorders in the child. In N. J. Lass, L. V. McReynolds, J. L. Northern, & D. E. Yoder (Eds.), *Handbook of speech-language pathology and audiology* (pp. 787–808). Philadelphia, PA: B. C. Decker.

Johnson, T. S., & Parrish, M. L. (1971). A behavior management approach to vocal nodules in children II: Report of cases. *Feedback, 4*, 11–12.

Johnson, W. (1944a). The Indians have no word for it: I. Stuttering in children. *Quarterly Journal of Speech, 30*, 330–337.

Johnson, W. (1944b). The Indians have no word for it: II. Stuttering in adults. *Quarterly Journal of Speech, 30*, 330–337.

Johnson, W., & Associates. (1959). *The onset of stuttering*. Minneapolis, MN: University of Minnesota Press.

Johnson, W., & Knott, J. R. (1936). The moment of stuttering. *Journal of Genetic Psychology, 46*, 475–479.

Johnson, W., & Leutenegger, R. R. (1955). *Stuttering in children and adults*. Minneapolis, MN: University of Minnesota Press.

Joint-Committee-on-Testing-Practices. (2004). Code of fair testing practices in education. National Council on Measurement in Education.

Jones, K. L. (2005). *Smith's recognizable forms of human malformations* (6th ed.). Philadelphia, PA: W. B. Saunders.

Judd-Wall, J. (1995). *Assistive technology screener*. Retrieved from http://taicenter.com/at screener.html

Justice, L. M. (Ed.) (2006). *Clinical approaches to emergent literacy intervention*. San Diego, CA: Plural.

Justice, L. M., Bowles, R., & Skibbe, L. (2006). Measuring preschool attainment of print concepts: A study of typical and at-risk 3- to 5-year-old children. *Language, Speech, and Hearing Services in Schools, 37*, 1–12.

Justice, L. M., Chow, S., Capellini, C., Flanigan, K., & Colton, S. (2003). Emergent literacy intervention for vulnerable preschoolers: Relative effects of two approaches. *American Journal of Speech-Language Pathology, 12*, 320–322.

Justice, L. M., & Ezell, H. K. (2004). Print referencing: An emergent literacy enhancement technique and its clinical applications. *Language, Speech, and Hearing Services in Schools, 35*, 185–193.

Kahane, J. C., & Mayo, R. (1989). The need for aggressive pursuit of healthy childhood voices. *Language, Speech, and Hearing Services in Schools, 20*, 102–107.

Kamhi, A. G., Pollock, K. E., & Harris, J. L. (1996). *Communication development and disorders in African American children*. Baltimore, MD: Paul H. Brookes.

Kaminski, R. A., & Good, R. H. (1996). Toward a technology for assessing basic literacy skills. *School Psychology Review, 25*, 215–227.

Kangas, K., & Lloyd, L. (1988). Early cognitive skills as prerequisites to augmentative and alternative communication use: What are we waiting for? *Augmentative and Alternative Communication, 4*, 211–221.

Kapantzoglou, M., Restropo, M. A., & Thompson, M. S. (2012). Dynamic assessment of world learning skills: Identifying language impairment in bilingual children. *Language, Speech, and Hearing Services in Schools, 43,* 81–96.

Karkos, P. D., Leong, S. C., Apostolidou, M. T., & Apostolidis, T. (2006). Laryngeal manifestations and pediatric laryngopharyngeal reflux. *American Journal of Otolaryngology-Head and Neck Medicine and Surgery, 27* (Suppl. 1), 200–203.

Karnell, M., Melton, S., Childes, J., Coleman, T., Dailey, S., & Hoffman, H. (2007). Reliability of clinician-based (GRBAS and CAPE-V) and patient-based (V-RQOL and IPVI) documentation of voice disorders. *Journal of Voice, 21,* 576–590.

Kaufman, A., & Kaufman, N. (1983). *Kaufman Assessment Battery for Children: Interpretive manual.* Circle Pines, MN: American Guidance Service.

Kaufman, J. (1995). *Kaufman Speech Praxis Test (KSPT).* Detroit, MI: Wayne State University Press.

Kaufman, J., Sataloff, R., & Touhill, R. (1996). Laryngopharyngeal reflux: Consensus conference report. *Journal of Voice, 10,* 215–216.

Kay-Raining Bird, E., & Vetter, R. S. (1994). Storytelling in Chippewa-Cree children. *Journal of Speech and Hearing Research, 37*(6), 1354–1368.

Kayser, H. (1989). Speech and language assessment of Spanish-English speaking children. *Language, Speech, and Hearing Services in Schools, 20,* 226–244.

Kayser, H. (1995). *Bilingual speech-language pathology: A Hispanic focus.* San Diego, CA: Singular.

Kayser, H. (2002). Bilingual language development and language disorders. In D. Battle (Ed.), *Communication disorders in multicultural populations* (3rd ed., pp. 205–232). Boston, MA: Butterworth-Heinemann.

Kelchner, L., de Alarcon, A., Weinrich, B., & Brehm, S. (2009). Special considerations in the management of the pediatric voice and airway patient. *Perspectives on Voice and Voice Disorders, 19*(3), 96–104.

Kelly, D. J., & Rice, M. L. (1986). A strategy for assessment of young children. *Language, Speech, and Hearing Services in Schools, 17,* 83–94.

Kelley, M. E., Shillingsburg, M. A., Castro, M. J., Addison, L. R., & LaRue, Jr., R. H. (2007).

Further evaluation of emerging speech in children with developmental disabilities: Training verbal behavior. *Journal of Applied Behavior Analysis, 40,* 431–445.

Kelley, E. M., Shillingsburg, M. A., Castro, M. J., Addison, L. R., LaRue, Jr., R. H., & Martins, M. P. (2007). Assessment of the functions of vocal behavior in children with developmental disabilities: A replication. *Journal of Applied Behavior Analysis, 40,* 571–576.

Kempster, G., Gerratt, B., Verdolini Abbott, K., Barkmeier-Kraemer, J., & Hillman, R. (2009). Clinical focus Consensus Auditory-Perceptual Evaluation of Voice: Development of a standardized clinical protocol. *American Journal of Speech-Language Pathology, 18,* 124–132. doi:10.1044/1058-0360(2008/08-0017

Kent, R. (1994). *Reference manual for communication sciences and disorders.* Austin, TX: Pro-Ed.

Khan, L. M. (2002). The sixth view: Assessing preschoolers' articulation and phonology from the trenches. *American Journal of Speech-Language Pathology, 11,* 250–254.

Khan, L. M., & Lewis, N. (2002). *The Khan-Lewis Phonological Assessment* (2nd ed.). Circle Pines, MN: American Guidance Service.

Kinzler, M., & Johnson, C. (1993). *Joliet 3-Minute Speech and Language Screen* (Revised). Austin, TX: Pro-Ed.

Knox, H. A. (1914). A scale based on the work at Ellis Island for estimating mental defect. *Journal of the American Medical Association, 62,* 741–747.

Kohnert, K. (2007). *Language disorders in bilingual children and adults.* San Diego, CA: Plural.

Koppenhaver, D., Evans, D., & Yoder, D. (1991). Childhood reading and writing experiences of literate adults with severe speech and motor impairments. *Augmentative and Alternative Communication, 7,* 20–33.

Koufman, J. A. (1991). The otolaryngologic manifestations of gastroesophageal reflux disease (GERD): A clinical investigation of 225 patients using ambulatory 24-hour pH monitoring and an experimental investigation of the role of acid and pepsin in the development of laryngeal injury. *Laryngoscope, 101*(53), 1–78.

Koufman, J. A. (2002a). Laryngopharyngeal reflux 2002: A new paradigm of airway disease. *Ear, Nose, and Throat Journal, 81*(9), 2–6.

Koufman, J. A. (2002b). Laryngopharyngeal reflux is different from classical gastroesophageal reflux disease. *Ear, Nose, and Throat Journal, 81*(9), 7–9.

Koufman, J. A., Amin, M. R., & Panetti, M. (2000). Prevalence of reflux in 113 consecutive patients with laryngeal and voice disorders. *Otolaryngology-Head and Neck Surgery, 123,* 385–388.

Koufman, J. A., Wiener, G. J., Wu, W. C., & Castell, D. O. (1988). Reflux laryngitis and its sequelae: The diagnostic role of 24-hour pH monitoring. *Journal of Voice, 2,* 78–79.

Kovach, T. M. (2009). *Augmentative and Alternative Communication Profile.* East Moline, IL: LinguiSystems.

Kratcoski, A. M. (1998). Guidelines for using portfolios in assessment and evaluation. *Language, Speech, and Hearing Services in Schools, 29*(1), 3–10.

Kravits, T. R., Kamps, D. M., Kemmerer, K., & Potucek, J. (2002). Brief report: Increasing communication skills for an elementary-aged student with autism using the Picture Exchange Communication System. *Journal of Autism and Developmental Disorders, 32,* 225–230.

Kreiman, J., & Gerratt, B. (2010). Perceptual assessment of voice quality: Past, present and future. *Percpectives on Voice and Voice Disorders, 20(2),* 62–67.

Krug, D., Arick, J., & Almond, P. (2008). *Autism Screening Instrument for Educational Planning-3rd Edition (ASIEP-3).* Austin, TX: Pro-Ed.

Kuhn, J., Toohill, R., & Ulualp, S. (1998). Pharyngeal acid reflux events in patients with vocal cord nodules. *Laryngoscope, 108,* 1146–1149.

Labov, W. (1972). *Language in the inner city: Studies in Black English vernacular.* Philadelphia, PA: University of Pennsylvania Press.

Laing, S. P. (2003). Assessment of phonology in preschool African American Vernacular English speakers using an alternate response mode. *American Journal of Speech-Language Pathology, 12,* 273–281.

LaFrance, D., Wildre, D. A., Normand, M. P., & Squires, J. L. (2009). Extending the assessment of functions of vocalization in children with limited verbal repertoires. *Analysis of Verbal Behavior, 25,* 19–32.

Laing, S. P., & Kamhi, A. (2003). Alternative assessment of language and literacy in culturally and linguistically diverse populations. *Language, Speech, and Hearing Services in Schools, 34*(1), 44–55.

Lamarre, J., & Holand, J. G. (1985). The functional independence of mands and tacts. *Journal of the Experimental Analysis of Behavior, 43,* 5–19.

Lambert, W. E. (1977). The effects of bilingualism on the individual: Cognitive and sociocultural consequences. In P. A. Hornby (Ed.), *Bilingualism: Psychological, social, and educational implications* (pp. 17–27). New York, NY: Academic Press.

Larsen, J. A., & Nippold, M. A. (Morphological analysis in school-age children: Dynamic assessment of a word learning strategy. *Language, Speech, and Hearing Services in Schools, 38,* 201–212.

Lass, N., Ruscello, D., Stout, L., & Hoffmann, F. (1991). Peer perceptions of normal and voice-disordered children. *Folia Phoniatrica, 34,* 29–35.

Lecoq, M., & Drape, F. (1996). Epidemiological survey of dysphonia in children at primary school. *Revue de Laryngologie Otologie Rhinologie, 117*(4), 323–325.

Leeper, L. H. (1992). Diagnostic examination of children with voice disorders: A low-cost solution. *Language, Speech, and Hearing Services in Schools, 23,* 353–360.

Leonard, L. B. (1991). Specific language impairment as a clinical category. *Language, Speech, and Hearing Services in Schools, 29,* 3–10.

Leonard, L. B. (1998). *Children with specific language impairment.* Cambridge, MA: MIT Press.

Lerman, D. C., Parten, M., Addison, L. R., Vorndran, C. M., Volkert, V. M., & Kodak, T. (2005). A methodology for assessing the functions of emerging speech in children with developmental disabilities. *Journal of Applied Behavior Analysis, 38,* 303–316.

Lewis, B. A. (2010). Genetic influence on speech sound disorders. In R. Paul & P. Flipsen, Jr., *Speech sound disorders in children* (pp. 51–70). San Diego, CA: Plural.

Lewis, B. A., & Freebairn, L. A. (1992). Residual effects of preschool phonology disorders in grade school, adolescence and adulthood. *Journal of Speech and Hearing Research, 35,* 819–831.

Lewis, B. A., Freebairn, L. A., Hansen, A. J., Iyengar, S. K., & Taylor, H. G. (2004a). Family pedigrees of children with suspected childhood apraxia of speech. *Journal of Communication Disorders, 37*(2), 157–175.

Lewis, B. A., Freebairn, L. A., Hansen, A. J., Iyengar, S. K., & Taylor, H. G. (2004b). School-age follow-up of children with childhood apraxia of speech. *Language, Speech, and Hearing Services in Schools, 35,* 122–140.

Lewis, B. A., O'Donnell, B., Freebairn, L. A., & Taylor, H. G. (1998). Spoken language and written expression—Interplay of delays. *American Journal of Speech-Language Pathology, 7*(3), 77–84.

Lidz, C. S. (1987). Historical perspectives. In C. S. Lidz (Ed.), *Dynamic assessment: An interactive approach to evaluating learning potential* (pp. 3–34). New York, NY: Guilford.

Lidz, C. S. (1991). *A practitioner's guide to dynamic assessment.* New York, NY: Guilford Press.

Lidz, C. S., & Peña, E. D. (1996). Dynamic assessment: The model, its relevance as a nonbiased approach, and its application to Latino American preschool children. *Language, Speech, and Hearing Services in Schools, 27,* 367–372.

Lidz, C. S., & Thomas, C. (1987). The preschool learning assessment device: Extension of a static approach. In C. S. Lidz (Ed.), *Dynamic assessment: An interactional approach to evaluating learning potential* (pp. 288–326). New York, NY: Guilford.

Lifter, K., & Bloom, L. (1989). Object knowledge and the emergence of language. *Infant Behavior and Development, 12,* 395–423.

Light, J., Beukelman, D. R., & Reichle, J. (2003). *Communicative competence for individuals who use AAC.* Baltimore, MD: Paul H. Brookes.

Light, J., Roberts, B., Dimarco, R., & Greiner, N. (1998). Augmentative and alternative communication to support receptive and expressive communication for people with autism. *Journal of Communicative Disorders, 31,* 153–180.

Lindsay, J. (2004). *The Hmong people in the U.S.* Retrieved from http://www.jefflindsay.com/Hmong_tragedy.html

Linville, S. E. (2002). Source characteristics of aged voice assessed from long-term average spectra. *Journal of Voice, 16,* 472–479.

Lippke, B. A., Dickey, S. E., Selmar, J. W., & Soder, A. L. (1997). *Photo Articulation Test* (3rd ed.). Austin, TX: Pro-Ed.

Little, J. P., Matthews, B. L., Glock, M. S., Koufman, J. A., Reboussin, D. M., Loughlin, C. J., & McGuirt, W. I. (1997). Extraesophageal pediatric reflux: 24-hour double-probe pH monitoring in 222 children. *Annals of Otology, Rhinology, and Laryngology, 169*(Suppl.), 1–16.

Lombardino, L. J., Lieberman, R. J., & Brown, J. C. (2005). *Assessment of Literacy and Language.* Boston, MA: Pearson.

Long, S. (1994). Language and bilingual-bicultural children. In V. A. Reed (Ed.), *An introduction to children with language disorders* (2nd ed.). New York, NY: Macmillan College.

Long, S. (2005a). Language and children with intellectual disabilities. In V. A. Reed (Ed.), *An introduction to children with language disorders* (3rd ed., pp. 220–252). Boston, MA: Allyn & Bacon.

Long, S. (2005b). Language and children with autism. In V. A. Reed (Ed.), *An introduction to children with language disorders* (3rd ed., pp. 253–273). Boston, MA: Allyn & Bacon.

Lonigan, C. J., Wagner, R. K., Torgesen, K., & Rashotte, C. A. (2007). *Test of Preschool Early Literacy.* Austin, TX: Pro-Ed.

Love, R. J. (2000). *Childhood motor speech disability* (2nd ed.). Boston, MA: Allyn & Bacon.

Lowe, R. J. (2000). *Assessment Link between Phonology and Articulation-Revised: (ALPHA-R).* Moline, IL: LinguiSystems.

Lynch, E., & Hanson, M. (1992). *Developing cross-cultural competence.* Baltimore, MD: Paul H. Brookes.

MacGinitie, W., MacGinitie, R., Marie, K., & Dreyer, L. (2000). *Gates-MacGinitie Reading Tests®* (4th ed.). Itasca, IL: Riverside.

Markwardt, F. J. (1998). *Peabody Individual Achievement Test-Revised-Normative Update (PIAT-R/NU).* Circle Pines, MN: American Guidance Service.

Maronian, N., Robinson, L., Waugh, P., & Hillel, A. (2004). A new electromyographic definition of laryngeal synkinesis. *Annals of Otology, Rhinology, and Laryngology, 113,* 877–886.

Marquardt, P. T., Sussman, H. M., & Davis, B. L. (2001). Developmental apraxia of speech: Advances in theory and practice. In D. Vogel & M. P. Cannito (Eds.), *Treating disordered speech motor control* (2nd ed.). Austin, TX: Pro-Ed.

Martin, R. R., & Haroldson, S. K. (1981). Stuttering identification: Standard definition and moment of stuttering. *Journal of Speech and Hearing Research, 24,* 59–63.

Marvin, C., & Mirenda, P. (1993). Home literacy experiences of preschoolers enrolled in Head Start and special education programs. *Journal of Early Intervention, 17*, 351–367.

Masaki, A. (2009). *Optimizing acoustic and perceptual assessment of voice quality in children with vocal nodules* (Doctoral dissertation). Retrieved from dspace.mit.edu/bitstream/handle/1721.1/54666/607313724.pdf

Mason, R. M., & Grandstaff, H. L. (1971). Evaluating the velopharyngeal mechanism in hypernasal speakers. *Language, Speech, and Hearing Services in Schools, 2*, 53–61.

Masterson, J., & Bernhardt, B. (2001). *Computerized articulation and phonology evaluation*. Austin, TX: Pro-Ed.

Masterson, J., & Pagan, F. (1994). *Interactive system for phonological analysis* [computer software]. San Antonio, TX: Psychological Corporation.

Matas, J. A., Mathy-Laikko, P., Beukelman, D. R., & Legresley, K. (1985). Identifying the nonspeaking population: A demographic study. *Augmentative and Alternative Communication, 1*, 17–31.

Mates, L. J. (1994). *Spanish Articulation Measures, Revised Edition (SAM)*. Oceanside, CA: Academic Communication Associates.

Mates, L. J. (1995a). *Bilingual Vocabulary Assessment Measure*. Oceanside, CA: Academic Communication Associates.

Mates, L. J. (1995b). *Spanish Language Assessment Procedures, Third Edition (SLAP)*. Oceanside, CA: Academic Communication Associates.

Mates, L. J., & Santiago, G. (1985). *Bilingual Language Proficiency Questionnaire*. Oceanside, CA: Academic Communication Associates.

McAllister, A., Sederholm, E., Sundberg, J., & Gramming, P. (1994). Relations between voice range profiles and physiological and perceptual voice characteristics in ten-year-old children. *Journal of Voice, 8*, 230–239.

McCauley, R. J. (1996). Familiar strangers: Criterion referenced measures in communication disorders. *Language, Speech, and Hearing Services in Schools, 27*, 122–131.

McCauley, R., & Swisher, L. (1984a). Psychometric review of language and articulation tests for preschool children. *Journal of Speech and Hearing Disorders, 49*(1), 34–42.

McCauley, R., & Swisher, L. (1984b). Use and misuse of norm-referenced tests in clinical assessment: A hypothetical case. *Journal of Speech and Hearing Disorders, 49*, 338–348.

McCune, L. (1995). A normative study of representational play at the transition to language. *Developmental Psychology, 31*, 198–206.

McFadden, T. U. (1996). Creating language impairment in typically achieving children: The pitfalls of "normal" normative samples. *Language, Speech, and Hearing Services in Schools, 27*(1), 3–9.

McGhee, R., Bryant, B., Larson, S., & Rivera, D. (1995). *Test of Written Expression (TOWE)*. Circle Pines, MN: AGS.

McGregor, K., Williams, D., Hearst, S., & Johnson, A. (1997). The use of contrastive analysis in distinguishing difference from disorder. *American Journal of Speech-Language Pathology, 6*, 45–56.

McInnes, A., & Manassis, K. (2005). When silence is not golden: An integrated approach to selective mutism. *Seminars in Speech and Language, 26*(3), 201–210.

McLaughlin, S. (2006). *Introduction to language development* (2nd ed.). Clifton Park, NY: Thomson Delmar Learning.

McLaughlin, S. F. (2010). Verbal Behavior by B. F. Skinner: Contributions to analyzing early language acquisition. *Journal of Speech-Language Pathology and Applied Behavior Analysis, 5*, 114–131.

McMurray, J. S. (2003). Disorders of phonation in children. *Pediatric Clinics of North America, 50*(2), 363–380.

McNamera, A. P., & Perry, C. K. (1994). Vocal abuse prevention practices: A national survey of school-based speech-language pathologists. *Language, Speech, and Hearing Services in Schools, 25*, 105–111.

McReynolds, L. V., & Engmann, D. L. (1974). An experimental analysis of the relationship between subject noun and object noun phrases. (ASHA Monograph No. 18). In L. V. McReynolds (Ed.), *Developing systematic procedures for training children's language* (pp. 30–46). Rockville, MD: American Speech-Language-Hearing Association.

Mecham, M. J. (1996). *Cerebral palsy* (2nd ed.). Austin, TX: Pro-Ed.

Mecham, M. J. (2003). *Utah Test of Language Development-4*. Austin, TX: Pro-Ed.

Medline Plus. (2006). *Croup*. Retrieved from http://www.nlm.nih.gov/medlineplus/ency/article

Meisels, S. J. (1991). Dimensions of early identification. *Journal of Early Identification, 15*, 26–35.

Miccio, A. W. (2002). Clinical problem solving: Assessment of the phonological disorders. *American Journal of Speech-Language Pathology, 11,* 221–229.

Michael, J. (2000). Implications and refinements of the establishing operation concept. *Journal of Applied Behavior Analysis, 33,* 401–410.

Millar, D., Light, J., & Schlosser, R. (2006). The impact of augmentative and alternative communication intervention on speech production of individuals with developmental disabilities: A research review. *Journal of Speech, Language, and Hearing Research, 49,* 248–264.

Millard, S. K., Nicholas, A., & Cook, F. M. (2008). Is Parent-Child Interaction Therapy effective in reducing stuttering? *Journal of Speech, Language, and Hearing Research, 51,* 636–650.

Miller, J. (1981). *Assessing language production in children.* Needham Heights, MA: Allyn & Bacon.

Miller, J., & Chapman, R. (1981). The relation between age and mean length of utterance in morphemes. *Journal of Speech and Hearing Research, 24,* 154–161.

Miller, S., Manhal, M., & Lee, L. (1991). Parental beliefs, parental accuracy, and children's cognitive performance: A search for causal relations. *Developmental Psychology, 27,* 267–276.

Mirenda, P. (2003). Toward functional augmentative and alternative communication for students with autism: Manual signs, graphic symbols, and voice output communication aids. *Language, Speech, and Hearing Services in Schools, 34,* 203–216.

Mirenda, P., Wilk, D., & Carson, P. (2000). A retrospective analysis of technology use patterns in students with autism over a five-year period. *Journal of Special Education Technology, 15,* 5–16.

Moats, L. (1995). *Spelling development, disability, and instruction.* Baltimore, MD: York.

Moerk, E. L. (2000). *The guided acquisition of first language skills.* Stamford, CT: Ablex.

Moore, G. P. (1982). Voice disorders. In G. H. Shames & E. H. Wiig (Eds.), *Human communication disorders: An introduction* (pp. 142–186). Columbus, OH: Charles E. Merrill.

Moran, M. J., & Pentz, A. L. (1987). Otolaryngologists' opinions of voice therapy for vocal nodules in children. *Language, Speech, and Hearing Services in Schools, 18,* 172–178.

Mori, K. (1999). Vocal fold nodules in children: Preferable therapy. *International Journal of Pediatric Otorhinolaryngology, 49,* 303–306.

Morris, H., & Spriestersbach, D. (1978). Appraisal of respiration and phonation. In F. Darley & D. Spriestersbach (Eds.), *Diagnostic methods in speech pathology* (pp. 200–212). New York, NY: Harper & Row.

Mufwene, S. S., Rickford, J. R., Bailey, G., & Baugh, J. (1998). *African American English: Structure, history, and use.* London, UK: Rutledge.

Myers, F. L., & St. Louis, K. O. (1992). *Cluttering: A clinical perspective.* Kibworth, UK: Far Communications.

Nancollis, A., Lawrie, B, & Dodd, B. (2005). Phonological awareness intervention and the acquisition of literacy skills in children from deprived social background. *Language, Speech, and Hearing Services in Schools, 36,* 325–335.

National Research Council and Institute of Medicine. (2000). *From neurons to neighborhoods: The science of early childhood development.* Committee on Integrating the Science of Early Childhood Development. J. P. Shonkoff & D. A. Phillips (Eds.), Board on Children, Youth, and Families, Commission on Behavioral and Social Sciences and Education. Washington, DC: National Academy Press.

Nelson, K. E. (1973). Structure and strategy in learning to talk. *Monographs of the Society for Research on Child Development, 38.*

Newcomer, P. (1999). *Standard Reading Inventory.* Austin, TX: Pro-Ed.

Newcomer, P., & Barenbaum, E. (2003). *Test of Phonological Awareness Skills.* Austin, TX: Pro-Ed.

Newcomer, P., & Hammill, D. (2008a). *Test of Language Development-Primary (TOLD-P:4).* Austin, TX: Pro-Ed.

Newcomer, P., & Hammill, D. (2008b). *Test of Language Development-Intermediate–(TOLD-I:4).* Austin, TX: Pro-Ed.

Nippold, M. A. (1990). Concomitant speech and language disorders in stuttering children: A critique of the literature. *Journal of Speech and Hearing Disorders, 55,* 51–60.

Nippold, M. A. (1996). Proverb comprehension in youth: The role of concreteness and familiarity. *Journal of Speech and Hearing Research, 39,* 166–176.

Nippold, M. A. (2007). *Later language development* (2nd ed.). Austin, TX: Pro-Ed.

Noens, I., van Berckelaer-Onnes, I., Verpoorten, R., & van Dujin, G. (2006). Forerunners in communication (ComFor). *Journal of Intellectual Disability Research, 50*(9), 621–632.

Notari, A., Cole, K., & Mills, P. (1992). Cognitive referencing: The (non)relationship between theory and application. *Topics in Early Childhood Education, 11*(4), 22–38.

Nugent, T. M., Shipley, K. G., & Provencio, D. O. (1991). *Spanish Test for Assessing Morphologic Production.* Oceanside, CA: Academic Communication Associates.

Observing the Classroom Environment. (2008). Pittsburg, PA: DynaVox Mayer-Johnson.

Oetting, J. B., & Pruitt, S. (2005). Southern African-American English use across groups. *Journal of Multilingual Communication Disorders, 3*(2), 136–144.

Oliver, C., Hall, S., & Nixon, J. (1999). A molecular to molar analysis of communicative and problem behaviors. *Research in Developmental Disabilities, 20*(3), 197–213

Olswang, L., & Bain, B. (1996). Assessment information for predicting upcoming change in language production. *Journal of Speech and Hearing Research 39,* 414–423.

Olswang, L., Bain, B., & Johnson, G. (1992). Using dynamic assessment with children with language disorders. In S. Warren & J. Reichle (Eds.), *Causes and effects in communication and language intervention* (pp. 187–216). Baltimore, MD: Paul H. Brookes.

O'Neill, D. K. (2007). The Language Use Inventory for young children: A parent-report measure of pragmatic language development for 18- to 47-month-old children. *Journal of Speech, Language, and Hearing Research, 50*(1), 214–228.

Onslow, M., Packman, A., & Harrison, E. (2003). *The Lidcombe Program of early stuttering intervention.* Austin, TX: Pro-Ed.

Owens, R. E. (2004). *Language disorders: A functional approach to assessment and intervention* (4th ed.). Boston, MA: Allyn & Bacon.

Owens, R. E. (2012). *Language development: An introduction* (8th ed.). Boston, MA: Allyn & Bacon.

Oxford advanced learner's dictionary. (7th ed.). 2005. Oxford, UK: Oxford University Press.

Palmer, D. C. (2006). On Chomsky's appraisal of Skinner's Verbal Behavior: A half-century of misunderstanding. *Behavior Analyst, 29,* 253–267.

Palmer, D. C. (2008). On Skinner's definition of verbal behavior. *International Journal of Psychology and Psychological Therapy, 8*(3), 295–307.

Paradis, J., & Genesee, F. (1996). Syntactic acquisition in bilingual children: Autonomous or interdependent? *Studies in Second Language Acquisition, 18,* 1–25.

Parette, P., VanBiervliet, A., & Hourcade, J. (2000) Family centered decision making in assistive technology. *Journal of Special Education Technology, 15,* 45–55.

Paul, D., & Roth, F. (2011). Guiding principles and clinical applications for speech-language pathology practice in early intervention. *Language, Speech, and Hearing Services in Schools, 42,* 320–330.

Paul, R. (2001). *Language disorders from infancy through adolescence: Assessment and intervention.* St. Louis, MO: Mosby-Yearbook.

Paul, R., & Flipsen, P., Jr. (2010). *Speech sound disorders in children.* San Diego, CA: Plural.

Paulson, L. H., Noble, L. A., Jepson, S., & van den Pol, R. (2001). *Building early literacy and language skills.* Longman, CO: Sopris West.

Pearson, B. Z., Velleman, S. L., Bryant, T. J., & Charko, T. (2009). Phonological milestones for African American English-speaking children learning Mainstream American English as a second dialect. *Language, Speech, and Hearing Services in Schools, 40,* 229–244.

Peña, E. D. (1996). Dynamic assessment: The model and its language applications. In P. Cole, P. Dale, & D. Thal (Eds.), *Assessment of communication and language.* Baltimore, MD: Paul H. Brookes.

Peña, E. D., Gillam, R. B., Malek, M., Ruiz-Felter, R., Resendiz, M., Fiestas, C., & Sabel, T. (2006). Dynamic assessment of school-age children's narrative ability: An experimental investigation of classification accuracy. *Journal of Speech, Language, and Hearing Research, 49,* 1037–1057.

Peña, E. D, Quinn, M., & Iglesias, A. (1992). The application of dynamic methods to language assessment: A non-biased procedure. *Journal of Special Education, 26,* 269–280.

Peña, E. D., Spaulding, T. J., & Plante, E. (2006). The composition of normative groups and diagnostic decision making: Shooting ourselves in the foot. *American Journal of Speech-Language Pathology, 15,* 247–254.

Peña-Brooks, A., & Hegde, M. N. (2007). *Assessment and treatment of articulation and phono-*

logical disorders in children (2nd ed.). Austin, TX: Pro-Ed.

Pence, K. L. (Ed.) (2007). *Assessment in emergent literacy.* San Diego, CA: Plural.

Pence, K. L., & Justice, L. M. (2012). *Language development from theory to practice* (2nd ed.). Upper Saddle River, NJ: Merrill Prentice-Hall.

Pendergast, K., Dickey, S. E., Selman, J. W., & Sorder, A. L. (1974). *Photo Articulation Test.* Danville, IL: Interstate.

Petursdottir, A. I., Carr, J. C., & Michael, J. (2005). Emergence of mands and tacts of novel objects among preschool children. *Analysis of Verbal Behavior, 21,* 59–74.

Phelphs-Terasaki, D., & Phelps-Gunn, T. (2007). *Test of Pragmatic Language-Second Edition.* Austin, TX: Pro-Ed.

Polloway, E. A., & Smith, T. (1992). *Language instruction for students with disabilities.* Denver, CO: Love Publishing.

Poole, I. (1934). Genetic development of consonant sounds in English. *Elementary English Review, 11,* 159–161.

Portney, L. G., & Watkins, M. P. (2000). *Foundations of clinical research: Applications to practice.* Upper Saddle River, NJ: Prentice-Hall.

Powell, M., Filter, M., & Williams, B. (1989). A longitudinal study of the prevalence of voice disorders in children from a rural school division. *Journal of Communication Disorders, 22,* 375–382.

Prater, R. J., & Swift, R. W. (1984). *Manual of voice therapy.* Boston, MA: Little, Brown & Co.

Prather, E. M., Hedrick, E. L., & Kerin, C. A. (1975). Articulation development in children aged two to four years. *Journal of Speech and Hearing Disorders, 40,* 179–191.

Prizant, B. (1983). Language acquisition and communicative behavior in autism: Toward an understanding of the "whole" of it. *Journal of Speech and Hearing Disorders, 48,* 296–307.

Pruitt, S., & Oetting, J. (2009). Past tense marking by African American English-speaking children reared in poverty. *Journal of Speech, Language, and Hearing Research, 52,* 2–15.

Psychological Corporation. (2002). *Early Reading Diagnostic Assessment-Revised.* San Antonio, TX: Author.

Pugliese, M. (2001). *Stages: Software solutions for special needs.* Newton, MA: Assistive Technologies.

Purcell, R. M., & Runyan, C. M. (1980). Normative study of speech rates of children. *Journal of the Speech and Hearing Association of Virginia, 21,* 6–14.

Qi, K. H., Kaiser, A. P., Milan, S. E., Yzquierdo, Z., & Hancock, T. B. (2003). The performance of low-income, African American children on the Preschool Language Scale-3. *Journal of Speech, Language, and Hearing Research, 46,* 576–590.

Ramig, L. O., Verdolini, K. (1998). Treatment efficacy: Voice disorders. *Journal of Speech and Hearing Research, 41,* 101–116.

Ramig, P. R. (1993). High reported spontaneous stuttering recovery rates: Fact or fiction? *Language, Speech, and Hearing Services in Schools, 24,* 156–160.

Ramos, M., & Ramos, J. (2007). *Test of Early Language Development-Third Edition: Spanish.* Austin, TX: Pro-Ed.

Raphael, L. J., Borden, G., & Harris, K. S. (2011). *Speech science primer* (6th ed.). Philadelphia, PA: Lippincott Williams & Wilkins.

Rast, M., & Meltzoff, A. (1995). Memory and representation in young children with Down syndrome: Exploring deferred imitation and object permanence. *Development and Psychopathology, 7,* 393–407.

Reed, V. A. (2005). *An introduction to children with language disorders* (3rd ed.). Boston, MA: Allyn & Bacon.

Reichle, J., Barrett, C., Tertile, R. R., & McQuarter, R. J. (1987). The effect of prior intervention to establish generalized requesting on the acquisition of object labels. *Augmentative and Alternative Communication, 3,* 3–11.

Reichle, J., & Karlan, G. (1985). Decision rules for the adoption of augmentative techniques. In R. L. Scheifelbusch & L. Lloyd (Eds.), *Language perspectives II.* Austin, TX: Pro-Ed.

Reichle, J., & Wacker, D. P. (1993). *Communicative alternatives to challenging behavior: Integrating functional assessment and intervention strategies.* Baltimore, MD: Paul H. Brookes.

Reid, K., Hresko, W. P., & Hammill, D. D. (2001). *Test of Early Reading Ability.* Austin, TX: Pro-Ed.

Repp, A. C., & Singh, N. N. (1990) (Eds.). *Perspectives on the use of aversive and nonaversive interventions for persons with developmental disabilities.* Sycamore, IL: Sycamore

Rescorla, L. (1989). The Language Development Survey: A screening tool for delayed language in toddlers. *Journal of Speech and Hearing Disorders, 54,* 587–599.

Rescorla, L., & Lee, L. (2001). Language impairment in young children. In T. Layton, E. Crais, & L. Watson (Eds.), *Handbook of early language impairment in children: Nature* (pp. 1–55). Clifton Park, NY: Delmar.

Rescorla, L., Roberts, J., & Dahlsgaard, K. (1997). Late talkers at 2: Outcomes at age 3. *Journal of Speech, Language, and Hearing Research, 40*, 556–566.

Rhyner, P. M., Kelly, D. J., Brantley, A. L., & Krueger, D. M. (1999). Screening low-income African American children using the BLT-2S and the SPELT-P. *American Journal of Speech-Language Pathology, 8*(1), 44–52.

Riccio, C. A., Imhoff, B., & Hasbrouck, J. E., & Davis, N. (2004). *Test of Phonological Awareness in Spanish.* Austin, TX: Pro-Ed.

Rice, M. L. (1989). Children's language acquisition. *American Psychologist, 44*, 149–156.

Rickford, J. R. (1999). *African American Vernacular English: Features, evolution, educational implications.* Malden, MA: Blackwell.

Robbins, A. M., & Osberger, M. J. (1992). *Meaningful use of speech scale.* Indianapolis, IN: Indiana University School of Medicine.

Robertson, C., & Salter, W. (1997). *Phonological Awareness Test.* East Moline, IL: LinguiSystems.

Robinson, J., T. L., & Crowe, T. A. (2002). Fluency disorders. In D. E. Battle (Ed.), *Communication disorders in multicultural populations* (pp. 267–297). Boston, MA: Butterworth-Heinemann.

Robinson-Zanartu, C. (1996). Serving Native American children and families: Considering cultural variables. *Language, Speech, and Hearing Services in Schools, 27*, 373–384.

Rodekohr, R., & Haynes, W. (2001). Differentiating dialect from disorder: A comparison of two processing tasks and a standardized language test. *Journal of Communicative Disorders, 34*, 255–272.

Roid, G. H., & Miller, L. J. (1997). *Examiner's manual: Leiter International Performance Scale-Revised.* Wood Dale, IL: Stoelting.

Roland, N., Bhalla, R., & Earis, J. (2004). The local side effects of inhaled corticosteroids: Current understanding and review of the literature. *Chest, 126*(1), 213–219.

Romski, M. A., & Sevcik, R. A. (1993). Language learning through augmented means: The process and its products. In A. P. Kaiser & D. B. Gray (Eds.), *Communication and language intervention series: Vol. 2. Enhancing children's communication: Research foundations for intervention.* Baltimore, MD: Paul H. Brookes.

Romski, M. A., Sevcik, R. A., & Pate, J. (1988). The establishment of symbolic communication in persons with severe mental retardation. *Journal of Speech and Hearing Disorders, 49*, 293–302.

Roseberry-McKibbin, C. (1994). Assessment and intervention for children with limited English proficiency and language disorders. *American Journal of Speech-Language Pathology, 3*(1), 77–88.

Roseberry-McKibbin, C. (2002). *Multicultural students with special language needs: Practical strategies for assessment and intervention* (2nd ed.). Oceanside, CA: Academic Communication Associates.

Roseberry-McKibbin, C. (2008). *Increasing language skills of students from low income backgrounds.* San Diego, CA: Plural.

Rosenbek, J. C., LaPointe, L. L., & Wertz, R. T. (1989). *Aphasia: A clinical approach.* Austin, TX: Pro-Ed.

Rothman, K. J., & Greenland, S. (1998). *Modern epidemiology* (2nd ed.). Philadelphia, PA: Lippincott Williams & Wilkins.

Rowland, C. (1996). *Communication matrix.* Portland, OR: Portland Health Sciences University.

Rowland, C. (2004). *Communication matrix.* Portland, OR: Portland Health Sciences University.

Rowland, C., & Schweigert, P. (1996). *Tangible Symbol Systems, Levels of Representation Pre-Test* [Videotape]. San Antonio, TX: Harcourt Assessment.

Rowland, C., & Schweigert, P. (2002). *Problem solving skills.* Portland, OR: Design to Learn.

Rowland, C., & Schweigert, P. (2003). Cognitive skills and AAC. In J. Light, D. R. Beukelman, & J. Reichle (Eds.), *Communicative competence for individuals who use AAC: From research to effective practice.* Baltimore, MD: Paul H. Brookes.

Ruben, R. J. (2000). Redefining the survival of the fittest: Communication disorders in the 21st century. *Laryngoscope, 110*(2), 241–245.

Ruddy, B., McCrea, C., Fischera, P., & Lehman, J. (2008). *Perceptions of school-aged children with voice disorders toward classroom participation and peer interaction* (Poster session). Retrieved from http://www.asha.org/Events/convention/handouts/2008/1932_Fischera_Jeff/

Ruscello, D. M., Lass, N. J., & Podbeseki, J. (1988). Listeners' perceptions of normal and voice-disordered children. *Folia Phoniatrica, 40,* 290–296.

Rvachew, S., & Brosseau-Lapre, F. (2012). *Developmental phonological disorders: Foundations of clinical practice.* San Diego, CA: Plural.

Salvia, J., & Ysseldyke, J. (1981). *Assessment in special and remedial education.* Boston, MA: Houghton-Mifflin.

Sandage, M. J., & Zelazny, S. K. (2004). Paradoxical vocal fold motion in children and adolescents. *Language, Speech, and Hearing Services in Schools, 35,* 353–362.

Sander, E. K. (1963). Frequency of syllable repetition and "stutterer" judgments. *Journal of Speech and Hearing Disorders, 28,* 19–30.

Sander, E. K. (1972). When are speech sounds learned? *Journal of Speech and Hearing Disorders, 37,* 55–63.

Saniga, R., & Carlin, M. (1993). Vocal abuse behaviors in young children. *Language, Speech, and Hearing Services in Schools, 24,* 79–83.

Sapor, S., Baker, K., Larson, C., & Ramig, L. (2000). Short-latency changes in voice F_o and neck surface EMG induced by mechanical perturbations of the larynx during sustained vowel phonation. *Journal of Speech, Language, and Hearing Research, 43,* 268–276.

Sataloff, R. T. (2005). *Clinical assessment of voice.* San Diego, CA: Plural.

Scarborough, H. (1998). Early identification of children at risk for reading disabilities: Phonological awareness and some other promising predictors. In B. Shapiro, P. Accoardo, & A. Capute (Eds.), *Specific reading disability: A view of the spectrum* (pp. 35–42). Timonium, MD: York Press.

Scheffner-Hammer, C., Pennock-Roman, M., Rzasa, S., & Tomblin, J. B. (2002). An analysis of the Test of Language Development: Primary for item bias. *American Journal of Speech-Language Pathology, 11,* 274–284.

Scherer, M. (1997). *Matching Assistive Technology and Child (MATCH).* Webster, NY: Institute for Matching Person & Technology.

Schlesinger, I. M. (1971). Production of utterances and language acquisition. In D. Slobin (Ed.), *The ontogenesis of grammar.* New York, NY: Academic Press.

Schlosser, R., McGhie-Richmond, D., Blackstien-Adler, S., Mirenda, P., Antonius, K., & Janzen, P. (2000). Training a school team to integrate technology meaningfully into the curriculum: Effects on student participation. *Journal of Special Education Technology, 15,* 31–44.

Schlosser, R., & Wendt, O. (2008). Effects of Augmentative and alternative communication intervention on speech production in children with autism: A systematic review. *American Journal of Speech-Language Pathology, 17,* 212–230.

Schraeder, T., Quinn, M., Stockman, I., & Miller, J. (1999). Authentic assessment as an approach to preschool speech-language screening. *American Journal of Speech-Language Pathology, 8,* 195–200.

Schuele, C. M., Skibbe, L. E., & Rao, P. K. S. (2007). Assessing phonological awareness. In K. L. Pence (Ed.), *Assessment of emergent literacy* (pp. 275–325). San Diego, CA: Plural.

Scott, A. (1998, October 19). Assessing and treating GER. *Advance for Speech-Language Pathologists and Audiologists,* pp. 16–17.

Secord, W. A. (1981). *T-MAC: Test of Minimal Articulation Competence.* San Antonio, TX: Psychological Corporation.

Secord, W. A., & Donohue, J. (2002). *Clinical Assessment of Articulation and Phonology (CAAP).* Greenville, SC: SuperDuper Publications.

Seikel, J. A., King, D. W., & Drumright, D. G. (2010). *Anatomy and physiology of speech, language, and hearing* (4th ed.). Clifton Park, NY: Thomson Delmar Learning.

Semel, E., Secord, W., & Wiig, E. H., (2004). *CELF-Preschool-Second Edition.* New York, NY: Harcourt Assessment.

Semel, E., Wiig, E. H., & Secord, W. (2003). *Clinical Evaluation of Language Fundamentals-Preschool (CELF-Preschool)* (2nd ed.). San Antonio, TX: Psychological Corporation.

Semel, E., Wiig, E. H., & Secord, W. (2004). *CELF-4 Screening Test.* New York, NY: Harcourt Assessment.

Senturia, B. H., & Wilson, F. B. (1968). Otorhinolaryngologic findings in children with voice deviation. Preliminary report. *Annals of Otology, Rhinology, and Laryngology, 77,* 1027–1042.

Seymour, H., Bland-Stewart, L., & Green, L. (1998). Differences versus deficit in child African-American English. *Language, Speech, and Hearing Services in Schools, 29,* 96–108.

Seymour, H., Roeper, T., & de Villiers, J. (2003) *Diagnostic Evaluation of Language Variation-Screening Test (DELV-Screening Test).* San Antonio, TX: Psychological Corporation.

Seymour, H., Roeper, T., & de Villiers, J. (2005) *Diagnostic Evaluation of Language Variation-(DELV)-Norm-Referenced*. San Antonio, TX: Psychological Corporation.

Seymour, N. H. (2004). A noncontrastive model for assessment of phonology. *Seminars in Speech and Language*, 25(1), 91–99.

Shah, R., Harvey Woodnorth, G., Glynn, A., & Nuss, R. (2005). Pediatric vocal nodules: Correlation with perceptual voice analysis. *International Journal of Pediatric Otorhinolaryngology*, 69, 903–909.

Shane, H. (1980). Approaches to assessing the communication of nonspeaking persons. In R. L. Schiefelbusch (Ed.), *Nonspeech language and communication: Analysis and intervention*. Baltimore, MD: University Park Press.

Shearer, W. (1972). The diagnosis and treatment of voice disorders in school children. *Journal of Speech and Hearing Disorders*, 37, 215–221.

Shipley, K. G. (1992). *Interviewing and counseling in communicative disorders: Principles and procedures*. New York, NY: Merrill/Macmillan.

Shipley, K. G., Stone, T. A., & Sue, M. B. (1983). *Test for Examining Expressive Morphology*. Tucson, AZ: Communication Skill Builders.

Shore, C. (1986). Combination play, conceptual development, and early mulitword speech. *Developmental Psychology*, 22, 184–190.

Shprintzen, J. R. (2000). *Syndrome identification for speech-language pathology*. San Diego, CA: Singular.

Shriberg, L. D., Aram, D. M., & Kwiatkowski, J. (1997). Developmental apraxia of speech: I. Descriptive and theoretical perspectives. *Journal of Speech and Hearing Research*, 40, 273–286.

Shriberg, L. D., & Kent, R. (2003). *Clinical phonetics* (3rd ed.). Boston, MA: Allyn & Bacon.

Shriberg, L. D., & Kwiatkowski, J. (1983). Computer-assisted Natural process analysis (NPA): Recent issues and data. *Seminars in Speech and Language*, 4, 397–406.

Shriberg, L. D., & Kwiatkowski, J. (1994). Developmental phonological disorders I: A clinical profile. *Journal of Speech and Hearing Research*, 37, 1100–1126.

Shriberg, L. D., Lewis, B. A., Tomblin, J. B., McSweeney, J. L., Karlsson, H. K., & Scheer, A. R. (2005). Toward diagnostic and phenotype markers for genetically transmitted speech delay. *Journal of Speech, Language, and Hearing Research*, 48, 834–852.

Shrivastav, R. (2002). Acoustic analysis of children's voices. *Voice and Voice Disorders*, 12(1), 11–12.

Sicherer, S., & Eggleston, P. (2007). Environmental Allergens. In P. Lieberman & J. Anderson (Eds.), *Allergic diseases: Diagnosis and treatment* (pp. 39–50). Totowa, NJ: Humana Press.

Sigafoos, J., Didden, R., & O'Reilly, M. (2003). Effects of speech output on maintenance of requesting and frequency of vocalizations in three children with developmental disabilities. *Augmentative and Alternative Communication*, 19, 37–47.

Silva, A. B., & Hotaling, A. J. (1994). Advances in pediatric gastroesophageal reflux disease. *Otolaryngology-Head and Neck Surgery*, 2, 508–514.

Silver, K. (2005). *Communication Assessment Record (CAR)*. London, UK: Jessica Kingsley.

Silverman, E., & Zimmer, C. (1975). Incidence of chronic hoarseness among school-age children. *Journal of Speech and Hearing Disorders*, 40, 211–215.

Silverman, F. H. (1980). *Communication for the speechless*. Englewood Cliffs, NJ: Prentice-Hall.

Silverman, F. H. (1995). *Communication for the speechless* (3rd ed.). Needham Heights, MA: Allyn & Bacon.

Simon, C. S. (1994). *Evaluating communicative competence: A functional pragmatic procedure* (Rev. ed.). Tucson, AZ: Communication Skill Builders.

Skinner, B. F. (1957). *Verbal behavior*. New York, NY: Appleton-Century-Crofts.

Small, L. H. (2005). *Fundamentals of phonetics* (2nd ed.). Boston, MA: Allyn & Bacon.

Smit, A. B. (1993a). Phonologic error distributions in the Iowa-Nebraska articulation norms project: Consonant singletons. *Journal of Speech-Language-Hearing Research*, 36, 533–547.

Smit, A. B. (1993b). Phonologic error distributions in the Iowa-Nebraska articulation norms project: Word-initial consonant clusters. *Journal of Speech-Language-Hearing Research*, 36, 533–547.

Smit, A. B. (2004). *Articulation and phonology resource guide for school-age children and adults*. Clifton Park, NY: Thomson Delmar.

Smit, A. B., & Hand, L. (1997). *Smit-Hand Articulation and Phonology Evaluation*. Los Angeles, CA: Western Psychological Corporation.

Smit, A. B., Hand, L., Freilinger, J. J., Bernthal, J. E., & Bird, A. (1990). The Iowa articulation norms project and its Nebraska replication. *Journal of Speech and Hearing Disorders, 55,* 779–798.

Smith, A., Denny, M., Shaffer, L., Kelly, E., & Hirano, M. (1996). Activity of intrinsic laryngeal muscles in fluent and disfluent speech. *Journal of Speech and Hearing Research, 39,* 329–348.

Smith, M., King, J., Elsherif, A., Muntz, H., Park, A., & Kouretas, P. (2009). Should all newborns who undergo patent ductus arteriosus ligation be examined for vocal fold mobility? *Laryngoscope, 119,* 1606–1609.

Smith, M., Marsh, J., Cotton, R., & Myer, C. (1993). Voice problems after pediatric laryngotracheal reconstruction: Videolaryngostroboscopic, acoustic, and perceptual assessment. *International Journal of Pediatric Otorhinolaryngology, 25*(1–3), 173–181.

Smith, M., & Sauder, C. (2009). Pediatric vocal fold paralysis/immobility. *Perspectives on Voice and Voice Disorders, 19*(3), 113–121.

Snell, M. (2002). Using dynamic assessment with learners who communicate nonsymbolically. *Augmentative and Alternative Communication, 18,* 163–176.

Snow, C., Burns, M. S., & Griffin, P. (1998). *Preventing reading difficulties in young children.* Washington, DC: National Academy Press.

Snow, C. E., Scarborough, H. S., & Burns, M. S. (1999). What speech-language pathologists need to know about early reading. *Topics in Language Disorders, 20*(1), 48–58.

Spaulding, T. J., Plante, E., & Farinella, K. A. (2006). Eligibility criteria for language impairment: Is the low end of normal appropriate? *Language, Speech, and Hearing Services in Schools, 37,* 61–72.

Spector, J. (1992). Predicting progress in beginning reading: Dynamic assessment of phonemic awareness. *Journal of Educational Psychology, 84,* 353–363.

Speech-Ease. (1985). *Speech-Ease Screening Inventory.* Austin, TX: Pro-Ed.

Squires, J., & Bricker, D. (1991). Impact of completing infant developmental questionnaires on at-risk mothers. *Journal of Early Intervention, 15*(2), 162–172.

Starkweather, C. W. (1987). *Fluency and stuttering.* Englewood Cliffs, NJ: Prentice-Hall.

Stathopoulos, E., Huber, J., & Sussman, J. (2011). Change in acoustic characteristics of the voice across the life span: Measures from individuals 4–93 years of age. *Journal*

of Speech, Language, and Hearing Research, 54, 1011–1021.

Stemple, J., Glaze, L., & Klaben, B. (2000). *Clinical voice pathology.* San Diego, CA: Singular.

Stemple, J., Glaze, L., & Klaben, B. (2010). *Clinical voice pathology* (4th ed.). San Diego, CA: Plural.

Stevens, N., & Isles, D. (2001). *Phonological Screening Assessment (PSA).* East Aurora, NY: Slosson.

Stevenson, H. W., & Newman, R. S. (1986). Long-term prediction of achievement and attitudes in mathematics and reading. *Child Development, 57,* 646–659.

St. Louis, K., Hansen, G., Buch, J., & Oliver, T. (1992). Voice deviations and coexisting communication disorders. *Language, Speech, and Hearing Services in Schools, 23,* 82–87.

Stockman, I. (1996a). Phonological development and disorders in African American children. In A. G. Kamhi, K. E. Pollock & J. L. Harris (Eds.), *Communication development and disorders in African American children* (pp. 117–153). Baltimore, MD: Paul H. Brookes.

Stockman, I. (1996b). The promises and pitfalls of language sample analysis as an assessment tool for linguistic minority children. *Language, Speech, and Hearing Services in Schools, 27,* 355–366.

Stockman, I. (2000). The new Peabody Picture Vocabulary Test - III: An Illusion of unbiased assessment. *Language, Speech, and Hearing Services in Schools, 31,* 340–353.

Stockman, I. (2006). Evidence for a minimal competence core of consonant sounds in the speech of African American children: A preliminary study. *Clinical Linguistics and Phonetics, 20*(10), 723–749.

Stockman, I. (2008). Toward validation of a minimal competence phonetic core for African American children. *Journal of Speech, Language, and Hearing Research, 51,* 1244–1262.

Stockman, I. (2010). A review of developmental and applied language research on African American children: From a deficit to difference perspective on dialectal differences. *Language, Speech, and Hearing Services in Schools, 41,* 23–38.

Stockman, I., Karasinski, L., & Guillory, B. (2008). The use of conversational repairs by African American preschoolers. *Language, Speech, and Hearing Services in Schools, 39,* 461–474.

Sulzby, E. (1985). Children's emergent reading of favorite storybooks: A developmental study. *Reading Research Quarterly, 20*, 458–481.

Taylor, O. (Ed.). (1983). *Nature of communication disorders in culturally and linguistically diverse populations*. Boston, MA: Little, Brown.

Taylor, O., & Payne, K. (1983). Culturally valid testing: A proactive approach. *Topics in Language Disorders, 3*, 8–20.

Teale, W. H., & Sulzby, E. (Eds.) (1986). *Emergent literacy: Writing and reading*. Norwood, NJ: Ablex.

Templin, M. C. (1957). *Certain language skills in children. Institute of Child Welfare Monograph Series No. 26*. Minneapolis, MN: University of Minnesota Press.

Templin, M. C., & Darey, F. L. (1969). *The Templin-Darley Test of Articulation: Manual and Discussion of Articulation Testing* (2nd ed.*)*. Iowa City, IA: Bureau of Educational Research and Service, University of Iowa.

Theis, S. (2010, November 23). Pediatric voice disorders: Evaluation and treatment. *ASHA Leader.* Retrieved from http://www.asha.org/Publications/leader/2010/101123/Pediatric-Voice-Disorders

Theis, S. (2011). Reflux in children and its effects on assessment and management of voice disorders from a speech-language pathologist's perspective. *Perspectives on Voice and Voice Disorders, 21*(3), 106–111.

Thomas-Tate, S., Washington, J., Craig, H., & Packard, M. (2006). Performance of African American preschool and kindergarten students on the Expressive Vocabulary Test. *Language, Speech, and Hearing Services in Schools, 37*, 143–149.

Tomblin, J. B., Morris, H. L., & Spriestersbach, D. C. (2002). *Diagnosis in speech-language pathology.* San Diego, CA: Singular.

Tomblin, J. B., Records, N. L., & Zhang, X. (1996). A system for the diagnosis of specific language impairment in kindergarten children. *Journal of Speech and Hearing Research, 39*, 1284–1294.

Torgesen, J. K., & Bryant, B. R. (2004). TOPA-2+ *Test of Phonological Awareness* (2nd ed.*)*. Austin, TX: Pro-Ed.

Trudeau, M. D. (1998). Paradoxical vocal cord dysfunction among juveniles. *Asha Newsletter, 8*(1), 11–13.

Twyman, J. S. (1996). The functional independence of impure mands and tacts of abstract stimulus properties. *Analysis of Verbal Behavior, 13*, 1–9.

Tyler, A. A. (2010). Subgroups, comorbidity, and treatment implications. In R. Paul, & P. Flipsen, Jr., *Speech sound disorders in children* (pp. 71–92). San Diego, CA: Plural.

Tyler, A., Lewis, K., Haskill, A., & Tolbert, L. (2002). Efficacy of a cross-domain effects of a morphosyntactic and phonologic intervention. *Language, Speech, and Hearing Services in Schools, 33*, 52–66.

Tyler, A. A., & Tolbert, L. C. (2002). Speech-language assessment in the clinical setting. *American Journal of Speech-Language Pathology, 11*, 215–220.

UC Davis Health System: Center for Voice and Swallowing. (2012). Laryngeal papilloma. Retrieved from http://www.ucdvoice.org/papilloma.html

Udvari, A., & Thousand, J. (1995). Promising practices that foster inclusive education. In R. Villa & J. Thousand (Eds.), *Creating an inclusive school*. Alexandria, VA: Association for Supervision and Curriculum Development.

UKAT Toolkit. (2002). Lexington: University of Kentucky Assistive Technology Project.

Ukrainetz, T., Harpell, S., Walsh, C., & Coyle, C. (2000). A preliminary investigation of dynamic assessment with Native American kindergartners. *Language, Speech, and Hearing Services in Schools, 31*, 142–154.

Ulualp, S., & Brodsky, L. (2005). Nasal pain disrupting sleep as a presenting symptom of extraesophageal acid reflux in children. *International Journal of Pediatric Otorhinolaryngology, 69*, 1555–1557.

Vandenplas, Y., & Sacre-Smits, L. (1987). Continuous 24-hour esophageal pH monitoring in 285 asymptomatic infants 0–15 months old. *Journal of Pediatric Gastrointestinal Nutrition, 6*, 220–224.

Vanderveldon, M., & Siegel, L. (1999). Phonological processing and literacy in AAC users and students with motor speech impairments. *Augmentative and Alternative Communication, 17*, 37–51.

van Keulen, J. E., Weddington, G. T., & DeBose, C. E. (1998). *Speech, language, learning, and the African American child*. Boston, MA: Allyn & Bacon.

van Kleeck, A. (1990). Emergent literacy: Learning about print before learning to read. *Topics in Language Disorders, 10*(2), 25–45.

van Kleeck, A. (1998). Preliteracy domains and stages: Laying the foundations for beginning reading. *Journal of Children's Communication Development, 20*, 33–51.

Van Ornum, W., Dunlap, L. L., & Shore, M. F. (2008). *Psychological testing across the life span.* Upper Saddle River, NJ: Prentice-Hall.

Van Riper, C. (1982). *The nature of stuttering* (2nd ed.). Englewood Cliffs, NJ: Prentice-Hall.

Vanryckeghem, M., & Brutten, G. (2007). *The KiddyCAT: A speech associated attitude test for preschoolers and kindergarteners.* San Diego, CA: Plural.

Vanryckeghem, M., Hylebos, C., Brutten, G., & Pearlman, M. (2001). The relationship between communication attitude and emotion of children who stutter. *Journal of Fluency Disorders, 26*, 1–15.

Vaughn-Cooke, F. (1987). Are Black and White vernaculars diverging? *American Speech, 62*, 12–32.

Wade, K., & Haynes, W. (1989). Dynamic assessment of spontaneous language and cue responses in adult-directed and child-directed play: A descriptive and statistical analysis. *Child Language Teaching and Therapy, 5*, 157–173.

Wagner, R., Torgesen, J., & Rashotte, C. (1999). *Comprehensive Test of Phonological Processing.* Austin, TX: Pro-Ed.

Wallace, G., & Hammill, D.(2002). *Comprehensive Receptive and Expressive Vocabulary-2 (CREVT-2).* Austin, TX: Pro-Ed.

Warr-Leeper, G. A., McShea, R. S., & Leeper, H. A. (1979). The incidence of voice and speech deviations in a middle school population. *Language, Speech, and Hearing Services in Schools, 10*, 14–20.

Washington, J. A. (1996). Issues in assessing the language abilities of African American children. In A. G. Kamhi, K. E. Pollock, P. H. Brookes, & J. L. Harris (Eds.), *Communication development and disorders in African American children.* Baltimore, MD: Brookes.

Washington, J. A., & Craig, H. K. (1992). Articulation test performances of low-income, African-American preschoolers with communication impairments. *Language, Speech, and Hearing Services in Schools, 23*, 203–207.

Washington, J. A., & Craig, H. K. (1999). Performance of at-risk African American preschoolers on the Peabody Picture Vocabulary Test-III. *Language, Speech, and Hearing Services in Schools, 30*, 75–82.

Washington, J. A., & Craig, H. K. (2002). Morphosyntactic forms of African American English used by young children and their caregivers. *Applied Psycholinguistics, 23*, 209–231.

Washington, J. A., & Craig, H. K. (2004). A language screening protocol for use with young African American children in urban settings. *American Journal of Speech-Language Pathology, 13*, 329–240.

Washington, J. A., Craig, H. K., & Kushmaul, A. J. (1998). Variable use of African American English across language sampling contexts. *Journal of Speech, Language, and Hearing Research, 41*, 1115–1124.

Watkins, R. V. (2005. Language abilities of young children who stutter. In E. Yairi & N. G. Ambrose (Eds.), *Early childhood stuttering* (pp.197–234). Austin, TX: Pro-Ed.

Weidemann, H. R., & Kunze, J. (1997). *Clinical syndromes* (3rd ed.). London, UK: Mosby-Wolfe.

Weiner, F. (1979). *Phonological process analysis.* Baltimore, MD: University Park Press.

Weiss, C. (1980). *Weiss Comprehensive Articulation Test (WCAT).* Austin, TX: Pro-Ed.

Weitzman, R. (2010). The bases for language repertoires: Functional stimulus-response relations. *Journal of Speech-Language Pathology and Applied Behavior Analysis, 5*(2), 132–149.

Wellman, B., Case, L., Mengert, I., & Bradbury, D. (1931). Speech sounds of young children. *State University of Iowa Studies in Child Welfare, 5*(2).

Westby, C. E. (2002). Multicultural issues in speech and language assessment. In J. B. Tomblin, H. L. Morris, & D. C. Spriestersbach (Eds.), *Diagnosis in speech-language pathology.* San Diego, CA: Singular.

Wetherby, A., & Prizant, B. (1992). Profiling young children's communicative competence. In S. Warres & J. Reichle (Eds.), *Causes and effects in communication and language intervention.* Baltimore, MD: Paul H. Brookes.

Wetherby, A., & Prizant, B. (2003). *Communication and Symbolic Behavior Scales Developmental Profile (CSBS DP).* Baltimore, MD: Paul H. Brookes.

Wheat, M. C., & Hudson, A. I. (1988). Spontaneous speaking fundamental frequency of 6-year-old Black children. *Journal of Speech and Hearing Research, 31*, 723–725.

Whited, R. E. (1979). Laryngeal dysfunction following prolonged intubation. *Annals of Otology, Rhinology, and Laryngology, 88,* 474–478.

Whited, R. E. (1984). A prospective study of laryngotracheal sequelae in long-term intubation. *Laryngoscope, 94,* 367–377.

Whitehurst, G. J., & Fischel, J. E. (2000). Reading and language impairments in conditions of poverty. In D. V. M. Bishop & L. B. Leonard (Eds.), *Speech and language impairments in children: Causes, characteristics, intervention and outcome* (pp. 53–71). Philadelphia, PA: Psychology Press.

Whitehurst, G. J., & Lonigan, C. J. (1998). Child development and emergent literacy. *Child Development, 69*(3), 848–872.

Whitehurst, G., & Lonigan, C. (2001). *Get ready to read!* Retrieved from http://www.getreadytoread.org

Wiig, E. H. (1990). *Wiig Criterion-Referenced Inventory of Language.* New York, NY: Harcourt Assessment.

Wiig, E. H., Secord, W. A., & Semel, E. (2006). *Clinical Evaluation of Language Fundamentals-Fourth Edition, Spanish (CELF-4 Spanish).* Boston, MA: Pearson.

Wiig, E. H., Secord, W. A., & Semel, E. (2009). *Clinical Evaluation of Language Fundamentals-Second Edition, Spanish (CELF Preschool-2 Spanish).* Boston, MA: Pearson.

Wilkinson, G. (1993). *Wide Range Achievement Test-Third Revision (WRAT-3).* Wilmington, DE: Jastak Associates.

Williams, A. L. (2002). Epiloque: Perspectives in the assessment of children's speech. *American Journal of Speech-Language Pathology, 11,* 259–263.

Williams, D. E., & Kent, L. R. (1958). Listener evaluations of speech interruptions. *Journal of Speech and Hearing Research, 1,* 124–131.

Williams, K. T. (2007). *Expressive Vocabulary Test-Second Edition (EVT).* Boston, MA: Pearson Assessment Group.

Williams, K. T. (2001). *Group Reading Assessment and Diagnostic Evaluation.* Circle Pines, MN: American Guidance Service.

Williams, P., & Stackhouse, J. (1998). Diadochokinetic skills: Normal and atypical performance in children aged 3–5 years. *International Journal of Language and Communication Disorders, 33*(Suppl.), 481–486.

Williams, W., Stemach, G., Wolfe, S., & Stanger, C. (1998). *Lifespace access profile.* Volo, IL: Don Johntson.

Willis, W. (1992). Families with African American roots. In E. W. Lynch & M. A. Hanson (Eds.), *Developing cross-cultural competence: A guide for working with young children and their families.* Baltimore, MD: Paul H. Brookes.

Wilson, D. K. (1987). *Voice problems of children* (3rd ed.). Baltimore, MD: Williams & Wilkins.

Wilson, J., Theis, S. M., & Wilson, E. M. (2009). Evaluation and management of vocal cord dysfunction in the athlete. *Current Sports Medicine Reports, 8*(2), 65–70.

Winokur, S. (1976). *A primer of verbal behavior.* Englewood Cliffs, NJ: Prentice-Hall.

Wintgens, A. (2005). Selective mutism in children. *Child Language Teaching and Therapy, 21*(2), 214–216.

Wisconsin Assistive Technology Initiative (WATI). (2004) *W.A.T.I. Assistive Technology Assessment.* Retrieved from http://www.wati.org/Products/products.html

Wolfram, R. W. (1994). The phonology of a sociocultural society: The case of African American Vernacular English. In J. E. Bernthal & N. W. Bankson (Eds.), *Child phonology: Characteristics, assessment, and intervention with special populations* (pp. 227–244). New York, NY: Thieme.

Wolfram, W. (1986). Language variation in the United States. In O. L. Taylor (Ed.), *Nature of communication disorders in culturally and linguistically diverse populations* (pp. 73–115). San Diego, CA: Singular.

Wong-Fillmore, L. W. (1991). A question of early childhood programs: English first or families first. *National Association of Bilingual Education News, 14*(7), 14–19.

Woodcock, R., McGrew, K., & Mather, N. (2007). *Woodcock-Johnson® III.* Itasca, IL: Riverside.

Woodcock, R. W. (1991). *Woodcock Language Proficiency Battery-Revised.* Allen, TX: DLM Teaching Resources.

Woodnorth, G. H. (2004) Assessing and managing medically fragile children: Tracheostomy and ventilator support. *Language, Speech, and Hearing Services in Schools, 35,* 363–372.

Wren, S., & Watts, J. (2002). *The Abecedarian Reading Assessment.* Austin, TX: Balanced Reading. Retrieved from: http://www.balancedreading.com

Wyatt, T. (1995). Language development in African American English child speech. *Linguistics and Education, 7,* 7–22.

Yairi, E., & Ambrose, N. G. (2005). *Early childhood stuttering.* Austin, TX: Pro-Ed.

Yates, A. (1987). Current status and future directions of research on the American Indian child. *American Journal of Psychiatry, 144*, 1135–1142.

Yellon, R. F. (1997). The spectrum of reflux-associated otolaryngologic problems in infants and children. *American Journal of Medicine, 105*(5A), 125–129S.

Yiu, E., Verdolini, K., & Chow, L. (2005). Electromyographic study of motor learning for a voice production task. *Journal of Speech, Language, and Hearing Research, 48*, 1254–1268.

Yoder, P. J., & Layton, T. L. (1988). Speech following sign language training in autistic children with minimal verbal language. *Journal of Autism and Developmental Disabilities, 18*, 217–229.

Yoder, P. J., Warren, S. F., & McCathren, R. B. (1998). Determining spoken language prognosis in children with developmental disabilities. *American Journal of Speech Language Pathology, 7*, 77–87.

Yorkston, K., & Karlan, G. (1986). Assessment procedures. In S. Blackstone (Ed.), *Augmentative communication: An introduction*. Rockville, MD: American Speech-Language-Hearing Association.

Zalesska-Krecicka, M., Krecicki, T., Iwanczak, B., Blitek, A., & Horobiowska, M. (2002). Laryngeal manifestations of gastroesophageal reflux disease in children. *Acta Otolaryngologica, 122*, 306–310.

Zbar, R. I., & Smith, R. J. (1996). Vocal fold paralysis in infants twelve months of age and younger. *Otolaryngology-Head and Neck Surgery, 114*, 18–21.

Zebrowski, P. M. (1997). Assisting young children who stutter and their families: Defining the role of the speech-language pathologist. *American Journal of Speech-Language Pathology, 6*, 19–28.

Zimmerman, G. N., Liljeblad, S., Frank, A., & Cleeland, C. (1983). The Indians have many terms for it: Stuttering among Bannock-Shoshone. *Journal of Speech and Hearing Research, 26*, 315–318.

Zimmerman, I., Steiner, V., & Evatt-Pond, R. (2002a). *Preschool Language Scale, Fourth Edition (PLS-4)-Spanish Edition*. San Antonio, TX: Psychological Corporation.

Zimmerman, I., Steiner, V., & Evatt-Pond, R. (2002b). *Preschool Language Scale, Fourth Edition (PLS-4)*. San Antonio, TX: Psychological Corporation.

Zraick, R., Kempster, G., Connor, N., Thibeault, S., Klaben, B., Bursac, Z., . . . Glaze, L. (2011). Research article establishing validity of the Consensus Auditory-Perceptual Evaluation of Voice (CAPE-V). *American Journal of Speech-Language Pathology, 20*, 14–22. doi:10.1044/1058-0360(2010/09-0105)

Zucker, T. A., & Grant, S. I. (2007). Assessing home support for literacy. In K. L. Pence (Ed.), *Assessment of emergent literacy* (pp. 81–187). San Diego, CA: Plural.

Index